Rheumatoid Arthritis: Current Status and Future Challenges

Rheumatoid Arthritis: Current Status and Future Challenges

Guest Editor

Blanca Hernández-Cruz

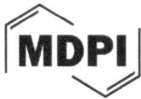

Basel • Beijing • Wuhan • Barcelona • Belgrade • Novi Sad • Cluj • Manchester

Guest Editor
Blanca Hernández-Cruz
Rheumatology Department
Virgen Macarena University
Hospital
Seville
Spain

Editorial Office
MDPI AG
Grosspeteranlage 5
4052 Basel, Switzerland

This is a reprint of the Special Issue, published open access by the journal *Journal of Clinical Medicine* (ISSN 2077-0383), freely accessible at: https://www.mdpi.com/journal/jcm/special_issues/5N2748R15T.

For citation purposes, cite each article independently as indicated on the article page online and as indicated below:

Lastname, A.A.; Lastname, B.B. Article Title. *Journal Name* **Year**, *Volume Number*, Page Range.

ISBN 978-3-7258-3195-1 (Hbk)
ISBN 978-3-7258-3196-8 (PDF)
https://doi.org/10.3390/books978-3-7258-3196-8

Cover image courtesy of Jorge Luis Rodas Flores

© 2025 by the authors. Articles in this book are Open Access and distributed under the Creative Commons Attribution (CC BY) license. The book as a whole is distributed by MDPI under the terms and conditions of the Creative Commons Attribution-NonCommercial-NoDerivs (CC BY-NC-ND) license (https://creativecommons.org/licenses/by-nc-nd/4.0/).

Contents

About the Editor vii

Preface ix

Raimon Sanmartí, Beatriz Frade-Sosa and Andres Ponce
The So-Called Pre-Clinical Rheumatoid Arthritis: Doubts, Challenges, and Opportunities
Reprinted from: J. Clin. Med. 2024, 13, 6387, https://doi.org/10.3390/jcm13216387 1

Loreto Carmona, Elena Aurrecoechea and María Jesús García de Yébenes
Tailoring Rheumatoid Arthritis Treatment through a Sex and Gender Lens
Reprinted from: J. Clin. Med. 2023, 13, 55, https://doi.org/10.3390/jcm13010055 7

Felipe Alexis Avalos-Salgado, Laura Gonzalez-Lopez, Sergio Gonzalez-Vazquez,
Juan Manuel Ponce-Guarneros, Aline Priscilla Santiago-Garcia,
Edna Lizeth Amaya-Cabrera, et al.
Risk Factors Associated with Adverse Events Leading to Methotrexate Withdrawal in Elderly
Rheumatoid Arthritis Patients: A Retrospective Cohort Study
Reprinted from: J. Clin. Med. 2024, 13, 1863, https://doi.org/10.3390/jcm13071863 23

Jesús Tornero Molina, Blanca Hernández-Cruz and Héctor Corominas
Initial Treatment with Biological Therapy in Rheumatoid Arthritis
Reprinted from: J. Clin. Med. 2023, 13, 48, https://doi.org/10.3390/jcm13010048 40

Alberto Calvo-Garcia, Esther Ramírez Herráiz, Irene María Llorente Cubas,
Blanca Varas De Dios, Juana Benedí González, Alberto Morell Baladrón
and Rosario García-Vicuña
The Real-World Effectiveness, Persistence, Adherence, and Safety of Janus Kinase Inhibitor
Baricitinib in Rheumatoid Arthritis: A Long-Term Study
Reprinted from: J. Clin. Med. 2024, 13, 2517, https://doi.org/10.3390/jcm13092517 52

Cristina Martinez-Molina, Anna Feliu, Hye S. Park, Ana Juanes, Cesar Diaz-Torne,
Silvia Vidal and Hèctor Corominas
Are There Sex-Related Differences in the Effectiveness of Janus Kinase Inhibitors in Rheumatoid
Arthritis Patients?
Reprinted from: J. Clin. Med. 2024, 13, 2355, https://doi.org/10.3390/jcm13082355 67

Shuhei Yoshida, Masayuki Miyata, Eiji Suzuki, Takashi Kanno, Yuya Sumichika,
Kenji Saito, et al.
Incidence Rates of Infections in Rheumatoid Arthritis Patients Treated with Janus Kinase or
Interleukin-6 Inhibitors: Results of a Retrospective, Multicenter Cohort Study
Reprinted from: J. Clin. Med. 2024, 13, 3000, https://doi.org/10.3390/jcm13103000 76

Javier Narváez
Moving forward in Rheumatoid Arthritis-Associated Interstitial Lung Disease Screening
Reprinted from: J. Clin. Med. 2024, 13, 5385, https://doi.org/10.3390/jcm13185385 88

Jorge Luis Rodas Flores, Blanca Hernández-Cruz, Víctor Sánchez-Margalet,
Ana Fernández-Reboul Fernández, Esther Fernández Panadero, Gracia Moral García
and José Javier Pérez Venegas
Neutropenia and Felty Syndrome in the Twenty-First Century: Redefining Ancient Concepts in
Rheumatoid Arthritis Patients
Reprinted from: J. Clin. Med. 2024, 13, 7677, https://doi.org/10.3390/jcm13247677 99

Lena L. N. Brandt, Hendrik Schulze-Koops, Thomas Hügle, Michael J. Nissen, Johannes von Kempis and Ruediger B. Mueller
Radiographic Progression in Patients with Rheumatoid Arthritis in Clinical Remission or Low Disease Activity: Results from a Swiss National Registry (SCQM)
Reprinted from: *J. Clin. Med.* **2024**, *13*, 7424, https://doi.org/10.3390/jcm13237424 . . . . **112**

Richard T. Meehan, Mary T. Gill, Eric D. Hoffman, Claire M. Coeshott, Manuel D. Galvan, Molly L. Wolf, et al.
Ultrasound-Guided Injections of HYADD4 for Knee Osteoarthritis Improves Pain and Functional Outcomes at 3, 6, and 12 Months without Changes in Measured Synovial Fluid, Serum Collagen Biomarkers, or Most Synovial Fluid Biomarker Proteins at 3 Months
Reprinted from: *J. Clin. Med.* **2023**, *12*, 5541, https://doi.org/10.3390/jcm12175541 . . . . **121**

About the Editor

Blanca Hernández-Cruz

Dr. Blanca Hernández-Cruz completed her medical studies at the Universidad Veracruzana de México in 1987. She specialized in Internal Medicine at the Salvador Zubirán National Institute of Medical Sciences and Nutrition and the National Autonomous University of Mexico in 1993 and specialized in Rheumatology at the same institution in 1995. She completed her master's degree in Medical Sciences at the National Autonomous University of Mexico in 2001 and completed her Medical Doctorate at the University of Seville in 2006.

From 1995 to 1999, she worked as a Rheumatologist and Researcher in the Department of Internal Medicine at the National Institute of Medical Sciences and Nutrition in Mexico City. She has been a resident of Spain since 1999, where she currently works at the Virgen Macarena University Hospital as a Rheumatologist in the Rheumatology Department.

Her research focuses on areas such as rheumatoid arthritis, biological therapies, clinimetrics, quality of life, gender perspective in immune-mediated diseases, and osteoporosis. She has than 60 publications to her name in indexed journals, with more than 2000 citations of her published work, and an H-index of 26.

In addition to her clinical and research roles, she worked as a tutor of rheumatology fellows from 2017 to 2023. She was awarded accreditation as a contracted professor by the Agency of Accreditation and Excellence of Spain in 2023.

She is responsible for the care of a large cohort of patients with inflammatory pathologies and osteoporosis. She is the coordinator of the Fracture Prevention Unit of the Virgen Macarena University Hospital. She has held accreditation as Excellent in Medical Attention by the Agency of Quality in Health of Andalucian since 2017.

She is also the spokesperson for the Spanish Society of Rheumatology, working as a health communicator with several communications to newspapers, medical journals, and the media.

Preface

The Special Issue attempts to tour various topics that are current in the management of rheumatoid arthritis patients. The scope ranges from preclinical forms and if we must treat it, as well as the gender differences that the clinician must keep in mind. In regard to DMARDs, one article is about therapeutic strategy and reviewing the data of efficacy using biologics in first line. Another focuses on methotrexate and adverse events. Other three articles focus on JAKi, persistence in real-world infections, and sex differences in clinical response to JAKi, respectively. Finally, radiographic progression and its clinical relevance, interstitial lung disease and neutropenia are the scope of the rest of the Special Issue.

As you can see in the expertise of our authors, they are researchers involved in the management of rheumatoid arthritis patients and made great efforts and a brilliant contribution to our Special Issue. The purpose of the issue was answering questions that arise daily for a clinician about several hot topics. I am sure that readers will be able to find answers, no matter what their particular interest may be.

Blanca Hernández-Cruz
Guest Editor

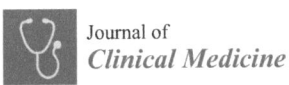

Editorial

The So-Called Pre-Clinical Rheumatoid Arthritis: Doubts, Challenges, and Opportunities

Raimon Sanmartí *, Beatriz Frade-Sosa and Andres Ponce

Arthritis Unit, Rheumatology Department, Hospital Clinic of Barcelona, 08036 Barcelona, Catalonia, Spain; frade@clinic.cat (B.F.-S.); aponce@clinic.cat (A.P.)
* Correspondence: sanmarti@clinic.cat

A Clinical Case of Possible Pre-Rheumatoid Arthritis

A 46-year-old female, a scientist working in a laboratory, presented in the Arthritis Unit with polyarthralgia of an intermittent course. She has a cousin with rheumatoid arthritis (RA) but denied other inflammatory rheumatic diseases in her family. She has a history of urticaria "a frigore". The current symptoms began one year ago with mild bilateral metatarsalgia, with a relapsing course. Three months before the first visit, she complained of bilateral shoulder pain, and three weeks later, polyarthralgia, particularly in her hands, without swelling, which improved after 2 weeks and was treated with ibuprofen. The joint pain disappeared but recurred after one month, affecting both hands, especially in the proximal interphalangeal (PIP) and metacarpophalangeal (MCP) joints. The symptoms predominated in the early morning, with mild morning stiffness (<60 min). Her family physician prescribed ibuprofen with partial improvement. Initial blood tests showed normal ESR and CRP values, negative rheumatoid factor (RF), and antinuclear antibodies (ANA) but high levels of anti-CCP antibodies (CCP2 test: 112 IU, normal value <3). The clinical exam at the first visit showed a positive squeeze test but no joint swelling. An ultrasonographic study of her hands and feet only disclosed mild peritendinitis without joint synovitis in the fifth PIP joint of the right hand. A diagnosis of arthralgia suspicious for progression to RA (clinically suspect arthralgia [CSA]), as established based on this clinical picture and the presence of anti-CCP antibodies. The probability of progression to clinical RA seems high in this individual. However, some doubts arise regarding the most appropriate management of the symptoms or the disease at this pre-arthritis stage. Some of the relevant questions are as follows:

Is This Individual Suffering from Inflammatory Arthralgia with a High Risk of Developing RA in the near Future? If So, Is This Risk Imminent? Can We Quantify This Risk?

Given the current knowledge, it is widely agreed among rheumatologists that this individual has inflammatory arthralgia, and the presence of an ACPA-positive test suggests a high risk of progression to RA, likely in the near future. This case represents a possible pre-clinical RA, although the diagnosis remains retrospective until persistent clinical arthritis develops. Such individuals have been described in the literature as suffering from inflammatory arthralgia, CSA, or even imminent RA [1,2]. In 2017, EULAR published recommendations for defining individuals with arthralgia suspicious for RA progression, emphasizing the type and characteristics of arthralgia (recent onset, symptoms predominating in the early morning, and affecting small joints of the hands) [3]. This definition requires the absence of clinical joint swelling, differentiating it from undifferentiated arthritis, where patients have clinical arthritis but do not meet criteria for RA or other inflammatory arthritis [4]. In this strict definition, the patient suffering from palindromic rheumatism, a form of intermittent arthritis/periarthritis without joint pain and swelling in the intercritical period, could not be classified as inflammatory arthralgia or CSA, although the risk of RA progression in these patients is quite high [5].

Citation: Sanmartí, R.; Frade-Sosa, B.; Ponce, A. The So-Called Pre-Clinical Rheumatoid Arthritis: Doubts, Challenges, and Opportunities. *J. Clin. Med.* **2024**, *13*, 6387. https://doi.org/10.3390/jcm13216387

Received: 27 September 2024
Accepted: 22 October 2024
Published: 25 October 2024

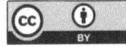

Copyright: © 2024 by the authors. Licensee MDPI, Basel, Switzerland. This article is an open access article distributed under the terms and conditions of the Creative Commons Attribution (CC BY) license (https://creativecommons.org/licenses/by/4.0/).

The question arises as to whether the risk for RA progression is imminent in these individuals. It is evident that in addition to the clinical phenotype (inflammatory arthralgia), the presence of an ACPA-positive test increases the probability of RA progression and likely decreases the latency period to persistent arthritis. Several studies have addressed this issue to quantify the risk, concluding that between 20% to 50% of individuals progress to RA after 2–3 years of follow-up [1,6–8]. The percentages may be higher if the individuals have other risk factors such as first-degree relatives with RA, overweight, tobacco smoking [9], high titers of ACPA, or the combination of other characteristic autoantibodies of RA, such as RF or anti-CarP [10]. However, it is important to note that most individuals do not progress to RA in the short term. Therefore, from a practical point of view, determining the exact risk in an individual patient is challenging, complicating the recommendation of a therapeutic strategy at this stage.

Why Does This Individual Have Joint Pain without Evidence of Inflammation at the Clinical Exam, Even Using Sensitive Imaging Techniques Such as Ultrasound or MRI?

As previously discussed, the definition of CSA or inflammatory arthralgia is based on the absence of synovitis at the physical examination. In some cases, the presence of inflammation may be very mild and difficult to recognize, especially given variability among rheumatologists in assessing clinical synovitis [11] This feature is more relevant in these patients, including those with early arthritis where signs of inflammation may be mild or subtle. However, studies confirm that a high percentage of these individuals present with synovitis when examined using imaging techniques such as MRI or ultrasound, which may explain the presence of joint pain or stiffness [12,13]. These techniques have higher sensitivity than clinical examination, though possible false positives may occur. In approximately half of the individuals with CSA, no clear evidence of imaging synovitis is found [12]. In these cases, no satisfactory explanation exists for the presence of persistent joint pain.

Pain is a complex and subjective symptom that may be influenced by psychological or social factors, but in patients with CSA, the pain is inflammatory and located in joints commonly affected by synovial inflammation. Therefore, it is possible that imaging techniques are not sufficiently sensitive to capture some degrees of synovitis that may have a clinical impact. It is possible that pathological studies of synovial tissue have detected relevant changes, perhaps only at the molecular level, in these individuals [14].

It has been suggested that in patients with ACPA-positive inflammatory arthralgia, autoantibodies "per se" may account for the induction of joint pain in the absence of synovial inflammation [15]. In a rat model, ACPA may induce the production of IL-8 by monocytes, a chemokine that may stimulate sensory neurons and induce joint pain [16]. However, this mechanism may explain pain in ACPA positive patients but does not account for inflammatory arthralgia in seronegative individuals.

What Is the Most Appropriate Management for This Individual at This Stage? What Is the Scientific Evidence for the Benefits of Antirheumatic Drugs in These Individuals? What Is the Drug of Choice?

There is no satisfactory answer to these questions. In clinical practice, it seems reasonable for patients with CSA with known risk factors to address these modifiable factors, such as avoiding tobacco consumption, reducing body weight, and maintaining good dental hygiene, although no scientific evidence exists about the exact clinical benefit in this population. However, should these individuals be treated with antirheumatic drugs beyond symptomatic treatments like analgesics, NSAIDs, or even low doses of glucocorticoids? Does the clinical picture of our patient, at risk for RA progression, warrant an antirheumatic drug intervention with synthetic or targeted disease-modifying antirheumatic drugs (DMARDs)?

This question lacks a definitive answer. The choice and use of drugs for our patient would likely differ among rheumatologists. Intensive drug treatment might seem more acceptable in the presence of synovitis determined via imaging techniques but may be met with reluctance in the absence of subclinical synovitis. Furthermore, the goal of therapeutic intervention needs clarification: should it focus on significant improvement in joint pain, disability, or achieving remission, or should it aim to delay or even prevent progression to RA?

The quality of life for RA patients has improved dramatically due to early treat-to-target strategies and the use of targeted therapies that efficiently control synovitis [17]. However, there is no cure for these patients once clinical arthritis develops. At the pre-rheumatoid stage, intensive therapeutic intervention may hypothetically reduce the risk of developing persistent clinical arthritis and provide a "cure", at least for some individuals. This potential window of opportunity is encouraging.

Recent years have seen several randomized clinical trials aimed at this objective in patients with inflammatory arthralgia, yielding heterogeneous results (Table 1) [18–23]. One issue with these studies is the variability in inclusion criteria, and all of them based their criteria for arthralgia on physician opinion or non-validated criteria. None of the studies used the EULAR criteria for arthralgia suspicious for progression to RA [3], as these studies were initiated before the publication of the EULAR recommendations. The study designs also varied based on other inclusion criteria, such as the presence of autoantibodies or synovitis detected by imaging techniques. All trials had a placebo control group and a maximum follow-up period of two years. A withdrawal period in the active arm was included to assess if clinical benefits persisted post-intervention. Three trials involved biologic drugs (abatacept in two and rituximab in one), while methotrexate, hydroxychloroquine, and atorvastatin were each tested in one trial. The latter two were canceled before study completion due to inefficacy [19,20]. The Treat Early trial found methotrexate beneficial for joint pain and disability but did not reduce RA progression compared to placebo at the study's end [21]. The trials with abatacept (ARIAA and APIPPRA) [22,23] observed positive effects in preventing or delaying RA progression even after the intervention period. However, a significant proportion of patients in the intervention arm developed RA, and many in the placebo arm did not progress to RA. A randomized trial in early-onset palindromic rheumatism (abatacept vs. hydroxychloroquine) is ongoing (EudraCT#: 2017-004543-20). Recent EULAR recommendations on clinical trials for pre-RA or undifferentiated arthritis and palindromic rheumatism were published after the design of these clinical trials [24].

Table 1. Summary of randomized clinical trials evaluating interventions in individuals at risk of rheumatoid arthritis progression.

Trial	Sample Size	Intervention	Dosage	Duration of Active Treatment	Inclusion Criteria	Total Duration of Follow-Up	Primary Outcome	Progression to RA (Active vs. Placebo *)
PRAIRI [18]	82	Rituximab	1000 mg, single-dose	29 months	Arthralgia; ACPA-positive and RF-positive; Subclinical synovitis by MRI or CRP > 0.6 mg/L	29 months	Reduction of ACPA Level > 50%	34% vs. 40%
STAPRA [19]	62	Atorvastatin	40 mg/day	36 months	Arthralgia; ACPA-positive and RF-positive or ACPA-positive with high levels (>3)	Not specified	Clinical Arthritis	29% vs. 19%
STOPRA [20]	144	Hydroxychloroquine	200–400 mg/day	12 months	High ACPA-positive; Subclinical synovitis by MRI	Not specified	2010 ACR/EULAR Criteria for RA; Clinical Arthritis with XR Erosion	34% vs. 36%
TREAT EARLIER [21]	236	Methotrexate	25 mg/week	12 months	Arthralgia; Subclinical synovitis on MRI	24 months	2010 ACR/EULAR Criteria for RA	19% vs. 18%
ARIAA [22]	100	Abatacept	125 mg/week	6 months	Arthralgia; ACPA-positive; Subclinical synovitis by MRI	18 months	Improvement in MRI Scores of Synovitis	35% vs. 57%
APIPPRA [23]	213	Abatacept	125 mg/week	12 months	Arthralgia; ACPA-positive and RF-positive or ACPA-positive with high titer (>3)	24 months	2010 ACR/EULAR Criteria for RA or Clinical Arthritis in >3 Joints	25% vs. 37%

* Note: "Active" refers to the intervention group and "Placebo" refers to the control group.

Several questions arise from these trials beyond population inclusion criteria, including the duration of drug therapy, the follow-up period, and the non-interventional periods. Is a 6-month course of abatacept sufficient, as in the ARIAA trial? Or is a single cycle of rituximab, as in the PRAIRI trial, adequate? Is intermittent or continuous drug use necessary to maintain the objective? What is the best drug for these at-risk individuals?

If the goal is to prevent disease progression rather than just improve clinical and functional outcomes, cell-modifying agents such as abatacept or rituximab may be more appropriate than methotrexate, the standard drug used for early RA. However, the challenge of stratifying and quantifying risk, coupled with the fact that many patients do not progress to RA, complicates the design of interventional trials. Moreover, participants may be reluctant to engage in trials for drugs that may raise concerns about adherence, tolerability, and serious adverse events, especially when the aim is to prevent a hypothetical but not certain adverse outcome [25].

Future Perspectives and Research Agenda

The current knowledge highlights significant doubts regarding the optimal management of individuals at risk for RA. However, theoretical intervention at this pre-RA stage might influence the progression to persistent and destructive polyarthritis such as RA. The critical question is whether therapeutic intervention during this "window of opportunity" should be uniform across the entire at-risk population or if it should target a specific subgroup that might benefit more clearly from this strategy. Stratification of at-risk individuals is essential to identify those with very high risk of progression and to avoid overtreatment. Efforts to develop and validate risk stratification scores for clinical practice are ongoing but require further validation [26,27].

A deeper understanding of the immunological mechanisms driving the progression from pre-RA to clinical RA is crucial. Such insights could lead to more rational drug and therapeutic strategies. For example, studies focusing on the types and characteristics of the immune response in seropositive patients (e.g., ACPA titers, isotype use, antigenic expansion, glycosylation, presence of other autoantibodies like RF or anti-CarP) or sensitive innovative imaging findings might better identify individuals with a favorable risk–benefit ratio for therapeutic intervention. Personalized or individualized medicine is vital for this population. Additionally, research into the effects of modifying risk factors such as obesity, smoking, exercise, dietary habits, and even the mucosal microbiome is of particular interest.

In conclusion, there is some scientific evidence suggesting that progression toward clinical arthritis may be delayed or prevented in individuals at risk for RA. However, there remains considerable uncertainty about the best strategy by which to achieve this goal. In the coming decade, new interventional clinical trials involving various antirheumatic drugs in well-defined at-risk populations will provide more insights into this intriguing question, potentially bringing us closer to a hypothetical cure for this disease or at least optimizing the management of our patients.

Conflicts of Interest: The authors declare no conflict of interest.

References

1. van Steenbergen, H.W.; Mangnus, L.; Reijnierse, M.; Huizinga, T.W.; van der Helm-van Mil, A.H.M. Clinical factors, anticitrullinated peptide antibodies and MRI-detected subclinical inflammation in relation to progression from clinically suspect arthralgia to arthritis. *Ann. Rheum. Dis.* **2016**, *75*, 1824–1830. [CrossRef] [PubMed]
2. Nam, J.L.; Hunt, L.; Hensor, E.M.; Emery, P. Enriching case selection for imminent RA: The use of anti-CCP antibodies in individuals with new non-specific musculoskeletal symptoms—A cohort study. *Ann. Rheum. Dis.* **2016**, *75*, 1452–1456. [CrossRef] [PubMed]
3. van Steenbergen, H.W.; Aletaha, D.; Beaart-van de Voorde, L.J.; Brouwer, E.; Codreanu, C.; Combe, B.; Fonseca, J.E.; Hetland, M.L.; Humby, F.; Kvien, T.K.; et al. EULAR definition of arthralgia suspicious for progression to rheumatoid arthritis. *Ann. Rheum. Dis.* **2017**, *76*, 491–496. [CrossRef] [PubMed]
4. Krabben, A.; Huizinga, T.W.; van der Helm-van Mil, A.H.M. Undifferentiated arthritis characteristics and outcomes when applying the 2010 and 1987 criteria for rheumatoid arthritis. *Ann. Rheum. Dis.* **2012**, *71*, 238–241. [CrossRef] [PubMed]

5. Sanmartí, R.; Frade-Sosa, B.; Morlà, R.; Castellanos-Moreira, R.; Cabrera-Villalba, S.; Ramirez, J.; Salvador, G.; Haro, I.; Cañete, J.D. Palindromic Rheumatism: Just a Pre-rheumatoid Stage or Something Else? *Front. Med.* **2021**, *8*, 657983. [CrossRef]
6. Rakieh, C.; Nam, J.L.; Hunt, L.; A Hensor, E.M.; Das, S.; Bissell, L.-A.; Villeneuve, E.; McGonagle, D.; Hodgson, R.; Grainger, A.; et al. Predicting the development of clinical arthritis in anti-CCP positive individuals with non-specific musculoskeletal symptoms: A prospective observational cohort study. *Ann. Rheum. Dis.* **2015**, *74*, 1659–1666. [CrossRef]
7. Gan, R.W.; Bemis, E.A.; Demoruelle, M.K.; Striebich, C.C.; Brake, S.; Feser, M.L.; Moss, L.; Clare-Salzler, M.; Holers, V.M.; Deane, K.D.; et al. The association between omega-3 fatty acid biomarkers and inflammatory arthritis in an anti-citrullinated protein antibody positive population. *Rheumatology* **2017**, *56*, 2229–2236. [CrossRef]
8. Novella-Navarro, M.; Plasencia-Rodríguez, C.; Nuño, L.; Balsa, A. Risk Factors for Developing Rheumatoid Arthritis in Patients with Undifferentiated Arthritis and Inflammatory Arthralgia. *Front. Med.* **2021**, *8*, 668898. [CrossRef]
9. de Hair, M.J.; Landewé, R.B.; van de Sande, M.G.; van Schaardenburg, D.; van Baarsen, L.G.; Gerlag, D.M.; Tak, P.P. Smoking and overweight determine the likelihood of developing rheumatoid arthritis. *Ann. Rheum. Dis.* **2013**, *72*, 1654–1658. [CrossRef]
10. Ponchel, F.; Duquenne, L.; Xie, X.; Corscadden, D.; Shuweihdi, F.; Mankia, K.; Trouw, L.A.; Emery, P. Added value of multiple autoantibody testing for predicting progression to inflammatory arthritis in at-risk individuals. *RMD Open* **2022**, *8*, e002512. [CrossRef]
11. Grunke, M.; Antoni, C.E.; Kavanaugh, A.; Hildebrand, V.; Dechant, C.; Schett, G.; Manger, B.; Ronneberger, M. Standardization of joint examination technique leads to asignificant decrease in variability among different examiners. *J. Rheumatol.* **2010**, *37*, 860–864. [CrossRef] [PubMed]
12. Molina Collada, J.; López Gloria, K.; Castrejón, I.; Nieto-González, J.C.; Rivera, J.; Montero, F.; González, C.; Álvaro-Gracia, J.M. Ultrasound in clinically suspect arthralgia: The role of power Doppler to predict rheumatoid arthritis development. *Arthritis Res. Ther.* **2021**, *23*, 299. [CrossRef] [PubMed]
13. Boeren, A.M.P.; Oei, E.H.G.; van der Helm-van Mil, A.H.M. The value of MRI for detecting subclinical joint inflammation in clinically suspect arthralgia. *RMD Open* **2022**, *8*, e002128. [CrossRef] [PubMed]
14. de Jong, T.A.; de Hair, M.J.H.; van de Sande, M.G.H.; Semmelink, J.F.; Choi, I.Y.; Gerlag, D.M.; Tak, P.P.; van Baarsen, L.G.M. Synovial gene signatures associated with the development of rheumatoid arthritis in at risk individuals: A prospective study. *J. Autoimmun.* **2022**, *133*, 102923. [CrossRef] [PubMed]
15. Catrina, A.I.; Svensson, C.I.; Malmström, V.; Schett, G.; Klareskog, L. Mechanisms leading from systemic autoimmunity to joint-specific disease in rheumatoid arthritis. *Nat. Rev. Rheumatol.* **2017**, *13*, 79–86. [CrossRef]
16. Wigerblad, G.; Bas, D.B.; Fernades-Cerqueira, C.; Krishnamurthy, A.; Nandakumar, K.S.; Rogoz, K.; Kato, J.; Sandor, K.; Su, J.; Jimenez-Andrade, J.M.; et al. Autoantibodies to citrullinated proteins induce joint pain independent of inflammation via a chemokine-dependent mechanism. *Ann. Rheum. Dis.* **2016**, *75*, 730–738. [CrossRef]
17. Di Matteo, A.; Bathon, J.M.; Emery, P. Rheumatoid arthritis. *Lancet* **2023**, *402*, 2019–2033. [CrossRef]
18. Gerlag, D.M.; Safy, M.; I Maijer, K.; Tang, M.W.; Tas, S.W.; Starmans-Kool, M.J.F.; van Tubergen, A.; Janssen, M.; de Hair, M.; Hansson, M.; et al. Effects of B-cell directed therapy on the preclinical stage of rheumatoid arthritis: The PRAIRI study. *Ann. Rheum. Dis.* **2019**, *78*, 179–185. [CrossRef]
19. van Boheemen, L.; Turk, S.; Beers-Tas, M.V.; Bos, W.; Marsman, D.; Griep, E.N.; Starmans-Kool, M.; Popa, C.D.; van Sijl, A.; Boers, M.; et al. Atorvastatin is unlikely to prevent rheumatoid arthritis in high risk individuals: Results from the prematurely stopped STAtins to Prevent Rheumatoid Arthritis (STAPRA) trial. *RMD Open* **2021**, *7*, e001591. [CrossRef]
20. Deane, K.D.; Striebich, C.; Feser, M.; Demoruelle, K.; Moss, L.; Bemis, E.; Frazer-Abel, A.; Fleischer, C.; Sparks, J.; Solow, E.; et al. Hydroxychloroquine Does Not Prevent the Future Development of Rheumatoid Arthritis in a Population with Baseline High Levels of Antibodies to Citrullinated Protein Antigens and Absence of Inflammatory Arthritis: Interim Analysis of the StopRA Trial. *Arthritis Rheumatol.* **2022**, *74* (Suppl. S9), 3180–3182.
21. Krijbolder, D.I.; Verstappen, M.; van Dijk, B.T.; Dakkak, Y.J.; Burgers, L.E.; Boer, A.C.; Park, Y.J.; de Witt-Luth, M.E.; Visser, K.; Kok, M.R.; et al. Intervention with methotrexate in patients with arthralgia at rik of rheumatoid arthritis to reduce the development of persistent arthritis and its disease burden (TREAT EARLIER): A randomised, double-blind, placebo-controlled, proof-of-concept trial. *Lancet* **2022**, *400*, 283–294. [CrossRef] [PubMed]
22. Rech, J.; Tascilar, K.; Hagen, M.; Kleyer, A.; Manger, B.; Schoenau, V.; Hueber, A.J.; Kleinert, S.; Baraliakos, X.; Braun, J.; et al. Abatacept inhibits inflammation and onset of rheumatoid arthritis in individuals at high risk (ARIAA): A randomised, international, multicentre, double-blind, placebo-controlled trial. *Lancet* **2024**, *403*, 850–859. [CrossRef] [PubMed]
23. Cope, A.P.; Jasenecova, M.; Vasconcelos, J.C.; Filer, A.; Raza, K.; Qureshi, S.; D'Agostino, M.A.; McInnes, I.B.; Isaacs, J.D.; Pratt, A.G.; et al. Abatacept in individuals at high risk of rheumatoid arthritis (APIPPRA): A randomised, double-blind, multicentre, parallel, placebo-controlled, phase 2b clinical trial. *Lancet* **2024**, *403*, 838–849. [CrossRef] [PubMed]
24. Mankia, K.; Siddle, H.J.; Kerschbaumer, A.; Rodriguez, D.A.; Catrina, A.I.; Cañete, J.D.; Cope, A.P.; Daien, C.I.; Deane, K.D.; El Gabalawy, H.; et al. EULAR points to consider for conducting clinical trials and observational studies in individuals at risk of rheumatoid arthritis. *Ann. Rheum. Dis.* **2021**, *80*, 1286–1298. [CrossRef]
25. Toyoda, T.; Mankia, K. Prevention of Rheumatoid Arthritis in At-Risk Individuals: Current Status and Future Prospects. *Drugs* **2024**, *84*, 895–907. [CrossRef]

26. Duquenne, L.; Hensor, E.M.; Wilson, M.; Garcia-Montoya, L.; Nam, J.L.; Wu, J.; Harnden, K.; Anioke, I.C.; Di Matteo, A.; Chowdhury, R.; et al. Predicting Inflammatory Arthritis in At-Risk Persons: Development of Scores for Risk Stratification. *Ann. Intern. Med.* **2023**, *176*, 1027–1036. [CrossRef]
27. van de Stadt, L.A.; Witte, B.I.; Bos, W.H.; van Schaardenburg, D. A prediction rule for the development of arthritis in seropositive arthralgia patients. *Ann. Rheum. Dis.* **2013**, *72*, 1920–1926. [CrossRef]

Disclaimer/Publisher's Note: The statements, opinions and data contained in all publications are solely those of the individual author(s) and contributor(s) and not of MDPI and/or the editor(s). MDPI and/or the editor(s) disclaim responsibility for any injury to people or property resulting from any ideas, methods, instructions or products referred to in the content.

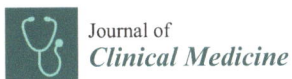

Review

Tailoring Rheumatoid Arthritis Treatment through a Sex and Gender Lens

Loreto Carmona [1,*], Elena Aurrecoechea [2] and María Jesús García de Yébenes [1]

[1] Instituto de Salud Musculoesquelética, 28045 Madrid, Spain
[2] Rheumatology Department, Hospital Sierrallana, Instituto de Investigación Valdecilla (IDIVAL), 39300 Torrelavega, Spain
* Correspondence: loreto.carmona@inmusc.eu

Abstract: Rheumatoid arthritis (RA) occurs more frequently in women than in men, and the studies that have addressed clinical and prognostic differences between the sexes are scarce and have contradictory results and methodological problems. The present work aims to evaluate sex- and gender-related differences in the clinical expression and prognosis of RA as well as on the impact on psychosocial variables, coping behavior, and healthcare use and access. By identifying between sex differences and gender-related outcomes in RA, it may be possible to design tailored therapeutic strategies that consider the differences and unmet needs. Being that sex, together with age, is the most relevant biomarker and health determinant, a so-called personalized medicine approach to RA must include clear guidance on what to do in case of differences.

Keywords: rheumatoid arthritis; sex; gender; personalized medicine

Citation: Carmona, L.; Aurrecoechea, E.; García de Yébenes, M.J. Tailoring Rheumatoid Arthritis Treatment through a Sex and Gender Lens. *J. Clin. Med.* **2024**, *13*, 55. https://doi.org/10.3390/jcm13010055

Academic Editor: Eugen Feist

Received: 14 November 2023
Revised: 13 December 2023
Accepted: 19 December 2023
Published: 21 December 2023

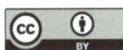

Copyright: © 2023 by the authors. Licensee MDPI, Basel, Switzerland. This article is an open access article distributed under the terms and conditions of the Creative Commons Attribution (CC BY) license (https://creativecommons.org/licenses/by/4.0/).

1. Introduction

Using 'sex' and 'gender' interchangeably is not ideal, although they pose close connections in biology and disease. Although it may be important to distinguish conceptually between sex and gender, the reality is that both concepts are intimately related, resulting in an interaction in which it is practically impossible to establish a clear line of separation between them. However, despite the difficulties in conceptualizing and operationalizing these concepts, the importance of including sex and gender in biomedical research has been stressed in recent years [1,2]. Sex is a biological reality, including genetics and hormones, that modifies disease pathophysiology, expression, and clinical effect and distribution of pharmaceuticals. Studying sex encompasses a focus on the impact of potential genetic, hormonal, anatomical, and physiological differences on health and disease. Gender can be defined as the behavioral, cultural, or psychological traits typically associated with one's sex resulting in a gendered division of labor, and socialization patterns that may impact an individual's well-being. Studying gender entails analyzing the role of gender identity, norms, relations, and institutional aspects as possible sources of health inequalities.

There is no universal standard for measuring gender, and some review studies have shown persistent inadequacies in the conceptual understanding and methodological operationalization of gender in the biomedical field [2]. Because gender is very context-specific and is exceedingly hard to quantify, gender has been used in place of sex, and typically operationalized as men/women, although solely biological phenomena are being studied [2,3]. Moreover, gender and sex are so entwined that it might be challenging to set them apart [4,5].

The sociocultural construction of gender influences the behavior of populations, clinicians, and patients through different mechanisms, such as discriminatory values, norms, and beliefs, differential exposure and disease susceptibility, and even possible bias in health systems and health research [5,6].

The lack of information on the effect of biological (sex) and sociocultural (gender) differences in health may be due to different factors. Prior to the 1980s, most medical research ignored women and females as subjects of inquiry except when investigating 'women's health issues'—that is, issues directly related to reproduction or disorders seen only or predominantly in women. In most instances, female bodies were assumed to operate in the same ways as male bodies, and findings from research conducted exclusively on men were often uncritically generalized to women [1]. On the other hand, the history of excluding females from clinical studies is reflected in the 1977 US Food and Drug Administration (FDA) guidelines advising that women of childbearing potential should be excluded from drug trials. These recommendations resulted in inadequate female representation in clinical trials for decades to protect pregnant women and their offspring [7]. Fortunately, a gender-based approach to medicine has emerged to recognize and analyze sex differences in anatomical, physiological, biological, and therapeutic aspects of disease, as well as to assess potential effects of gender roles on other aspects of disease [8].

1.1. Gender and Chronic Diseases

Sex and gender are strong risk factors for practically every disease through genetic, epigenetic, and hormonal effects influencing physiology, illness, and drug metabolism, and social constructs of gender affecting behaviors, health engagement, and, subsequently, health [6].

As to chronic or noncommunicable diseases (NCD), the Global Burden of Disease (GBD) study has revealed several gender disparities, both in terms of mortality and morbidity burden, in cardiovascular disease (CVD), cancer, diabetes, renal disease, asthma, autoimmune diseases, migraine, spondyloarthritis, multiple sclerosis, Alzheimer's disease, epilepsy, stroke, autism, depression, anxiety, and others [9,10]. Achieving equitable improvements in NCD morbidity and death requires recognizing and resolving these disparities.

1.2. Gender and Rheumatoid Arthritis

Rheumatoid arthritis (RA) is a chronic inflammatory autoimmune disease characterized by symmetrical polyarthritis that leads to progressive joint destruction and disability, plus damage to other organs and tissues. As in the majority of autoimmune conditions, RA occurs more frequently in women than in men (around three to one) [11], and there might be some sex differences in symptom severity and disease course, as well as in the effect of treatment and survival [12].

Female and male immune systems are different as they are affected by the distribution of hormones, the presence of two X chromosomes versus only one, and a singular response to environmental factors [11]. Several genes on the X chromosome regulate innate and adaptative immune responses. In addition, sex hormones are immunoregulatory, participate in the secretion of cytokines and chemokines, interact with inflammatory mediators, and play an essential role in pathobiological differences [13,14]. The role of environmental factors, including those in the psychosociological sphere, is less clear, probably reflecting the complex interaction among genes, hormones, and environment in autoimmunity [11,13].

Women with RA show a higher disease activity than their counterparts and respond worse to synthetic and biological disease-modifying therapies [14]. Also, pregnancy or childbearing desire influences the strategy for RA management. Consequently, to enhance treat-to-target performance, there is an ongoing demand for a precise reference to sex and gender issues in RA research. A more thorough understanding of the potential variables affecting sexual dimorphism in RA susceptibility, presentation pattern, disease activity, and outcome may result in more individualized treatment plans that minimize the illness's burden [8].

The objective of this review is to analyze the impact of sex and gender on different aspects of RA to propose a sex- and gender-tailored approach to the management of RA.

2. Susceptibility to RA

Autoimmune diseases like RA show gender differences in incidence and immune response [15]. Different mechanisms for sex differences in autoimmunity have been proposed.

2.1. Genetic

Numerous immune-related genes are encoded on the X chromosome, and their overexpression may have sex-dependent effects on the immunological response. Men have one maternal X and one paternal Y chromosome, whereas women have two X chromosomes. In the early stages of development, one X chromosome is randomly silenced in females to prevent the double dose of X chromosome-derived proteins. Nevertheless, some X-linked genes are overexpressed in females due to incomplete X chromosomal inactivation, which allows 15% of the genes to elude inactivation [11].

The immune response is regulated by genetic factors, which could also account for the variations in RA susceptibility across sexes. The MHC, in particular class II alleles with a "shared epitope" (SE), and other non-MHC loci that seem to be sex influenced determine the genetic risk for RA [16]. For example, there is a direct correlation between the number of DR4 alleles of HLA and the frequency of RA in females [17]. Single nucleotide polymorphisms (SNPs) in cell-mediated immune-response genes may affect women and men differently. At least partially, they may account for sex differences in susceptibility to RA [18]. Immunoglobulin Fc receptors connect cellular and humoral immune responses. Male–female variations in RA may also be influenced by the sex connection of some SNPs of the Fc receptor-like genes (FCRL) [19]. MicroRNAs, short noncoding RNA molecules, regulate various processes, including the immune response. Dysregulation of microRNAs has been associated with autoimmune diseases, such as RA. MicroRNAs influence the expression of multiple protein-encoding genes at the posttranscriptional level. Women may be more susceptible to RA due to variations in the expression of X-chromosome-linked microRNAs or the genotype of certain microRNAs [11,20,21]. IL-4 promotes RA development via cytokine–receptor interaction, Th1 and Th2 cell differentiation, Th17 cell differentiation, T-cell receptor signaling pathway, cancer pathways, and hematopoietic cell lineage; curiously, IL-4 gene expression is lower in women with RA than in men [22].

2.2. Hormonal

The higher frequency of RA among women, especially before menopause, and the effect of pregnancy and oral contraception suppressing RA point out hormonal and reproductive factors [23,24]. Sex hormones may impact the development, risk, and course of autoimmune illnesses and several aspects of immune-system function. While testosterone and progesterone naturally depress the immune system, estrogens, especially 17-β estradiol (E2) and prolactin, operate as enhancers of humoral immunity at least, upregulating the production of immunoglobulins and downregulating inflammatory responses [11]. The inverse correlation between RA severity and androgen levels could be a reason why RA is less severe in men [25].

2.3. Gut Microbiota

Both the immune system and the gut microbiota have an impact on innate and adaptive immunological responses. This interaction may have significant effects on the emergence of inflammatory diseases. Several research studies using animal models have demonstrated the role of gut bacteria in sex bias in autoimmune disorders [11].

2.4. Lifestyle

Different studies have demonstrated that smoking is the strongest environmental factor in RA development. Smoking may induce citrullination of peptide antigens, and shared epitope alleles interact with smoking in the triggering of anticitrulline immunity that may lead to ACPA-positive RA. The risk of RA associated with smoking is generally higher among men than among women [26,27].

Population-based studies have shown a biological effect modification of gender on the smoking–RA association, such that smoking is a strong risk factor for RA in men and not so strong in women. The immunologic cascade triggered by smoking and leading to RA is modulated differently in men and in women. This effect is probably due to hormonal differences in the modulation of the immune cascade activated by smoking, leading to rheumatoid factor (RF) production and clinical RA [28]. Genetic and immunological factors may also play a role in the association between tobacco and AR, especially in genetically predisposed individuals. Persistent inflammation due to oxidative stress, proinflammatory state, autoantibody production, and epigenetic effects might be implicated in the autoimmunity of RA. Some studies also provide evidence that clinical responses to anti-TNF drugs used to treat RA may be adversely affected by smoking, and smoking may be related to extra-articular manifestations in RA [29].

In the context of environmental and lifestyle factors, obesity as a potential risk factor for the development of RA has been an area of interest for many years. Epidemiologic studies have shown a complex interaction between RA and obesity. Obesity would contribute to the development of seronegative RA, especially in younger women, although others suggested a decreased risk of RA among men, and observed associations may also be affected by residual confounding [26]. Different biologic mechanisms have been proposed to explain this association. Because adipose tissue is proinflammatory, obesity may also be an environmental risk factor for RA, with sex-specific effects. One large population-based case-control study demonstrated an association between obesity and RA, primarily for men with early disease onset [30]. Adipose tissue is an active secretory organ producing numerous bioactive molecules that regulate carbohydrate and lipid metabolism, immune function, and inflammation. Obesity produces chronic inflammation, and adipose tissue secretes different proinflammatory and anti-inflammatory factors, including the adipokines leptin, adiponectin, resistin, and visfatin as well as cytokines and chemokines, like TNF-a, IL-6, and others. An additional mechanism is based on the relationship between obesity and sex hormones. Obese men and women have higher serum levels of estrogens and androgens. Estrogen not only stimulates antibody (and autoantibody) production but also has a role in the breakdown of B-cell tolerance [31]. Indeed, obesity may also be associated with more severe or more refractory inflammation through increased levels of the inflammatory adipocytokines or decreased levels of the anti-inflammatory adipocytokine adiponectin [26].

Lastly, dysregulations of neuroendocrine-immune networks may underlie the gender-specific link that has also been observed between the onset of RA and childhood trauma, especially in women. Large prospective studies are necessary to elucidate the association between early-life stress and the risk for RA in genetically vulnerable individuals [32].

Despite a lack of consensus on how sexual dimorphism may affect the pattern and burden of disease, gender may indirectly increase RA susceptibility by influencing environmental and behavioral factors, which are known to be implicated in seropositive RA pathogenesis, in addition to the direct pathogenic effect of sex hormones on the immune system [8].

3. Disease Expression in Men and Women

The effect of the HLA-DRB1 shared epitope on RA susceptibility differs between men and women, thus raising the possibility of modifying disease expression by sex. Globally, the RA phenotype seems to be more severe in women than men, and women develop anti-CCP antibodies more frequently than men [33]. Women are also known to generally report more symptoms and poorer scores on most questionnaires, potentially affecting disease activity measures, treatment, or response to treatment between men and women [8,34,35].

The QUEST-RA study, a large multinational cohort, also showed gender differences in disease characteristics, including nodules (more common in men) and erosive disease (more prevalent in women) [34]. A study in Ecuador ($n = 100$) observed significant clinical differences, with men showing less disease activity—by physician's assessment, painful and swollen joint counts, ESR, DAS28—than women, and lower functional and severe disability by HAQ-DI [25]. In a cross-sectional population-based study of 1128 RA patients from Latin America and Caribe (LAC), RA women showed a younger age at onset, longer disease duration, and higher prevalence of poly-autoimmunity and abdominal obesity. They were more likely to perform more household activities than men, whereas extra-articular manifestations were more frequent in men without differences in time to treatment. Some of these characteristics could explain the high rates of disability and worse prognosis observed in women with RA in these regions.

There are, however, some inconsistencies across studies. A retrospective study comparing the pattern of disease involvement in 438 Greek patients with early RA confirmed that women are affected more frequently and at a younger age than men. However, apart from a higher ESR, there were no significant differences in other clinical and laboratory parameters [36]. These results are similar to those obtained in the Spanish GENIRA study with 70 men and 70 women, in which no significant differences in disease activity—measured either by joint counts, physician or patient global scores, inflammatory markers, such as ESR or CRP, or by composite indices, such as DAS28- were observed [37].

Although differences can be attributed to biological factors, they could also be due to social factors related to gender rather than sex. The complexity of gender differences in health extends beyond notions of either physical or social disadvantages [38].

4. Prognosis and Mortality

Different outcome studies have shown gender differences in the disease course and prognosis of RA. Women seem to have a more aggressive early disease than men [39], and longitudinal studies have observed a more significant improvement in disease activity, function, and pain with time and treatment in men than in women [40]. The analysis of the long-term course of RA in the BARFOT (better antirheumatic pharmacotherapy) RA-inception cohort showed that being a woman was an independent predictor of persistent disease, defined as the absence of remission (DAS-28 < 2.6). However, this difference was unclear because most disease-related variables did not differ between women and men at the follow-up visits, indicating no gender bias in the measures of disease activity [41]. Female sex has also been described as the most powerful predictor of disability and data from early RA cohorts, with adverse HAQ trajectories more frequently seen in females [42]. Evidence points to similar disease activity in the early stages of the disease, followed by a worse clinical course among women over time, with lower remission rates, and these differences appear more pronounced in early RA [43].

In addition to disease progression, sex also appears to have a differential effect on RA mortality, although the literature data are not always consistent. Some studies show higher mortality rates in younger males but also a rapid increase in female mortality with age; this might be explained by specific hormonal protection of younger women, whose benefits are lost with menopause [39]. Prospective inception cohorts have shown that male sex is an independent predictor of long-term mortality [44,45]. Similarly, an Australian study covering trends from 1980 to 2015 found an increase in mortality among male patients compared with females, despite adequate treatment options, probably concerning differences in the CV risk profile [46]. However, other authors could not detect differences in RA mortality by gender. In a comprehensive review of 25 articles, Anderson et al. did not observe a clear association between sex and mortality in RA [47].

5. Comorbidity

Comorbidities pose a significant challenge in rheumatic diseases because of their impact on management and outcome. Independently of medication (glucocorticoids) and traditional risk factors (smoking), chronically active inflammation also predisposes to the development of comorbidity. The population-based international COMORA study showed that the diseases most frequently associated with RA are CVD, depression, asthma, solid neoplasms, and chronic obstructive pulmonary disease [48]. Gender differences in comorbidity can be summarized as a higher frequency of diabetes mellitus, peptic ulcer, and CV and respiratory diseases in men, with no significant impact on RA-related disability and QoL, and depression and osteoporosis being more frequent in women [37].

5.1. Depression

Depression is threefold more common in RA than in the general population and has a clear correlation with pain, fatigue, physical disability, and, consequently, poor quality of life (QoL). Women with RA are more frequently diagnosed with depression than men with RA. In turn, depression is independently associated with worse outcomes, other comorbidities, and mortality [37].

5.2. Cardiovascular Disease

Cardiovascular diseases are one of the most frequent comorbidities in RA and the leading cause of death [45,46]. Inflammation is, in addition to traditional risk factors, responsible for the development of accelerated atherosclerosis and heart disease. Cross-sectional studies comparing the CV risk profile by gender in low-activity RA without a history of CV disease have shown a higher atherosclerotic burden in male RA patients versus females, reflected by more increased carotid artery intima thickness, risk of 10-year CV death, atherogenic index, and NT-proBNP levels. However, men also smoke more and have lower HDL cholesterol levels, so the effect of classical CV risk factors cannot be ruled out [49]. Another possibility could be the documented underestimation of CV risk in women with RA using algorithms designed for the general population, such as the SCORE [50]. The measurement of structural vascular disease may be a more reliable option. Flow-mediated diameter percent change of the brachial artery is considered the gold standard of endothelial function and the best estimate of CV events risk. A prospective study showed a safer cardiovascular profile in RA females with better endothelial function than men. This may be surprising considering that women tend to have a more aggressive course, but this could be due to the beneficial effect of estrogens on endothelial function [51].

5.3. Osteoporosis

Osteoporosis is frequent in RA with the ongoing inflammatory process, low body mass index, lack of exercise, chronic use of glucocorticoids, and menopausal status [37]. Premenopausal women with RA also have more frequent osteoporosis than age-matched controls, and the same stands for men with RA. Oelzner et al. evaluated the frequency of osteoporosis by densitometry in a group of 551 RA patients. The results confirmed significant differences in the frequency of osteoporosis between postmenopausal women (55.7%), men (50.5%), and premenopausal women (18%). On the other hand, the relevance of the risk factors for osteoporosis was different in postmenopausal women (older age, high cumulative glucocorticoid dose, low BMI, and long disease duration). In contrast, the risk factors in premenopausal women and men are low BMI and high cumulative glucocorticoid dose, confirming the dependence of risk factors on gender and menopausal state [52].

5.4. Periodontitis

Periodontal disease is more prevalent in patients with active RA than in healthy individuals, and its severity is also associated with the severity of RA. The study of periodontal disease, using self-completed questionnaires, in 5600 Japanese RA patients in the IORRA cohort showed that 18.3% of patients reported a recent diagnosis of periodontitis, and 20.4% had a history of periodontitis. As in other comorbidities, the risk of periodontal disease also shows differences by sex, with women showing a higher risk, especially if aged and smokers [53].

6. Objective and Subjective Measures

Many indices are available to monitor RA, such as the DAS28 (with ESR or CRP), the Clinical Disease Activity Index (CDAI), or the Simplified Disease Activity Index (SDAI).

They are all potentially influenced by sex and age, plus other factors such as body mass index (BMI) [54]. In general, women score more poorly than men, probably owing to higher "normal" levels of ESR and higher counts of tender joints (TJC) [34]. Women have higher mean ESR levels than men due to persistent ferropenic anemia hormonal factors. In older patients, the hormonal influences specific to women disappear, and older women are then affected by the same factors as older men [45]. On the other hand, sex differences in DAS28 may lead to a bias in assessing disease activity and response to treatment [55].

Nishino et al. assessed the effect of sex on composite measures in a large study [54]. They showed that sex differences in the composite measurements (DAS28-ESR, DAS28-CRP CDAI, and SDAI) are only observed in remission based on DAS28-ESR, and this effect is mainly due to sex-related variability on ESR [56]. The score of the composite measures might be comparable between sexes, but not so the components; DAS28-CRP and SDAI may yield similar average scores despite a higher TJC28 and a lower CRP in women than in men. They suggest that almost 12% of men with RA could mistakenly be classified as in remission based on DAS28-ESR [54].

In addition to the sex effect on DAS28-ESR due to male–female differences in ESR, significantly higher SDAI and CDAI values have also been observed in women, probably because of a higher TJC and patient global assessment (PtGA) [57]. Both TJC and PtGA are affected by pain. Even though the mechanisms behind gender differences in pain perception are not fully clear, females are more sensitive to pain and report more daily pain than males [12,58,59]. A biopsychosocial perspective can explain these variations. Biologically, women may be more or less sensitive to pain than men. Women's hormonal status may condition the processing of nociceptive stimuli by the central nervous system. Depression and other psychological variables, such as pain sensitivity, can also affect how someone perceives pain. Lastly, variations in socialization and sociocultural norms concerning the attention to and expression of pain may be the cause of gender disparities in pain perception [12,60]. Thus, gender differences may be due to the specific components of the indices, e.g., pain, and not to different degrees of inflammation [54,57,60,61]. Interestingly, differences in activity may not be accompanied by changes in the presence of radiographic erosions [57].

Both versions of DAS are used interchangeably to assess disease activity, treatment response, and treat-to-target approaches. However, the effect of sex on ESR may lead to discordance between the DAS28-CRP and DAS28-ESR. Discrepancies are more pronounced in older patients, women, and those at lower disease activity levels. The consequences of these effects can be significant, such as the availability of biological treatment or precluding the comparison of studies that have adopted different versions of DAS28. To avoid these limitations, a gender-stratified adjustment of the DAS28-CRP has been proposed to improve interscore agreement with DAS28-ESR. This adjustment allows us to consider observed biological differences in ESR levels between males and females [56].

The QUEST-RA study also showed sex differences in the relationship between DAS28 and body mass index (BMI). DAS28 scores increased with BMI only in women, and high BMI was associated with increased disease activity in RA [34,62]. Gender differences in the relationship between BMI and activity have also been observed using RAPID3 (routine assessment of patient index data) as the measure of activity. In a cross-sectional study of 451 RA patients, only female sex was found to have disease activity significantly associated with increasing BMI. The mean RAPID3 score values for each BMI category were statistically higher for females versus men [63]. The variation in the average amount of fat that a man and a female can have with the same BMI may cause sex variances in the association between BMI and disease activity. Males typically contribute more muscle mass to their BMI than females, who, in general, have a higher proportion of fat and a lower proportion of muscle mass. This could account for a rise in the proinflammatory state that causes disease activity to be higher in females than males [63].

Common depressive symptoms are more frequent in women, as already mentioned, and may affect all disease-activity metric scores (pain, global assessment and function, physician global assessment, and tender points), except the DAS, joint swelling, and serum biomarkers [37]. Finally, the higher HAQ score observed in women, even adjusting for disease severity, could be related to the underscoring of disability or greater muscle strength in men or a higher impact of pain on HAQ scores in women [61], men overestimating their functional capacity, or women having higher pain scores [59].

Table 1 shows the main objective and subjective differences in the indices and their components.

Table 1. Differences in indices and their components by sex and gender.

Objective Measures: Differences by Sex	Subjective Measures: Differences by Gender
DAS-28	PtGA
CDAI	Pain
SDAI	Depression
RAPID-3	HAQ
ESR	Quality of life
TJC	
BMI	

7. Effect of Drugs

Empirical evidence points to female–male differences in biological treatment outcomes, which are probably multifactorial. Sex may influence effectiveness and safety through the effect of hormones on immune function, differences in drug pharmacokinetics and pharmacodynamics, and outcome measures [7,12]. In addition to sex, gender-related factors may also play a role in the effect of drugs. Understanding biological responses to drugs, especially adverse effects, in women relative to men has been negatively impacted by the underrepresentation of women in clinical trials. Also, social norms have caused disparities in health-seeking behavior and reporting, e.g., women report and experience more unfavorable effects than men due to higher perceived burdens, such as hair loss [7,64,65].

Prospective early RA cohorts are the best design to determine whether differences between sexes are present in the early stages of the disease or if they appear later. In a prospective DMARD-naïve early RA cohort ($n = 292$), Jawaheer et al. showed comparable disease activity early in the disease, followed by a worse course among women over time. The rate of change in activity scores was significantly influenced by gender, even after adjusting by other covariables like ESR, pain, function, or global health. At the same time, an increase in inflammation markers (ESR and CRP) was observed among women after six months, when disease activity scores started to diverge between men and women. It is possible that women are not as responsive to anti-inflammatory medication as men, which might explain the short-lived amelioration in levels of inflammatory markers. This increase in inflammation markers could be related to increased TJC and patient global scores and physician global assessment, observed after six months, and eventually higher disease activity among women [43].

The same authors investigated sex differences in response to anti-TNF in early (≤ 2 years since diagnosis) versus established RA in patients from the DANBIO registry. The outcome measure was EULAR response at 48 months. Among patients who initiated therapy within two years of diagnosis, men achieved better and faster EULAR responses than women (an interaction effect between sex and time was present). This gender difference in treatment response was not seen in patients who initiated anti-TNF therapy more than two years after diagnosis, suggesting that disease duration at baseline may determine the sex differences in response to treatment [66].

The effect of gender on the response to rituximab (RTX) shows inconsistent evidence. The British Society for Rheumatology Biologics Register showed a lower response rate in women than in men after six months of RTX treatment [67]. On the contrary, the French Autoimmunity and Rituximab registry showed that, after 12 months, remission rates (DAS28-ESR < 2.6) were higher in men if they had failed previously with anti-TNF but higher in women if they were anti-TNF naïve, suggesting that sex is probably not the determinant of response, but previous anti-TNF exposure [68].

As to the effect of gender on the response to abatacept, this was studied in the French Orencia and Rheumatoid arthritis registry but failed to detect any difference in response or remission rates, or even time to achieve them, between men and women after adjustment by age, disease duration, seropositivity, current DMARDs, previous anti-TNF, corticoid use, and disease activity, although the DAS28-ESR, TJC, and PtGA remained higher in women [69].

In a registry of 1912 RA patients who started biologic therapy, Lesuis et al. studied disease characteristics at the time of biologic initiation. The results confirmed gender differences in ESR, PtGA, TJC, HAQ, DAS28-ESR, and DAS28-CRP. However, no significant differences were observed in the prescribed biological treatment or the need for concurrent therapy with steroids, nonsteroidal anti-inflammatory drugs, or conventional DMARDs, with data equal to those observed in the GENIRA study [37]. According to their results, gender imbalance occurs only in subjective measures, such as pain, functional status, and QoL. These results may imply that subjective measurements are somewhat disregarded during the therapeutic decision-making process, which may point to female patients receiving insufficient care [59].

A meta-analysis by Fang et al. evaluated the impact of sex on the clinical response to six biological products ($n = 5874$) and found no significant differences in the ACR20 response rate between men and women. Interestingly, the analysis of subcomponents showed high heterogeneity between studies. Unfortunately, this meta-analysis did not evaluate gender differences in the treatment responses by subgroups of early and established RA [70]. We could not identify any study regarding differences in response or biological effect to jakinibs by sex.

8. Life Impact

There is a relationship between physical health and psychological well-being, although this link is far from perfect. Some individuals can maintain a high QoL, whereas others become depressed, and over time, many individuals tend to adapt to their condition such that psychological well-being improves even though physical debilitation may remain. Gender can be a potentially significant moderator in this process. Understanding the mechanisms by which gender operates can allow differential interventions to help men and women with RA achieve optimal QoL.

The gendered process appears to influence the psychological well-being of RA patients. Women have more depressive symptoms, higher levels of negative affect, somatic complaints, more passive coping strategies, and less socialization than men. Differential socialization patterns, leading to passive coping behaviors, may explain the observed gender differences in depressive symptoms. Women may be more likely to respond to stressful events by focusing internally on symptoms and their consequences [3].

The patient's perception of their disease directly impacts their behavior, treatment compliance, and outcome. The social process also affects gender differences in adherence to treatment and illness perception. In a cross-sectional study of 320 RA patients, nonadherence was significantly associated with stress, disease activity, functional measures, and deformity, and female gender was an independent predictor of nonadherent behavior and more negative illness perception [71].

Women with RA show more depression, higher levels of disability (HAQ), and poorer QoL (SF36) than men. This may not be explained by overt disease-related biological differences but rather by differences in the patient's comorbidity profile. As already mentioned, depressed RA patients have poorer long-term outcomes, more comorbidities, and increased mortality rates. Emotional responses to a physical illness characterized by pain and weakness are understandable, and somatic symptoms of depression might be expected as part of RA [37,72]. Differences in emotional distress between men and women with RA are mainly explained by functional ability and pain, as well as the characteristics of their paid work, with no independent effect for sex. Consequently, among employed RA patients with high levels of functional disability, gender is not a risk factor for emotional distress [73].

9. Coping

In general, RA is perceived by the patient as a source of chronic stress due to the associated limitations and symptoms. Stress coping strategies refer to the cognitive and behavioral efforts a person develops with specific demands of oneself or the environment. The inability to cope with stress results in a breakdown in health because of the depletion of the body's hormonal and immune resources. The right way to cope with stress is of particular importance in chronically ill patients, and incompetent coping can contribute to the lack of effectiveness of the therapy [74,75].

The International Classification Functioning (ICF) emphasizes that contextual factors, which include both personal (gender) and environmental factors (healthcare system and attitudes of others), influence daily functioning. The perspectives of patients with RA, in terms of the impact of their chronic disease on everyday activities, are probably different. In general, societal expectations of women's occupations and daily activities differ from those of men. Everyday activities mediate personal meaning and reflect one's performance capacities, but continuing to perform these activities might be challenged due to the impact of RA. However, it may also depend on contextual factors, such as gender, individual and societal attitudes, health and social care systems, and policies. Masculinity is associated with competitiveness, self-control, strength, body performance, and productivity, whereas the caring role is more assigned to women. Men with a disability are more likely than women to fail to meet these social and cultural expectations and put first their paid work commitments over their health concerns. On the other hand, emotion regulation is a psychological determinant of health and is associated with psychological well-being, social and physical functioning, and disease severity. Compared to men, women with RA have a higher emotional orientation and reported stronger relationships between emotion regulation and the affective dimension of perceived health [76,77].

Gender differences were not found in the qualitative study of the situation-specific methods used to manage participation restrictions resulting from RA. However, women tend to offer more varied descriptions of their problems, especially in the domains of the ICF of domestic life and self-care. In contrast, men seldom report participation restrictions concerning domestic work, and these results could be explained, at least partly, by the existence of traditional gender roles. However, equity is developing when comparing most reported activities in which situation-specific coping was used by both women and men, namely, in remunerative employment and recreation and leisure [78].

In RA patients, depressive symptoms increase over time and with increased levels of pain, functional disability, and household work disability. Social status can contribute to depressive symptoms in different ways, including a sense of control, the ability to maintain the expectations of core social roles, and the ability to garner coping resources in the face of stressors. These findings illustrate the ongoing significance of social inequality for individuals with RA and offer additional confirmation of the necessity of comprehending and addressing variations in people's capacities for coping with RA-related stressors [79].

10. Intersections of Gender

Studies on gender differences in pathological processes are complex due to the difficulty of measuring gender. The difficulty is even more significant in cases of sex–gender intersection. Hormone-replacement therapy, medication, and surgery can alter a transgender person's hormonal status, which can, in turn, impact negatively on their health, e.g., increasing their risk of CV events [7].

Transgender and gender-diverse individuals (TGGD) have a gender identity that differs from their assigned sex at birth. They may affirm this identity through lifestyle modifications, gender-affirming hormone therapy (GAHT), or gender-affirmation surgery (GAS). There is not enough information on the epidemiology, pathophysiology, and clinical course of rheumatic diseases in transgender individuals. In 2022, Mathias et al. published an article with retrospective data on TGGD and a literature review of this population. In a retrospective analysis of 1053 patients seen in a rheumatology department over two years, seven TGGD patients (one RA) with rheumatic diseases were identified. The literature review found 11 studies with a total of 13 transgender patients (one RA).

The effect of GAHT on rheumatic disease possibly differs between estrogens and androgens, as most patients on exogenous testosterone experienced either no disease changes or improvement in disease activity. In contrast, most patients on exogenous estrogen experienced a possible acceleration of disease activity. The effect may also differ among different autoimmune diseases. The existence of a direct causation between the initiation of GAHT and the development or worsening of arthritis should be taken with caution due to the study's limitations, mainly related to multiple confounders and probable publication bias. Higher-powered prospective studies are needed, and a registry would be valuable [80].

11. Gender and Health Services

Despite the importance of health care in patients with RA, little attention has been paid to whether there is differential access to or use of health care between men and women. Looking at differential access to health care by gender is not straightforward. Different factors are related, such as intrinsic patterns of healthcare use in men and women, socioeconomic barriers [77], and attitudes and behaviors [12].

The pattern of health care in RA patients is multifactorial and mainly explained by need-related factors, which supports the principle of equity. However, some gender differences have been observed. Women's sex is an independent determinant of overall care. It increases the probability of receiving allied health and home care after adjusting for other characteristics, such as disease activity, duration, comorbidity, and functional status [81]. Concerning patient empowerment, younger and more educated women show a greater need for information and involvement in treatment decisions [82,83].

A delay in referral to subspecialty care puts patients at risk for delayed treatment and, thus, potentially worse outcomes. A retrospective analysis of a population-based cohort of incident RA has not shown differences between males and females in median time from first joint swelling to fulfillment of ACR/EULAR classification criteria, without gender impact on the time to the first DMARD therapy. However, among seronegative patients, there was a delay in meeting the 2010 criteria for females compared with males, with a longer time to start corticosteroid therapy in women. In patients with early seronegative disease, symptoms in females could be more often attributed to fibromyalgia, other noninflammatory conditions, or other rheumatic diseases [84].

Some authors have suggested that gender differences in RA may be due to differences in treatment prescription between men and women. A retrospective analysis of RA patients has not shown gender differences in the medication of MTX, dose, route of administration, time from disease onset, and percentage of patients receiving suboptimal doses. Overall, the data indicate that gender does not influence MTX therapy assigned by treating rheumatologists [85].

The gender of the attending physician may also play an essential role in health-care delivery. Female patients are more likely to obtain formal health care, provide more psychosocial information during a consultation than male patients, and show more preference for female physicians. In contrast, female physicians pay more attention to the psychosocial aspects of the complaints and use more gender-specific communication strategies than male physicians [77].

While it is evident that a gender bias characterizes RA reporting, perhaps there is also a gap in the evaluation of disease activity related to the different genders of the rheumatologist. In the analysis of 154 patients and their physicians, Duca et al. showed that subjective measures of global health status (GH) and disease activity are generally higher when collected by a female examiner. Female examiners recorded a more significant disease activity and a worse health status in both genders, with both male and female patients scoring higher levels of disease activity when evaluated by the female examiner compared to the male one. This observation is primarily attributable to variations of the GH and PtGA scores reported by patients, according to the absence of significant differences in the physical examination (TJC and SJC) performed by the examiners. Considering the chronic course of the disease, the physician–patient relationship is central in managing RA patients. Female physicians tend to exhibit higher emotional intensity in the physician–patient relationship. In this context, the higher emotional involvement between female physicians and patients may justify the higher values of PROs reported to the female examiner. Bearing in mind the impact of emotional well-being on the perceived disease activity, female physicians may better identify the subjective nature of complaints reported. This allows a more objective assessment of the global disease activity, especially in female patients [86].

12. Conclusions

A review of the impact of sex and gender on RA is presented. Although it is difficult to establish a clear line of separation between both concepts, sex seems to be more related to susceptibility, comorbidity (cardiovascular, osteoporosis, and periodontal disease), and objective measures (ESR, TJC, and BMI). In contrast, the influence of gender could be greater on environmental and behavioral risk factors, depression, subjective measures (pain, PtGA, HAQ, and QoL), life impact, and use of health services. Finally, it could be a mixed effect (sex and gender) on disease expression and the effect of drugs.

Gender medicine is a new paradigm focused on the differences between men and women in health and disease. RA might be triggered by a complex interaction between genetic, hormonal, environmental, and behavioral factors, all of which may be affected by sex. Comorbidities, reproductive issues, and measurement of disease activity all might affect treatment choices. Without a sex- and gender-sensitive and equitable approach to the management of RA, disparities in outcomes will persist.

Implementing sex and gender differences in scientific reports might be essential to equality and inclusivity. There is a critical need for research that addresses the biological (i.e., sex) as well as sociocultural (i.e., gender) causes of male–female disparities in immunotherapy responses, toxicities, and outcomes. Studies are also needed to define the influences of both patient and physician gender and their mutual interaction on the management of patients with RA.

Accounting for sex- and gender-related factors on health is an important challenge in research. The definition of research questions, experimental models, and statistical analysis should incorporate the complex, dynamic, and context-dependent constructs of sex and gender.

Author Contributions: Conceptualization: L.C. and E.A.; writing-original draft preparation: M.J.G.d.Y. All authors have contributed to the search for evidence and writing. All authors have read and agreed to the published version of the manuscript.

Funding: This research received no external funding.

Institutional Review Board Statement: Not applicable.

Informed Consent Statement: Not applicable.

Data Availability Statement: Not applicable.

Acknowledgments: Jaime Calvo contributed to setting the seed of this article as thesis supervisor of Elena Aurrecoechea and principal investigator of the GENIRA study.

Conflicts of Interest: The authors declare no conflict of interest.

References

1. Ritz, S.A.; Greaves, L. Transcending the Male-Female Binary in Biomedical Research: Constellations, Heterogeneity, and Mechanism When Considering Sex and Gender. *Int. J. Environ. Res. Public Health* **2022**, *19*, 4083. [CrossRef] [PubMed]
2. Van den Hurk, L.; Hiltner, S.; Oertelt-Prigione, S. Operationalization and Reporting Practices in Manuscripts Addressing Gender Differences in Biomedical Research: A Cross-Sectional Bibliographical Study. *Int. J. Environ. Res. Public Health* **2022**, *19*, 14299. [CrossRef] [PubMed]
3. Dowdy, S.W.; Dwyer, K.A.; Smith, C.A.; Wallston, K.A. Gender and psychological well-being of persons with rheumatoid arthritis. *Arthritis Care Res.* **1996**, *9*, 449–456. [CrossRef] [PubMed]
4. Bewley, S.; McCartney, M.; Meads, C.; Rogers, A. Sex, gender, and medical data. *BMJ* **2021**, *372*, n735. [CrossRef] [PubMed]
5. Shannon, G.; Jansen, M.; Williams, K.; Cáceres, C.; Motta, A.; Odhiambo, A.; Eleveld, A.; Mannell, J. Gender equality in science, medicine, and global health: Where are we at and why does it matter? *Lancet* **2019**, *393*, 560–569. [CrossRef] [PubMed]
6. Mauvais-Jarvis, F.; Bairey Merz, N.; Barnes, P.J.; Brinton, R.D.; Carrero, J.J.; DeMeo, D.L.; De Vries, G.J.; Epperson, C.N.; Govindan, R.; Klein, S.L.; et al. Sex and gender: Modifiers of health, disease, and medicine. *Lancet* **2020**, *396*, 565–582. [CrossRef] [PubMed]
7. Klein, S.L.; Morgan, R. The impact of sex and gender on immunotherapy outcomes. *Biol. Sex Differ.* **2020**, *11*, 24. [CrossRef] [PubMed]
8. Favalli, E.G.; Biggioggero, M.; Crotti, C.; Becciolini, A.; Raimondo, M.G.; Meroni, P.L. Sex and Management of Rheumatoid Arthritis. *Clin. Rev. Allergy Immunol.* **2019**, *56*, 333–345. [CrossRef]
9. Ngaruiya, C. When women win, we all win-Call for a gendered global NCD agenda. *FASEB Bioadv.* **2022**, *4*, 741–757. [CrossRef]
10. Machluf, Y.; Chaiter, Y.; Tal, O. Gender medicine: Lessons from COVID-19 and other medical conditions for designing health policy. *World J. Clin. Cases* **2020**, *8*, 3645–3668. [CrossRef]
11. Ortona, E.; Pierdominici, M.; Maselli, A.; Veroni, C.; Aloisi, F.; Shoenfeld, Y. Sex-based differences in autoimmune diseases. *Ann. Ist. Super. Sanita* **2016**, *52*, 205–212. [CrossRef] [PubMed]
12. Maranini, B.; Bortoluzzi, A.; Silvagni, E.; Govoni, M. Focus on Sex and Gender: What We Need to Know in the Management of Rheumatoid Arthritis. *J. Pers. Med.* **2022**, *12*, 499. [CrossRef] [PubMed]
13. Klein, S.L.; Flanagan, K.L. Sex differences in immune responses. *Nat. Rev. Immunol.* **2016**, *16*, 626–638. [CrossRef]
14. Morgacheva, O.; Furst, D.E. Women are from venus, men are from Mars: Do gender differences also apply to rheumatoid arthritis activity and treatment responses? *J. Clin. Rheumatol.* **2012**, *18*, 259–260. [CrossRef] [PubMed]
15. Gabriel, S.E. The epidemiology of rheumatoid arthritis. *Rheum. Dis. Clin. N. Am.* **2001**, *27*, 269–281. [CrossRef] [PubMed]
16. Furuya, T.; Salstrom, J.L.; McCall-Vining, S.; Cannon, G.W.; Joe, B.; Remmers, E.F.; Griffiths, M.M.; Wilder, R.L. Genetic dissection of a rat model for rheumatoid arthritis: Significant gender influences on autosomal modifier loci. *Hum. Mol. Genet.* **2000**, *9*, 2241–2250. [CrossRef] [PubMed]
17. Khan, M.A.; Yamashita, T.S.; Reynolds, T.L.; Wolfe, F.; Khan, M.K. HLA-DR4 genotype frequency and gender effect in familial rheumatoid arthritis. *Tissue Antigens* **1988**, *31*, 254–258. [CrossRef]
18. Caliz, R.; Canet, L.M.; Lupianez, C.B.; Canhao, H.; Escudero, A.; Filipescu, I.; Segura-Catena, J.; Soto-Pino, M.J.; Exposito-Ruiz, M.; Ferrer, M.A.; et al. Gender-specific effects of genetic variants within Th1 and Th17 cell-mediated immune response genes on the risk of developing rheumatoid arthritis. *PLoS ONE* **2013**, *8*, e72732. [CrossRef]
19. Chen, J.Y.; Wang, C.M.; Wu, Y.J.; Kuo, S.N.; Shiu, C.F.; Chang, S.W.; Lin, Y.T.; Ho, H.H.; Wu, J. Disease phenotypes and gender association of FCRL3 single-nucleotide polymorphism -169T/C in Taiwanese patients with systemic lupus erythematosus and rheumatoid arthritis. *J. Rheumatol.* **2011**, *38*, 264–270. [CrossRef]
20. Khalifa, O.; Pers, Y.M.; Ferreira, R.; Senechal, A.; Jorgensen, C.; Apparailly, F.; Duroux-Richard, I. X-Linked miRNAs Associated with Gender Differences in Rheumatoid Arthritis. *Int. J. Mol. Sci.* **2016**, *17*, 1852. [CrossRef]
21. Zhou, X.; Zhu, J.; Zhang, H.; Zhou, G.; Huang, Y.; Liu, R. Is the microRNA-146a (rs2910164) polymorphism associated with rheumatoid arthritis? Association of microRNA-146a (rs2910164) polymorphism and rheumatoid arthritis could depend on gender. *Jt. Bone Spine* **2015**, *82*, 166–171. [CrossRef] [PubMed]
22. Yu, C.; Liu, C.; Jiang, J.; Li, H.; Chen, J.; Chen, T.; Zhan, X. Gender Differences in Rheumatoid Arthritis: Interleukin-4 Plays an Important Role. *J. Immunol. Res.* **2020**, *2020*, 4121524. [CrossRef] [PubMed]
23. Brennan, P.; Silman, A. Why the gender difference in susceptibility to rheumatoid arthritis? *Ann. Rheum. Dis.* **1995**, *54*, 694–695. [CrossRef] [PubMed]
24. Danneskiold-Samsoe, B.; Bartels, E.M.; Dreyer, L. Gender differences in autoimmune diseases illustrated by arthritis. *Ugeskr. Laeger* **2007**, *169*, 2440–2442.
25. Intriago, M.; Maldonado, G.; Cárdenas, J.; Ríos, C. Clinical Characteristics in Patients with Rheumatoid Arthritis: Differences between Genders. *Sci. World J.* **2019**, *2019*, 8103812. [CrossRef] [PubMed]
26. George, M.D.; Baker, J.F. The Obesity Epidemic and Consequences for Rheumatoid Arthritis Care. *Curr. Rheumatol. Rep.* **2016**, *18*, 6. [CrossRef] [PubMed]
27. Hedström, A.K.; Stawiarz, L.; Klareskog, L.; Alfredsson, L. Smoking and susceptibility to rheumatoid arthritis in a Swedish population-based case-control study. *Eur. J. Epidemiol.* **2018**, *33*, 415–423. [CrossRef]

28. Krishnan, E. Smoking, gender and rheumatoid arthritis-epidemiological clues to etiology. Results from the behavioral risk factor surveillance system. *Jt. Bone Spine* **2003**, *70*, 496–502. [CrossRef]
29. Chang, K.; Yang, S.M.; Kim, S.H.; Han, K.H.; Park, S.J.; Shin, J.I. Smoking and rheumatoid arthritis. *Int. J. Mol. Sci.* **2014**, *15*, 22279–22295. [CrossRef]
30. Ljung, L.; Rantapaa-Dahlqvist, S. Abdominal obesity, gender and the risk of rheumatoid arthritis—A nested case-control study. *Arthritis Res. Ther.* **2016**, *18*, 277. [CrossRef]
31. Dar, L.; Tiosano, S.; Watad, A.; Bragazzi, N.L.; Zisman, D.; Comaneshter, D.; Cohen, A.; Amital, H. Are obesity and rheumatoid arthritis interrelated? *Int. J. Clin. Pract.* **2018**, *72*, e13045. [CrossRef] [PubMed]
32. Spitzer, C.; Wegert, S.; Wollenhaupt, J.; Wingenfeld, K.; Barnow, S.; Grabe, H.J. Gender-specific association between childhood trauma and rheumatoid arthritis: A case-control study. *J. Psychosom. Res.* **2013**, *74*, 296–300. [CrossRef] [PubMed]
33. Goeldner, I.; Skare, T.L.; de Messias Reason, I.T.; Nisihara, R.M.; Silva, M.B.; da Rosa Utiyama, S.R. Association of anticyclic citrullinated peptide antibodies with extra-articular manifestations, gender, and tabagism in rheumatoid arthritis patients from southern Brazil. *Clin. Rheumatol.* **2011**, *30*, 975–980. [CrossRef] [PubMed]
34. Sokka, T.; Toloza, S.; Cutolo, M.; Kautiainen, H.; Makinen, H.; Gogus, F.; Skakic, V.; Badsha, H.; Peets, T.; Baranauskaite, A.; et al. Women, men, and rheumatoid arthritis: Analyses of disease activity, disease characteristics, and treatments in the QUEST-RA study. *Arthritis Res. Ther.* **2009**, *11*, R7. [CrossRef] [PubMed]
35. Van Vollenhoven, R.F. Sex differences in rheumatoid arthritis: More than meets the eye. *BMC Med.* **2009**, *7*, 12. [CrossRef] [PubMed]
36. Voulgari, P.V.; Papadopoulos, I.A.; Alamanos, Y.; Katsaraki, A.; Drosos, A.A. Early rheumatoid arthritis: Does gender influence disease expression? *Clin. Exp. Rheumatol.* **2004**, *22*, 165–170. [PubMed]
37. Aurrecoechea, E.; Llorca Diaz, J.; Diez Lizuain, M.L.; McGwin, G., Jr.; Calvo-Alen, J. Gender-associated comorbidities in rheumatoid arthritis and their impact on outcome: Data from GENIRA. *Rheumatol. Int.* **2017**, *37*, 479–485. [CrossRef]
38. Barragan-Martinez, C.; Amaya-Amaya, J.; Pineda-Tamayo, R.; Mantilla, R.D.; Castellanos-de la Hoz, J.; Bernal-Macias, S.; Rojas-Villarraga, A.; Anaya, J.M. Gender differences in Latin-American patients with rheumatoid arthritis. *Gend. Med.* **2012**, *9*, 490–510.e5. [CrossRef]
39. Da Silva, J.A.; Hall, G.M. The effects of gender and sex hormones on outcome in rheumatoid arthritis. *Baillieres Clin. Rheumatol.* **1992**, *6*, 196–219. [CrossRef]
40. Nilsson, J.; Andersson, M.L.E.; Hafström, I.; Svensson, B.; Forslind, K.; Ajeganova, S.; Leu Agelii, M.; Gjertsson, I. Influence of Age and Sex on Disease Course and Treatment in Rheumatoid Arthritis. *Open Access Rheumatol.* **2021**, *13*, 123–138. [CrossRef]
41. Svensson, B.; Andersson, M.; Forslind, K.; Ajeganova, S.; Hafström, I. Persistently active disease is common in patients with rheumatoid arthritis, particularly in women: A long-term inception cohort study. *Scand. J. Rheumatol.* **2016**, *45*, 448–455. [CrossRef] [PubMed]
42. Twigg, S.; Hensor, E.M.A.; Freeston, J.; Tan, A.L.; Emery, P.; Tennant, A.; Morgan, A.W. Effect of Fatigue, Older Age, Higher Body Mass Index, and Female Sex on Disability in Early Rheumatoid Arthritis in the Treatment-to-Target Era. *Arthritis Care Res.* **2018**, *70*, 361–368. [CrossRef] [PubMed]
43. Jawaheer, D.; Maranian, P.; Park, G.; Lahiff, M.; Amjadi, S.S.; Paulus, H.E. Disease progression and treatment responses in a prospective DMARD-naive seropositive early rheumatoid arthritis cohort: Does gender matter? *J. Rheumatol.* **2010**, *37*, 2475–2485. [CrossRef] [PubMed]
44. Kapetanovic, M.C.; Lindqvist, E.; Geborek, P.; Saxne, T.; Eberhard, K. Long-term mortality rate in rheumatoid arthritis patients with disease onset in the 1980s. *Scand. J. Rheumatol.* **2011**, *40*, 433–438. [CrossRef] [PubMed]
45. Radovits, B.J.; Fransen, J.; van Riel, P.L.; Laan, R.F. Influence of age and gender on the 28-joint Disease Activity Score (DAS28) in rheumatoid arthritis. *Ann. Rheum. Dis.* **2008**, *67*, 1127–1131. [CrossRef] [PubMed]
46. Almutairi, K.B.; Inderjeeth, C.A.; Preen, D.B.; Keen, H.I.; Nossent, J.C. Mortality Trends among Patients with Rheumatoid Arthritis in Western Australia. *Rheumatol. Ther.* **2023**, *10*, 1021–1037. [CrossRef] [PubMed]
47. Anderson, S.T. Mortality in rheumatoid arthritis: Do age and gender make a difference? *Semin. Arthritis Rheum.* **1996**, *25*, 291–296. [CrossRef]
48. Dougados, M.; Soubrier, M.; Antunez, A.; Balint, P.; Balsa, A.; Buch, M.H.; Casado, G.; Detert, J.; El-Zorkany, B.; Emery, P.; et al. Prevalence of comorbidities in rheumatoid arthritis and evaluation of their monitoring: Results of an international, cross-sectional study (COMORA). *Ann. Rheum. Dis.* **2014**, *73*, 62–68. [CrossRef]
49. Targonska-Stepniak, B.; Biskup, M.; Biskup, W.; Majdan, M. Gender Differences in Cardiovascular Risk Profile in Rheumatoid Arthritis Patients with Low Disease Activity. *Biomed. Res. Int.* **2019**, *2019*, 3265847. [CrossRef]
50. Rohrich, D.C.; van de Wetering, E.H.M.; Rennings, A.J.; Arts, E.E.; Meek, I.L.; den Broeder, A.A.; Fransen, J.; Popa, C.D. Younger age and female gender are determinants of underestimated cardiovascular risk in rheumatoid arthritis patients: A prospective cohort study. *Arthritis Res. Ther.* **2021**, *23*, 2. [CrossRef]
51. Adawi, M.; Gurovich, B.; Firas, S.; Watad, A.; Bragazzi, N.L.; Amital, H.; Sirchan, R.; Blum, A. Gender differences in cardiovascular risk of patients with rheumatoid arthritis. *QJM* **2019**, *112*, 657–661. [CrossRef]
52. Oelzner, P.; Schwabe, A.; Lehmann, G.; Eidner, T.; Franke, S.; Wolf, G.; Hein, G. Significance of risk factors for osteoporosis is dependent on gender and menopause in rheumatoid arthritis. *Rheumatol. Int.* **2008**, *28*, 1143–1150. [CrossRef] [PubMed]

53. Furuya, T.; Inoue, E.; Tanaka, E.; Maeda, S.; Ikari, K.; Taniguchi, A.; Yamanaka, H. Age and female gender associated with periodontal disease in Japanese patients with rheumatoid arthritis: Results from self-reported questionnaires from the IORRA cohort study. *Mod. Rheumatol.* **2020**, *30*, 465–470. [CrossRef] [PubMed]
54. Nishino, T.; Hashimoto, A.; Tohma, S.; Matsui, T. Comprehensive evaluation of the influence of sex differences on composite disease activity indices for rheumatoid arthritis: Results from a nationwide observational cohort study. *BMC Rheumatol.* **2023**, *7*, 4. [CrossRef] [PubMed]
55. Castrejon Fernandez, I.; Martinez-Lopez, J.A.; Ortiz Garcia, A.M.; Carmona Ortells, L.; Garcia-Vicuna, R.; Gonzalez-Alvaro, I. Influence of gender on treatment response in a cohort of patients with early rheumatoid arthritis in the area 2 of Madrid. *Reumatol. Clin.* **2010**, *6*, 134–140. [CrossRef]
56. Hamann, P.D.H.; Shaddick, G.; Hyrich, K.; Green, A.; McHugh, N.; Pauling, J.D.; Group, B.R.C. Gender stratified adjustment of the DAS28-CRP improves inter-score agreement with the DAS28-ESR in rheumatoid arthritis. *Rheumatology* **2019**, *58*, 831–835. [CrossRef] [PubMed]
57. Rintelen, B.; Haindl, P.M.; Maktari, A.; Nothnagl, T.; Hartl, E.; Leeb, B.F. SDAI/CDAI levels in rheumatoid arthritis patients are highly dependent on patient's pain perception and gender. *Scand. J. Rheumatol.* **2008**, *37*, 410–413. [CrossRef] [PubMed]
58. Fillingim, R.B.; King, C.D.; Ribeiro-Dasilva, M.C.; Rahim-Williams, B.; Riley, J.L., 3rd. Sex, gender, and pain: A review of recent clinical and experimental findings. *J. Pain.* **2009**, *10*, 447–485. [CrossRef]
59. Lesuis, N.; Befrits, R.; Nyberg, F.; van Vollenhoven, R.F. Gender and the treatment of immune-mediated chronic inflammatory diseases: Rheumatoid arthritis, inflammatory bowel disease and psoriasis: An observational study. *BMC Med.* **2012**, *10*, 82. [CrossRef]
60. Affleck, G.; Tennen, H.; Keefe, F.J.; Lefebvre, J.C.; Kashikar-Zuck, S.; Wright, K.; Starr, K.; Caldwell, D.S. Everyday life with osteoarthritis or rheumatoid arthritis: Independent effects of disease and gender on daily pain, mood, and coping. *Pain* **1999**, *83*, 601–609. [CrossRef]
61. Ahlmen, M.; Svensson, B.; Albertsson, K.; Forslind, K.; Hafstrom, I.; Group, B.S. Influence of gender on assessments of disease activity and function in early rheumatoid arthritis in relation to radiographic joint damage. *Ann. Rheum. Dis.* **2010**, *69*, 230–233. [CrossRef] [PubMed]
62. Jawaheer, D.; Olsen, J.; Lahiff, M.; Forsberg, S.; Lahteenmaki, J.; da Silveira, I.G.; Rocha, F.A.; Magalhaes Laurindo, I.M.; Henrique da Mota, L.M.; Drosos, A.A.; et al. Gender, body mass index and rheumatoid arthritis disease activity: Results from the QUEST-RA Study. *Clin. Exp. Rheumatol.* **2010**, *28*, 454–461. [PubMed]
63. Iqbal, S.M.; Burns, L.; Grisanti, J. Effect of Body Mass Index on the Disease Activity of Patients with Rheumatoid Arthritis in a Gender-Specific Manner and the Association of Respective Serum C-Reactive Protein Levels with the Body's Inflammatory Status. *Cureus* **2020**, *12*, e9417. [CrossRef] [PubMed]
64. Colombo, D.; Zagni, E.; Nica, M.; Rizzoli, S.; Ori, A.; Bellia, G. Gender differences in the adverse events' profile registered in seven observational studies of a wide gender-medicine (MetaGeM) project: The MetaGeM safety analysis. *Drug Des. Devel. Ther.* **2016**, *10*, 2917–2927. [CrossRef] [PubMed]
65. De Vries, S.T.; Denig, P.; Ekhart, C.; Burgers, J.S.; Kleefstra, N.; Mol, P.G.M.; van Puijenbroek, E.P. Sex differences in adverse drug reactions reported to the National Pharmacovigilance Centre in the Netherlands: An explorative observational study. *Br. J. Clin. Pharmacol.* **2019**, *85*, 1507–1515. [CrossRef] [PubMed]
66. Jawaheer, D.; Olsen, J.; Hetland, M.L. Sex differences in response to anti-tumor necrosis factor therapy in early and established rheumatoid arthritis—Results from the DANBIO registry. *J. Rheumatol.* **2012**, *39*, 46–53. [CrossRef] [PubMed]
67. Soliman, M.M.; Hyrich, K.L.; Lunt, M.; Watson, K.D.; Symmons, D.P.; Ashcroft, D.M. Effectiveness of rituximab in patients with rheumatoid arthritis: Observational study from the British Society for Rheumatology Biologics Register. *J. Rheumatol.* **2012**, *39*, 240–246. [CrossRef] [PubMed]
68. Couderc, M.; Gottenberg, J.E.; Mariette, X.; Pereira, B.; Bardin, T.; Cantagrel, A.; Combe, B.; Dougados, M.; Flipo, R.M.; Le Loet, X.; et al. Influence of gender on response to rituximab in patients with rheumatoid arthritis: Results from the Autoimmunity and Rituximab registry. *Rheumatology* **2014**, *53*, 1788–1793. [CrossRef]
69. Nourisson, C.; Soubrier, M.; Mulliez, A.; Baillet, A.; Bardin, T.; Cantagrel, A.; Combe, B.; Dougados, M.; Flipo, R.M.; Schaeverbeke, T.; et al. Impact of gender on the response and tolerance to abatacept in patients with rheumatoid arthritis: Results from the 'ORA' registry. *RMD Open* **2017**, *3*, e000515. [CrossRef]
70. Fang, L.; Sonvg, X.; Ji, P.; Wang, Y.; Maynard, J.; Yim, S.; Sahajwalla, C.; Xu, M.; Kim, M.J.; Zhao, L. Impact of Sex on Clinical Response in Rheumatoid Arthritis Patients Treated with Biologics at Approved Dosing Regimens. *J. Clin. Pharmacol.* **2020**, *60* (Suppl. 2), S103–S109. [CrossRef]
71. Hashmi, F.; Haroon, M.; Ullah, S.; Asif, S.; Javed, S.; Tayyab, Z. Stress at Home and Female Gender Are Significantly Associated with Non-adherence and Poor Illness Perception among Patients with Rheumatoid Arthritis. *Cureus* **2022**, *14*, e25835. [CrossRef] [PubMed]
72. Aurrecoechea, E.; Llorca Diaz, J.; Diez Lizuain, M.L.; McGwin, G., Jr.; Calvo-Alen, J. Impact of Gender in the Quality of Life of patients with Rheumatoid Arthritis. *J. Arthritis* **2015**, *4*, 1–7.
73. Fifield, J.; Reisine, S.; Sheehan, T.J.; McQuillan, J. Gender, paid work, and symptoms of emotional distress in rheumatoid arthritis patients. *Arthritis Rheum.* **1996**, *39*, 427–435. [CrossRef]

74. Peláez-Ballestas, I.; Boonen, A.; Vázquez-Mellado, J.; Reyes-Lagunes, I.; Hernández-Garduño, A.; Goycochea, M.V.; Bernard-Medina, A.G.; Rodríguez-Amado, J.; Casasola-Vargas, J.; Garza-Elizondo, M.A.; et al. Coping strategies for health and daily-life stressors in patients with rheumatoid arthritis, ankylosing spondylitis, and gout: STROBE-compliant article. *Medicine* **2015**, *94*, e600. [CrossRef] [PubMed]
75. Wróbel, A.; Barańska, I.; Szklarczyk, J.; Majda, A.; Jaworek, J. Relationship between perceived stress, stress coping strategies, and clinical status in patients with rheumatoid arthritis. *Rheumatol. Int.* **2023**, *43*, 1665–1674. [CrossRef]
76. Stamm, T.A.; Machold, K.P.; Smolen, J.; Prodinger, B. Life stories of people with rheumatoid arthritis who retired early: How gender and other contextual factors shaped their everyday activities, including paid work. *Musculoskelet. Care* **2010**, *8*, 78–86. [CrossRef] [PubMed]
77. Van Middendorp, H.; Geenen, R.; Sorbi, M.J.; Hox, J.J.; Vingerhoets, A.J.; van Doornen, L.J.; Bijlsma, J.W. Gender differences in emotion regulation and relationships with perceived health in patients with rheumatoid arthritis. *Women Health* **2005**, *42*, 75–97. [CrossRef]
78. Ostlund, G.; Bjork, M.; Thyberg, I.; Valtersson, E.; Sverker, A. Women's situation-specific strategies in managing participation restrictions due to early rheumatoid arthritis: A gender comparison. *Musculoskelet. Care* **2018**, *16*, 251–259. [CrossRef]
79. McQuillan, J.; Andersen, J.A.; Berdahl, T.A.; Willett, J. Associations of Rheumatoid Arthritis and Depressive Symptoms over Time: Are There Differences by Education, Race/Ethnicity, and Gender? *Arthritis Care Res.* **2022**, *74*, 2050–2058. [CrossRef]
80. Mathias, K.; Mathias, L.; Amarnani, A.; Samko, T.; Lahita, R.G.; Panush, R.S. Challenges of caring for transgender and gender diverse patients with rheumatic disease: Presentation of seven patients and review of the literature. *Curr. Opin. Rheumatol.* **2023**, *35*, 117–127. [CrossRef]
81. Jacobi, C.E.; Triemstra, M.; Rupp, I.; Dinant, H.J.; Van Den Bos, G.A. Health care utilization among rheumatoid arthritis patients referred to a rheumatology center: Unequal needs, unequal care? *Arthritis Rheum.* **2001**, *45*, 324–330. [CrossRef]
82. Marrie, R.A.; Walker, J.R.; Graff, L.A.; Patten, S.B.; Bolton, J.M.; Marriott, J.J.; Fisk, J.D.; Hitchon, C.; Peschken, C.; Bernstein, C.N.; et al. Gender differences in information needs and preferences regarding depression among individuals with multiple sclerosis, inflammatory bowel disease and rheumatoid arthritis. *Patient Educ. Couns.* **2019**, *102*, 1722–1729. [CrossRef]
83. Neame, R.; Hammond, A.; Deighton, C. Need for information and for involvement in decision making among patients with rheumatoid arthritis: A questionnaire survey. *Arthritis Rheum.* **2005**, *53*, 249–255. [CrossRef] [PubMed]
84. Pytel, A.; Wrzosek, Z. Estimation of patient knowledge on rheumatoid arthritis in the range of their own disease—Preliminary study. *Adv. Clin. Exp. Med.* **2012**, *21*, 343–351. [PubMed]
85. Coffey, C.M.; Davis, J.M., 3rd; Crowson, C.S. The impact of gender on time to rheumatoid arthritis classification: A retrospective analysis of a population-based cohort. *Rheumatol. Int.* **2019**, *39*, 2025–2030. [CrossRef] [PubMed]
86. Giusti, A.; Epis, O.M.; Migliore, A.; Ricioppo, A.; Sainaghi, P.P.; Di Matteo, L.; Massarotti, M.S.; Govoni, M.; Mazzone, A.; Traballi, G.; et al. The effect of gender on methotrexate prescription attitudes in Italian rheumatoid arthritis patients: The MARI study. *Clin. Exp. Rheumatol.* **2019**, *37*, 1003–1009.

Disclaimer/Publisher's Note: The statements, opinions and data contained in all publications are solely those of the individual author(s) and contributor(s) and not of MDPI and/or the editor(s). MDPI and/or the editor(s) disclaim responsibility for any injury to people or property resulting from any ideas, methods, instructions or products referred to in the content.

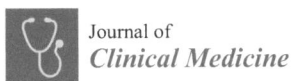

Article

Risk Factors Associated with Adverse Events Leading to Methotrexate Withdrawal in Elderly Rheumatoid Arthritis Patients: A Retrospective Cohort Study

Felipe Alexis Avalos-Salgado [1,2,†], Laura Gonzalez-Lopez [1,2,3,4,†], Sergio Gonzalez-Vazquez [5], Juan Manuel Ponce-Guarneros [2,4,6], Aline Priscilla Santiago-Garcia [1,2], Edna Lizeth Amaya-Cabrera [7], Reynaldo Arellano-Cervantes [1,2,8], J. Ahuixotl Gutiérrez-Aceves [1,2], Miriam Fabiola Alcaraz-Lopez [9], Cesar Arturo Nava-Valdivia [10], Fabiola Gonzalez-Ponce [2], Norma Alejandra Rodriguez-Jimenez [2,4], Miguel Angel Macias-Islas [11], Edgar Ricardo Valdivia-Tangarife [11], Ana Miriam Saldaña-Cruz [2,4], Ernesto German Cardona-Muñoz [2,4] and Jorge Ivan Gamez-Nava [1,2,3,4,*,‡] on behalf of Research Group for Factors Related to Therapeutic Outcomes in Autoimmune Diseases

1. Programa de Doctorado en Farmacología, Centro Universitario de Ciencias de la Salud, Universidad de Guadalajara, Guadalajara 44340, Mexico; felipe.asalgado@alumnos.udg.mx (F.A.A.-S.); ahuixotl.gutierrez@alumnos.udg.mx (J.A.G.-A.)
2. Research Group for Factors Related to Therapeutic Outcomes in Autoimmune Diseases, Centro Universitario de Ciencias de la Salud, Universidad de Guadalajara, Guadalajara 44340, Mexico; fabiola.gonzalez@academicos.udg.mx (F.G.-P.); norma.rodriguezj@academicos.udg.mx (N.A.R.-J.); german.cardona@academicos.udg.mx (E.G.C.-M.)
3. Programa de Maestria en Salud Publica, Departamento de Salud Pública, Centro Universitario de Ciencias de la Salud, Universidad de Guadalajara, Guadalajara 44340, Mexico
4. Instituto de Terapéutica Experimental y Clínica, Departamento de Fisiología, Centro Universitario de Ciencias de la Salud, Universidad de Guadalajara, Guadalajara 44340, Mexico
5. Hospital General Regional 110, Instituto Mexicano del Seguro Social, Guadalajara 44716, Mexico
6. Instituto Mexicano del Seguro Social, Unidad de Medicina Familiar No. 97, Magdalena 46474, Mexico
7. Departamento de Reumatología, Hospital Civil Fray Antonio Alcalde, Guadalajara 45019, Mexico; edna.amaya.cabrera@gmail.com
8. Departamento de Ciencias del Movimiento Humano, Centro Universitario de Ciencias de la Salud, Universidad de Guadalajara, Guadalajara 44340, Mexico
9. Departamento de Medicina Interna-Reumatología, Hospital General Regional Núm. 46, Instituto Mexicano del Seguro Social, Guadalajara 44910, Mexico
10. Departamento de Microbiología y Patología, Centro Universitario de Ciencias de la Salud, Universidad de Guadalajara, Guadalajara 44340, Mexico
11. Departamento de Neurociencias, Centro Universitario de Ciencias de la Salud, Universidad de Guadalajara, Guadalajara 44340, Mexico; miguelangelmacias@hotmail.com (M.A.M.-I.)

* Correspondence: ivangamezacademicoudg@gmail.com
† These authors contributed equally to this work and should be considered as first authors.
‡ Collaborators/Membership of the Group/Team Name is provided in the Acknowledgments.

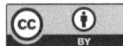

Abstract: Background: Rheumatoid arthritis (RA) in elderly population represents a challenge for physicians in terms of therapeutic management. Methotrexate (MTX) is the first-line treatment among conventional synthetic-disease-modifying anti-rheumatic drugs (cs-DMARDs); however, it is often associated with adverse events (AEs). Therefore, the objective of this study was to identify the incidence and risk factors of MTX discontinuation due to AEs in elderly patients with RA in a long-term retrospective cohort study. **Methods:** Clinical sheets from elderly RA patients taking MTX from an outpatient rheumatology consult in a university centre were reviewed. To assess MTX persistence, we used Kaplan–Meir curves and Cox regression models to identify the risk of withdrawing MTX due to adverse events. **Results:** In total, 198 elderly RA patients who reported using MTX were included. Of them, the rates of definitive suspension of MTX due to AEs were 23.0% at 5 years, 35.6% at 10 years and 51.7% at 15 years. The main organs and system involved were gastrointestinal (15.7%) and mucocutaneous (3.0%). Factors associated with withdrawing MTX due to AEs were MTX dose $\geq$ 15 mg/wk (adjusted HR: 2.46, 95% CI: 1.22–4.96, $p = 0.012$); instead, the folic acid supplementation was protective for withdrawal (adjusted HR: 0.28, 95% CI: 0.16–0.49, $p < 0.001$).

Conclusions: Higher doses of MTX increase the risk of withdrawals in elderly RA, while folic acid supplementation reduces the risk. Therefore, physicians working in therapeutic management for elderly patients using MTX must focus on using lower MTX doses together with the concomitant prescription of folic acid.

Keywords: rheumatoid arthritis in elderly; methotrexate; adverse events; withdrawals; treatment persistence; retrospective cohort studies

1. Introduction

Rheumatoid arthritis (RA) is a systemic, autoimmune inflammatory disease that affects synovial joints, causing chronic pain, bone erosions and disability [1]. The RA prevalence ranges from 0.5 to 1% worldwide [2]. Early onset of pharmacological treatment with conventional synthetic disease-modifying anti-rheumatic drugs (cs-DMARDs), constitutes the corner stone of the therapy directed to control the disease activity and decrease the progression of the disease. Methotrexate (MTX) is the synthetic DMARD prescribed as the first line of treatment [3,4]. MTX is a folic acid analog which exerts its therapeutic effects by inhibiting dihydrofolate reductase (DHFR), leading to decreased levels of tetrahydrofolate (THF), a vital component in purine synthesis. This depletion of purine nucleotides, including aminoimidazole carboxamide ribonucleotide transformylase (AICART), disrupts the synthesis of purines, crucial for cell proliferation. Consequently, methotrexate impedes the hyperactive immune response characteristic of RA, reducing inflammation and joint damage [5]. In many countries, including Mexico, MTX is the cs-DMARD most often prescribed to treat RA in around 70% of the patients [6]. However, most of the patients using MTX correspond to persons between the 4th and 5th decade of life and the information derived from using this drug in elderly patients is still limited, while in non-elderly RA patients, there is a wide variability in the time of using MTX [7–11]. The lack of persistence is one of the main factors that limits the effectiveness of MTX, and frequently, the withdrawals of the drug are caused by adverse events (AEs), which, depending on their severity, can lead to treatment discontinuation, from causing distress for the patient (mild) to more serious health complications (severe) [12]. Various factors associated with AEs that lead to MTX discontinuation have been investigated: increased body mass index (BMI) [13], higher pain perception [13], increased ALT levels [13], MTX dose [14], disease duration [14], lack of folate supplementation [14], age [14,15], sex [15], etc.

The World Health Organization (WHO) estimates that between 2015 and 2050, the proportion of the global population aged 60 years and older will nearly double. [16]. The presence of RA in elderly individuals is an important challenge for rheumatologists, internal medicine specialists and primary-care physicians. Studies performed in outpatient rheumatology clinics indicate that at least 20% of the patients with RA are older than 60 years [17]. However, the literature regarding the behavior of MTX and other drugs in this population is scarce. To date, there are few studies that have assessed MTX withdrawal due to adverse events in the elderly RA population during long-term therapy. Therefore, the present study aimed to identify the incidence and risk factors for withdrawals of MTX due to adverse events in elderly patients with RA in a long-term retrospective cohort study.

2. Materials and Methods

2.1. Study Design and Clinical Setting

Study design: retrospective cohort study. Three trained researchers performed a systematic assessment of clinical charts from elderly patients with RA from a 1000-patient cohort study who attended an outpatient rheumatology consultation therapeutic university centre from 1 January 1980 to 31 December 2016. The referred center mostly accommodates patients from Jalisco state in Mexico. The study was performed from September 2021 to January 2023.

2.2. Inclusion, Exclusion and Elimination Criteria

We included patients with RA diagnosed by a rheumatologist meeting the American Rheumatism Association 1987 revised criteria for RA [18]. These patients were ≥60 years old at the time of the first consult with the rheumatologist, were prescribed oral MTX for treating the joint manifestations of RA and had more than one visit to the rheumatologist for clinical assessment of evolution and response to treatment.

Patients with only one clinical visit were excluded. Other exclusion criteria were if at the baseline patients had any of the following conditions: cancer, chronic kidney disease (stage 3D or higher), liver diseases, hepatic insufficiency, active infectious diseases, untreated immunodeficiency, interstitial pneumonitis, pulmonary fibrosis, recent vaccination or hypersensitivity, alongside patients with overlapping syndrome (presence of RA plus symptoms of systemic lupus erythematosus, systemic scleroderma, and polymyositis).

2.3. Ethics

This study was approved by the following committees: Ethics in Research committee (CEI-CUCS) and Committee of Research (CI-CUCS) at the University Centre of Health Sciences (CUCS), University of Guadalajara, approval code CI-04021. This research protocol followed the Ethical Principles for Medical Research Involving Human Subjects described in the Helsinki Declaration [19].

2.4. Study Development

Demographic and clinical data were ascertained by three trained researchers who reviewed elderly RA patients' clinical charts who attended the public hospital. Information recollected was classified as:

(a) Sociodemographic variables: gender, age, type of insurance, body mass index (BMI), alcohol consumption, smoking;
(b) Comorbid diseases: hypertension, diabetes mellitus type 2, obesity, depression and other comorbid diseases;
(c) Disease characteristics: disease duration, articular and extraarticular manifestations, functional classification;
(d) Pharmacological treatment (cs-DMARDS use, Methotrexate, Sulfasalazine, Antimalarials, other cs-DMARDS), persistence of treatment (years), combined cs-DMARD therapy—use of 2 or more cs-DMARDs simultaneously—and any other drug prescribed, such as glucocorticoids, non-steroidal anti-inflammatory drugs, analgesics, painkillers, antiacids, or antihypertensives, alongside folic acid supplementation;
(e) Safety: adverse events that led to MTX discontinuation alongside MTX dose and usage time at the time of their appearance. Only adverse events that led patients to stop their MTX treatment for more than 90 days were counted. Additionally, these were classified based on the organ and system affected and the specific type of event.
(f) Adverse events were considered as reported by the rheumatologist in the clinical charts at the time of each visit. Because this is a retrospective cohort, we were unable to identify the adverse events using prespecified definitions; however, the guidelines/recommendations to identify adverse events associated with MTX in our institution are described briefly as follows:

- Gastritis, gastropathies and gastrointestinal manifestations. These included gastric or duodenal mucosal injury, nausea, vomiting, mucosal ulcers, loss of appetite and epigastralgia.
- Transaminitis (elevated transaminases): presence of alanine transaminase (ALT) and aspartate transaminase (AST), higher than upper limits of normal (ULN) cutoff values of the reference laboratory; the normal values in our laboratory were as follows: ALT: normal range 5–50 IU/L; AST: normal range 10 to 34 IU/L. Severe transaminitis was considered an increase of ALT or AST > 3-fold ULN in two consecutive visits.

- Diagnosis of bleeding diverticulitis was performed by gastroenterologist based on symptoms of recurrent mild abdominal pain and distension plus rectal bleeding, corroborated with diverticula images in abdominal CT scan.
- Oral ulcers: symptoms of painful and observation of well-defined small ulcers (yellow or white rounded by erythema) in mouth and throat plus diverse difficulty in swallowing food with presence of small mucosal erosions/ulcerations on oral mucosa and/or tongue. Chronologically associated with MTX use and disappearing after this DMARD withdrawn (corroborated by dermatologist).
- Alopecia and hair loss: hair loss temporally correlated with the use of MTX, disappeared when MTX was withdrawn (corroborated by dermatologist).
- Abnormal blood counts; definitions:
    - Anemia: hemoglobin level of <115 g/L;
    - Leukopenia: peripheral blood leukocyte count $< 3.0 \times 10^9$/L;
    - Neutropenia: neutrophil count of $<1.8 \times 10^9$/L;
    - Lymphopenia: lymphocytes count $< 1.1 \times 10^9$/L;
    - Thrombocytopenia: platelet count of $<100 \times 10^9$/L;
    - Thrombocytosis: platelet count of $>450 \times 10^9$/L.
- Interstitial pneumopathy: persistent symptoms of dyspnea and dry cough, plus findings of scattered or diffuse and patchy, ground glass opacity with images of reticular involvement identified by high resolution computed tomography (HRCT) and corroborated by a pneumologist. Pulmonary fibrosis was diagnosed by findings of honeycombing images (clustered cystic airspaces) located in subpleural region, with well-defined walls and diameters >0.5 cm, observed in HRCT corroborated by radiologist and pneumologist.
- Dermatosis attributable to MTX: cutaneous lesions of erythematous indurated papules located on proximal areas of the extremities with a direct chronologic correlation with MTX therapy corroborated by dermatologist. These lesions disappeared when MTX was withdrawn and had response to corticosteroids (topical or systemics).
- Weakness as persistent symptoms of fatigue or tiredness.
- Weight loss: >10% in kilograms, obtained from the difference between weight in the last visit (index visit)—weight in the previous visit.
- Recurrent infections: corroborated by persistent positive cultures or other accepted method.
- Urinary lithiasis: presence of stones observed in kidney or urinary tract using ultrasound or computed tomography (CT).

2.5. Statistical Analysis

The incidence rate for adverse events that led to MTX suspension was computed, and each adverse event was reported based on the organ and system affected along with their specific description. Independent Student's *t*-tests were used for comparisons of quantitative variables between groups; chi-square tests (or Fischer exact tests if required) were used for comparisons of proportions between groups. The cumulative drug survival probability of MTX treatment persistence was analyzed using the Kaplan–Meier method, where the reasons for censoring were the MTX continuation at the end of the study or loss to follow-up, and plots were used to determine the incidence density of MTX discontinuation due to AEs. Univariate and multivariate Cox proportional hazards regression models were used to assess potential predictors for MTX discontinuation due to AEs. The significance level was set at $p \leq 0.05$. The analyses were performed using the statistical software SPPS Statistics Version 24.

3. Results

From the cohort of 1000 RA patients, 355 patients were ≥60 years old and were screened for inclusion in the study. Of them, 133 patients were excluded because MTX was not prescribed during the follow-up, and 26 additional patients were excluded because they were prescribed biological therapy alongside MTX. Therefore, 198 elderly RA patients met the inclusion criteria and were included in the study.

Table 1 describes the sociodemographic and disease characteristics of the 198 elderly RA patients included in this study. Most of them were females (84.8%), with a mean age of 66.8 ± 5.6 years. The median RA disease duration was 1 year at the cohort onset, and 40.9% had a positive rheumatoid factor (RF). Of them, 65.7% had extraarticular manifestations, the three most frequent being anemia (35.4%), secondary Sjogren syndrome (34.8%) and rheumatoid nodules (23.7%).

Table 1. Characteristics of patients with rheumatoid arthritis.

	n = 198 (100.0)
Female gender, n (%)	168 (84.8)
Age (yrs), mean ± SD	66.8 ± 5.6
BMI *, mean ± SD	27.5 ± 5.7
Smoking, n (%)	6 (3.0)
Alcohol abuse, n (%)	4 (2.0)
Comorbidities, n (%)	153 (77.3)
Number of comorbidities, median (range)	1 (0.0, 4.0)
Overweight or Obesity, n (%)	118 (59.6)
Arterial Hypertension, n (%)	91 (46.0)
Osteoporosis, n (%)	57 (28.8)
Type 2 Diabetes Mellitus, n (%)	35 (17.1)
Clinical depression, n (%)	19 (9.6)
RA duration (yrs) up to onset of MTX treatment, median (range)	1.0 (0.0, 39.0)
Steinbroker's functional class, n (%)	
- Functional class I, n (%)	49 (24.7)
- Functional class II–IV, n (%)	149 (75.3)
Pain score (VAS ** 0–100), mean ± DS	72.5 ± 15.7
Morning stiffness (>1 h), n (%)	108 (54.5)
Positive RF ***, n (%)	81 (40.9)
Extraarticular manifestations, n (%):	130 (65.7)
Anemia, n (%)	70 (35.4)
Sjogren syndrome, n (%)	69 (34.8)
Rheumatic nodules, n (%)	47 (23.7)
Neuropathies, n (%)	39 (19.7)
Pneumopathies, n (%)	4 (2.0)

Abbreviations: * BMI: Body mass index, ** VAS: Visual analogue scale, *** RF: Rheumatoid factor. Qualitative variables are expressed as frequencies and percentages, and quantitative variables as means and standard deviations (SDs) or as medians with minimum and maximum values (range).

3.1. Pharmacological Treatment

Table 2 describes the pharmacological treatment prescribed by the rheumatologist at baseline. Monotherapy with MTX at the beginning of their treatment was reported in 120 patients (60.6%), while 78 patients (39.3%) used combined therapy since the onset of treatment, the most frequent combination being MTX plus Sulfasalazine (SSZ) (19.2%) and MTX plus Chloroquine (CHL) (8.6%). Polypharmacy (≥5 drugs taken simultaneously by ≥90 days) including all the drugs taken by the patients at the baseline was observed in almost all the patients (94.9%). Folate supplementation was prescribed for 77.8% of the patients. The MTX dose is reported as the last dosage reported.

Table 2. Baseline pharmacological treatment.

	n = 198 (100.0)
Methotrexate as monotherapy, n (%)	120 (60.6)
Combined therapy, n (%)	78 (39.3)
MTX dose (mg)/wk, mean ± SD	13.6 ± 3.6
Usage duration (yrs), median (min., max.)	5 (0.01, 15.00)
Combined therapy MTX plus:	
Sulfasalazine, n (%)	38 (19.2)
Azathioprine, n (%)	17 (8.6)
Leflunomide, n (%)	9 (4.5)
Chloroquine, n (%)	4 (2.0)
SSZ + CHQ, n (%)	5 (2.5)
AZA + LEF, n (%)	2 (1.0)
Other combinations *, n (%)	3 (1.5)
Glucocorticoids, n (%)	169 (85.4)
NSAIDs, n (%)	189 (95.5)
Analgesics, n (%)	156 (78.8)
Other drugs:	
Omeprazole, n (%)	130 (65.7)
Antiresorptive, n (%)	46 (23.2)
Antihypertensives, n (%)	43 (21.7)
Antidiabetic drugs, n (%)	16 (8.1)
Num. of drugs used at the same time, mean ± SD	8.3 ± 2.6
Polypharmacy (≥5 or more drugs), n (%)	188 (94.9)
Folic acid supplementation, n (%)	154 (77.8)

Abbreviations: MTX: Methotrexate, SSZ: Sulfasalazine, CHQ: Chloroquine, AZA: Azathioprine, LEF: Leflunomide, NSAIDs: Non-steroidal anti-inflammatory drug. Qualitative variables are expressed as frequencies and percentages, and quantitative variables as medians (ranges) or means and standard deviations (SDs). * Other combinations: MTX + SSZ + CHQ (0.5%), MTX + SSZ + LEF (0.5%) and MTX + CHQ + LEF (0.5%).

3.2. Changes of MTX Monotherapy to MTX Combined Therapy during the Follow-Up

The rate of using MTX as monotherapy decreased during the follow-up. After 5 years, 105 patients remained in the cohort; 44.8% patients used monotherapy with MTX and 55.2% combined therapy, the most frequent combinations being MTX plus SSZ (21.0%) and MTX plus Leflunomide (LEF) (9.5%). After 10 years, only 44 patients remained in the cohort; 29.5% patients used monotherapy with MTX and 70.5% combined therapy, the most used combination being MTX plus SSZ (22.7%). At 15 years, only 12 patients remained in the study; 30.6% were using MTX monotherapy and 55.1% combined therapy, with MTX plus SSZ (24.5%) as the most frequent combination of cs-DMARDs.

3.3. Adverse Events Leading to Suspension of MTX

Table 3 describes the adverse events that led to the suspension of MTX. During follow-up, 64/198 patients (32.3%) suspended MTX; of those, 54 (27.3%) withdrawals were due to adverse events, 5 (2.5%) were due to drug shortage and only 2 patients (1.0%) suspended MTX due to inefficacy. For the adverse events motivating definitive suspension of MTX, for 54 (27.3%), the main organs/systems involved were gastrointestinal (15.7%), mucocutaneous (3.0%), hepatic (2.5%) and constitutional symptoms (2.0%). In data that are not shown in tables, 16 patients (29.6%) had severe adverse events, such as: transaminasemia, bleeding diverticulitis and upper digestive tract bleeding, interstitial pneumopathy and/or pulmonary fibrosis, and severe infections.

Table 3. Classification of adverse events reported that led to discontinuation.

Patients Who Discontinued MTX Due to AEs	n = 54 (100.0)
Main organs and systems with AEs	
Gastrointestinal, n (%)	31 (57.4)
Mucocutaneous, n (%)	6 (11.1)
Hepatic, n (%)	5 (9.2)
Constitutional symptoms, n (%)	4 (7.4)
Recurrent infections, n (%)	3 (5.5)
Hematologic, n (%)	2 (3.7)
Pulmonary, n (%)	2 (3.7)
Renal, n (%)	1 (1.8)
Specific adverse event	
Epigastralgia and/or Gastritis	18 (33.3)
Nausea, vomiting, gastric intolerance and/or diarrhea	10 (18.5)
Transaminitis	5 (9.2)
Bleeding diverticulitis and upper digestive tract bleeding	5 (9.2)
Oral ulcers and/or Alopecia/hair loss	5 (9.2)
Leukopenia and/or lymphopenia	2 (3.7)
Interstitial pneumopathy/pulmonary fibrosis	2 (3.7)
Weakness and weight loss	2 (3.7)
Dermatosis	1 (1.8)
Tuberculosis infection.	1 (1.8)
Hepatitis C infection	1 (1.8)
Recurrent infections	1 (1.8)
Urinary lithiasis	1 (1.8)

Qualitative variables are expressed as frequencies and percentages, and quantitative variables as medians (ranges) or means and standard deviations (SDs).

3.4. Rate of MTX Withdrawal

The patients using MTX were followed up for a total of 1155.20 person-years (mean: 6.1 ± 4.9 years, median: 5.0 years). Density incidence of MTX suspension caused by adverse events was 0.040 per 1000 person-years. Figure 1 shows Kaplan–Meier survival curves of the time to MTX withdrawal, in which the cumulative incidence of MTX suspension was 23.0% after 5 years, 35.6% after 10 years and 51.7% after 15 years.

Table 4 shows a comparison of variables observed at baseline between patients who discontinued MTX with those who continued MTX. There were no differences in epidemiological variables (such as: age, BMI and comorbidities), nor variables associated with RA (tender joint count, swollen joint count, morning stiffness or extraarticular manifestations) between these groups. Patients who discontinued MTX had higher doses of this DMARD compared to patients who did not discontinue that DMARD ($p = 0.006$). Instead, patients who did not discontinue MTX had higher frequency of using folic acid supplements compared to those who discontinued MTX ($p < 0.001$). Patients who continued MTX had a longer time of using this DMARD compared to those who withdrew MTX ($p < 0.001$).

In Figure 2B1–B4, we showed different risk factors associated with MTX discontinuation by Kaplan–Meier analyses: Figure 2B1 describes the relation of suspension due to AEs with higher MTX doses (≥ 15 mg/wk). Patients with higher doses of MTX had significantly higher rate of suspension for MTX due to AEs ($p < 0.001$).

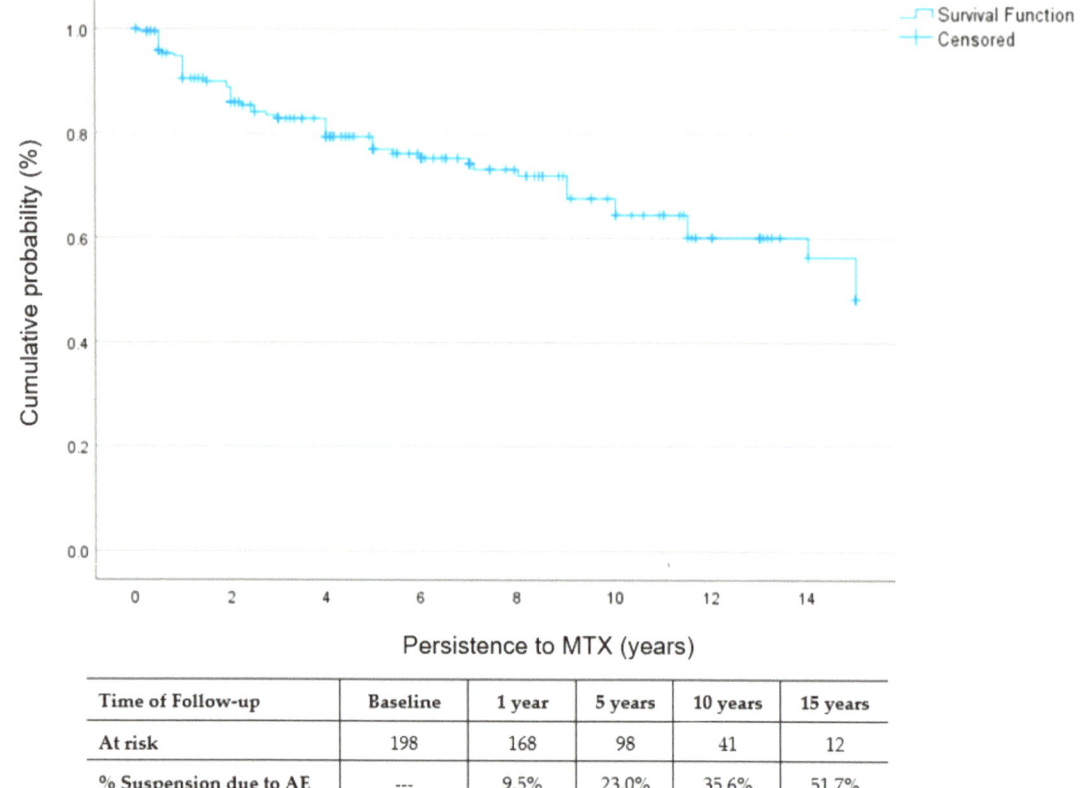

Time of Follow-up	Baseline	1 year	5 years	10 years	15 years
At risk	198	168	98	41	12
% Suspension due to AE	---	9.5%	23.0%	35.6%	51.7%

Figure 1. Persistence of MTX.

Table 4. Comparison of variables between RA patients with MTX withdrawals due to adverse events (AEs) vs. RA patients who continued MTX.

Variable, n (%)	MTX Withdrawals * n = 54 (100.0)	MTX (Non-Withdrawals) n = 144 (100.0)	p
Age (yrs), mean ± SD	65.6 ± 5.0	67.2 ± 5.7	0.08
BMI, mean ± SD	28.2 ± 7.5	27.2 ± 4.5	0.3
Num. comorbidities, mean ± SD	1.2 ± 1.1	1.3 ± 0.9	0.6
Arterial Hypertension, n (%)	25 (46.3)	66 (45.8)	0.9
RA duration before MTX, mean ± DS	5.6 ± 8.7	5.3 ± 7.9	0.8
Pain score (VAS 0–100 mm), mean ± DS	74.2 ± 14.6	73.3 ± 14.0	0.7
Tender joints count, mean ± DS	10.3 ± 5.9	10.4 ± 6.0	0.8
Swollen joints count, mean ± DS	9.9 ± 4.4	9.3 ± 4.1	0.4
Morning stiffness (>1 h), n (%)	30 (55.6)	78 (54.2)	0.8
Extraarticular manifestations, n (%):	40 (74.1)	90 (62.5)	0.1

Table 4. Cont.

Variable, n (%)	MTX Withdrawals * n = 54 (100.0)	MTX (Non-Withdrawals) n = 144 (100.0)	p
Sjogren syndrome, n (%)	14 (9.7)	7 (13.0)	0.5
Rheumatic nodules, n (%)	13 (24.1)	34 (23.6)	0.9
RF, n (%)	23 (42.6)	58 (40.3)	0.7
MTX dose (mg/wk), mean ± SD	14.2 ± 2.1	12.0 ± 2.2	0.006
Time of using MTX (years), mean ± SD	4.1 ± 4.0	6.4 ± 4.4	<0.001
Combined therapy **, n (%)	21 (38.9)	57 (39.6)	0.9
Glucocorticoids, n (%)	50 (92.6))	119 (82.6)	0.07
Polypharmacy (≥5 or more drugs), n (%)	50 (92.6)	138 (95.8)	0.3
Folic acid supplementation, n (%)	30 (55.6)	124 (86.1)	<0.001

Abbreviations: RA: Rheumatoid Arthritis, MTX: Methotrexate, BMI: Body Mass Index, VAS: Visual Analogue Scale, RF: Rheumatoid Factor * MTX withdrawals due to AEs. ** Combined therapy was considered as patients with MTX + at least 1 or more DMARDs. All variables were reported at cohort onset excepting: (1) MTX dose: this variable was reported as the last dose before suspending the drug (in patients with MTX suspension), or as the last MTX dose registered in the clinical chart in those patients who did not discontinue this drug; (2) Time of using MTX, this variable was reported computing the years of using that DMARD until drug suspension; in those who continued MTX this variable was computed as the total time since MTX onset until the last visit. Comparisons between proportions were performed using chi-square test and comparisons between means were performed using Student t-tests.

Figure 2B2 shows the comparison between survival on taking MTX in patients using folate supplementation vs. patients without it. Patients receiving folate supplementation had significantly lower rate of suspension for MTX due to AEs ($p < 0.001$). Figure 2B3 evaluates the effect of having gastropathy at baseline. Patients with gastropathy had significantly higher rate of suspension for MTX due to AEs ($p = 0.016$).

Other risk factors were evaluated, such as the number of DMARDs at the beginning of the treatment, the presence of comorbidities, anemia and BMI >25 (Overweight to obesity, Figure 2B4); though none of these reported an effect over MTX survival.

Table 5 shows the results of the multivariate Cox risk analysis. In the model, we included as time-dependent variable: MTX withdrawals due to adverse events. Covariables (potential confounders) tested in the unadjusted model (enter method) were female sex, overweight/obesity, presence of two or more comorbidities, tender joints count, swollen joints count, use of two or more DMARDs (MTX plus at least another DMARD), MTX dose equal to or higher than 15 mg/wk and folic acid supplementation. The risk model showed significant relations between MTX survival and the MTX dose ≥ 15 mg/wk (HR = 2.76, 95% CI: 1.33, 5.74, $p = 0.006$) and folic acid supplementation (HR = 0.27, 95% CI: 0.15, 0.49, $p < 0.001$), whereas no statistical associations were observed with the rest of covariables. In the second analysis, adjusting by stepwise method these potential confounders, in the model, only 2 variables remained significantly associated with risk of MTX withdrawals due to adverse events: MTX dose ≥ 15 mg/wk increasing the risk of MTX suspension (aHR = 2.46, 95% CI: 1.22, 4.96, $p = 0.012$) and folic acid supplementation as protective factor (aHR = 0.28, 95% CI: 0.16, 0.49, $p < 0.001$).

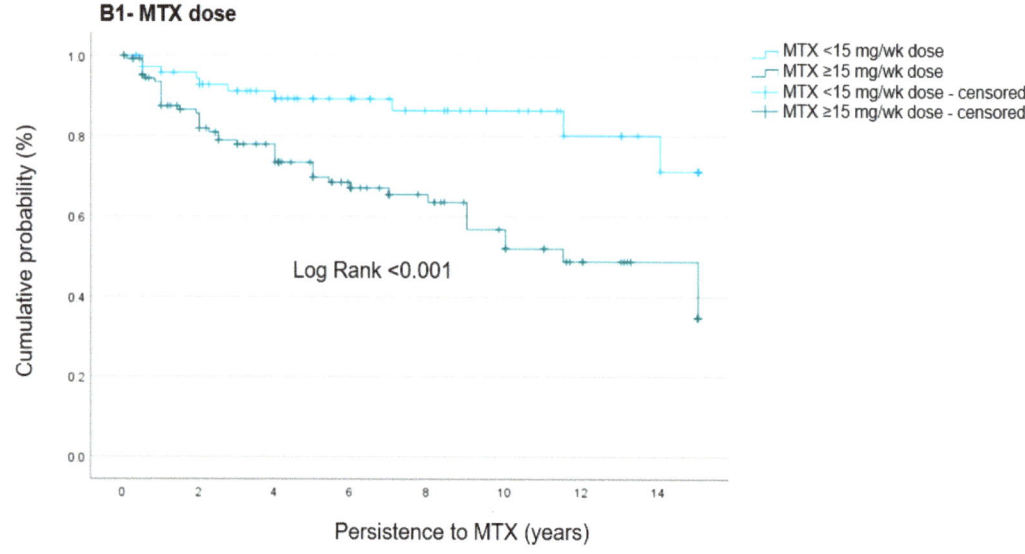
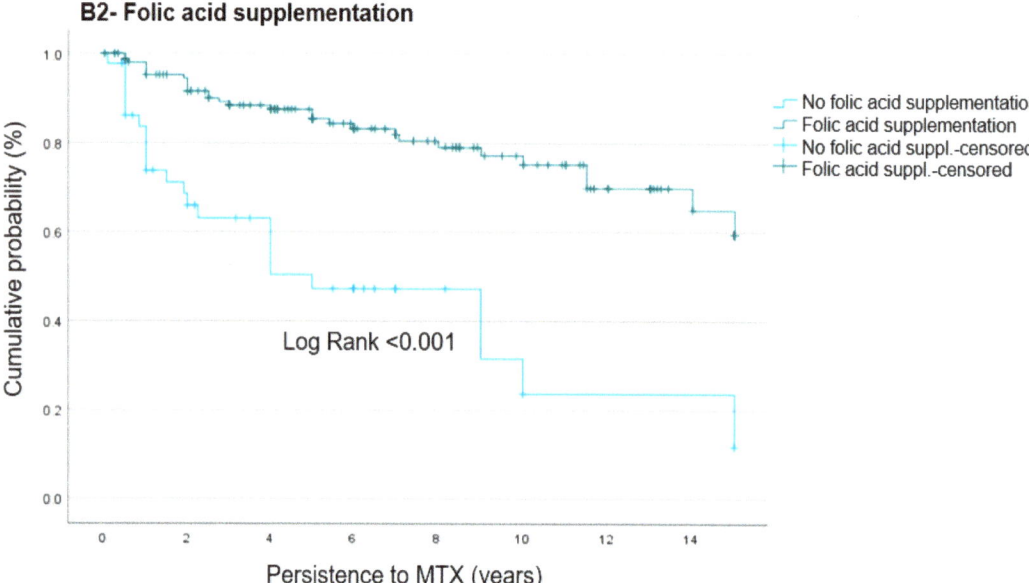

Figure 2. *Cont.*

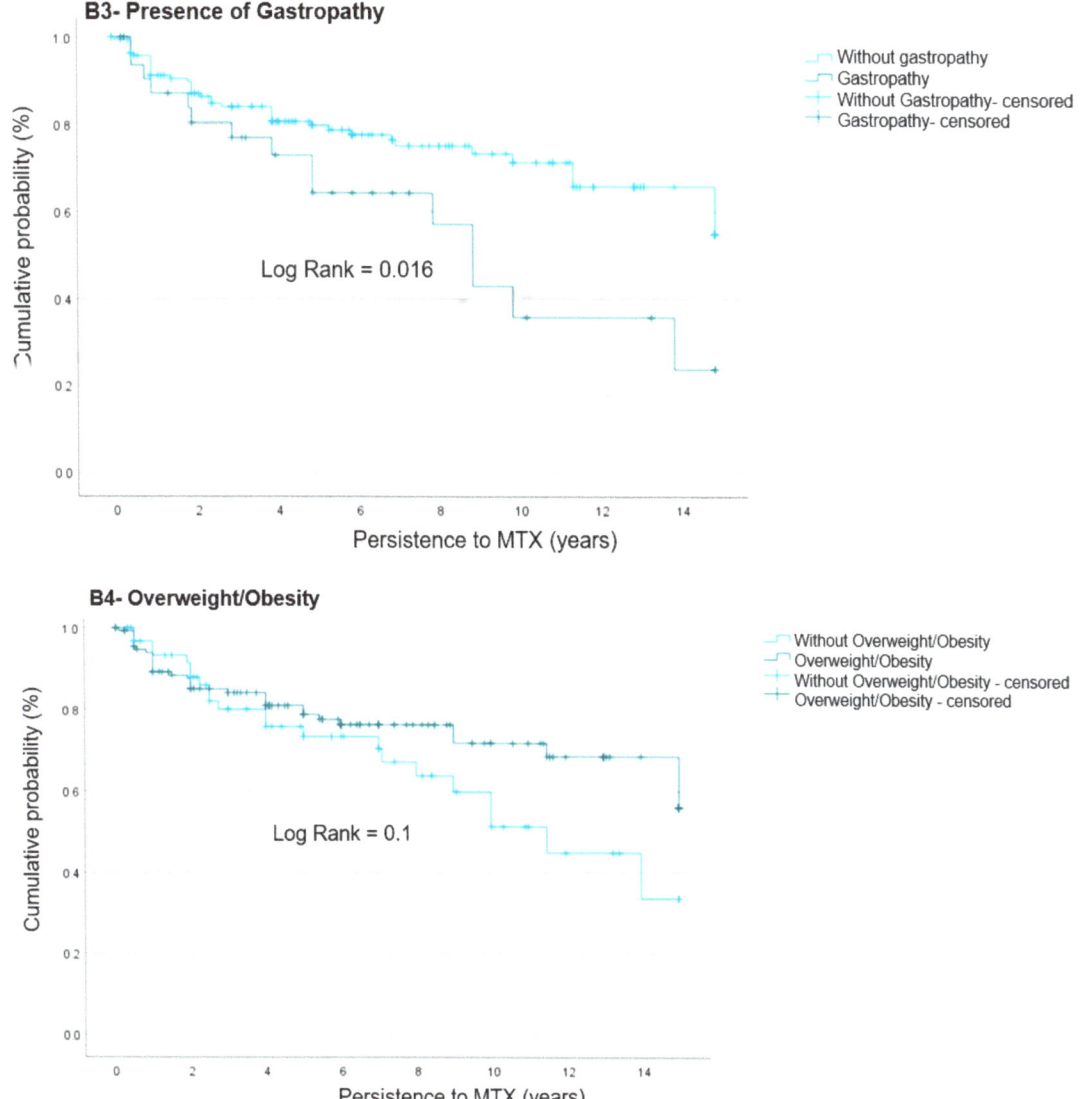

Figure 2. B1–B4: Risk factors of MTX discontinuation due to adverse events.

Table 5. Risk factors for MTX suspension due to adverse events in elderly patients with rheumatoid arthritis.

	MTX Treatment Suspension Due to Adverse Events					
	Unadjusted			Adjusted		
	Enter Method			Stepwise Method		
	HR	95% CI	*p*-Value	aHR	95% CI	*p*-Value
Female sex	1.03	0.47–2.28	0.9	--	--	--
Overweight/obesity	0.75	0.41–1.36	0.3	--	--	--
≥2 Comorbidities	0.70	0.33–1.46	0.3	--	--	--

Table 5. *Cont.*

	MTX Treatment Suspension Due to Adverse Events					
	Unadjusted			Adjusted		
	Enter Method			Stepwise Method		
	HR	95% CI	*p*-Value	aHR	95% CI	*p*-Value
Tender joints	0.98	0.93–1.03	0.6	--	--	--
Swollen joints	1.05	0.98–1.13	0.1	--	--	--
≥2 DMARDs *	0.78	0.43–1.41	0.4	--	--	--
MTX dose ≥ 15 mg/wk	2.76	1.33–5.74	0.006	2.46	1.22–4.96	0.012
Folic acid usage	0.27	0.15–0.49	<0.001	0.28	0.16–0.49	<0.001

Abbreviations: BMI: Body mass index. DMARDs: Disease-modifying antirheumatic drugs. MTX: Methotrexate. * For covariates the use of MTX plus one or more DMARDS (SSZ, CLQ, AZA and/or LEF) was considered as ≥2 DMARDs. aHR: Adjusted hazard ratio. 95 CI: 95% Confidence interval. Crude HRs were obtained using the enter method. aHR was obtained using the stepwise method. Variables excluded from the final model were female sex, ≥25 BMI, ≥2 comorbidities, tender joints, swollen joints and ≥2 DMARDs.

4. Discussion

This study identified that the incidence rates of definitive suspension of MTX due to AEs were 9.5% at 1 year, 23.0% at 5 years, 35.6% at 10 years and 51.7% at 15 years from initiating the drug. The main risk factor that increased the probability of MTX suspension due to AEs was the use of higher doses of MTX (≥15 mg/wk), whereas the use of folic acid acted as a protective factor against suspension due to AEs. The most frequent cause of MTX definitive suspension in RA elderly patients was adverse events, mainly gastrointestinal and mucocutaneus effects.

4.1. MTX Persistence

In the present study, we identified that 59.1% of elderly patients had MTX prescribed as a monotherapy at baseline and 29.7% in combined therapy. Monotherapy with MTX is more frequently indicated in elderly patients compared to young patients where the use of combined therapy with cs-DMARDS seems to be more frequently prescribed. In elderly RA patients, a concern is the increasing of side effects by pharmacological interactions of the high number of drugs used to treat comorbidities; therefore, it is more usual in our centers to prescribe MTX monotherapy in this population compared to younger RA patients. This therapeutic behavior has been reported by other studies: Tutuncu Z et al. compared in a cross-sectional design the information of two databases in different populations defined by age: the first was the information derived from the elderly-onset rheumatoid arthritis (EORA) database and the second derived from information of the younger-onset rheumatoid arthritis (YORA) database; these authors described a higher proportion of using MTX monotherapy in elderly RA compared to younger RA patients where the utilization of combined therapy was more usual (p = 0.005) [20]. Mathieu S et al. followed for five years French RA patients, stratified in three different age groups: >50, 50 to 64, and 65 to 74 years old, observing a higher prevalence (68.4%) of MTX monotherapy in their elderly group (65 to 74 years old), observing higher rates of MTX suspension correlated with the increase of other cs-DMARDS co-utilization, although the oldest group showed a higher persistence to RA treatment regardless of the number of drugs received [21]. Similarly, in our study, we did not identify statistical differences in the rate of suspension of MTX by AEs when it was used in combined therapy compared against use of MTX monotherapy.

We identified a low rate (9.5%) of MTX suspension due to AEs at 1 year of treatment; however, it increased to 23.0% at 5 years, and continued increasing to almost one of three patients (35.6%) at 10 years, and lastly, around one of each two patients (51.7%) suspended treatment at 15 years. Two studies performed in Danish and French RA patients identified a similar rate of MTX suspension at 5 years of treatment onset [15,21]. Bliddal H. et al. found a rate of MTX suspension in Danish RA patients (mean age 59.8 ± 14.4 years) similar to the one observed by us, of 25% at 5 years [15]. Mathieu S et al. observed in French

RA patients, stratified in three groups as stated above, the rate of MTX suspension of 25% at 5 years, showing a higher retention rate in the oldest group [21]. Other authors have reported higher rates of MTX suspensions in their cohorts. Alarcon G.S. et al. reported a 55% rate of suspending MTX at 5 years due to toxicity in North American RA patients (mean age: 61.2 ± 12.4 years) [9]. Scully C.J. et al., in North American RA patients (mean age: 51 ± 12 years), observed that almost four of five patients (71.5%) suspended MTX at 5 years [22]. Lastly, Ideguchi H et al. reported that in Japanese RA patients (mean age 57.6 ± 11.4 years), there was a 40% rate of MTX suspension at 5 years [14]. Rate of MTX suspension due to AEs at 10 years was 35.6%, similar to those reported in Danish patients by Bliddal H, observing that at 10 years, 35% of patients stopped MTX treatment [15]. Other cohorts reported higher rates of suspension at 10 years. Hoesktra M et al. reported that in Dutch RA patients (median age: 59.7), at 9 years, the rate of MTX withdrawal was 50% [10]; Alarcon G.S. et al. observed a higher discontinuation rate of 70% in RA patients after 10 years (mean age: 61.2 ± 12.4) [8]. Lastly, to the best of our knowledge, we could not identify a cohort with a follow-up of 15 years of elderly patients, where one of each two patients (51.7%) had suspended treatment at the end of the study period.

4.2. Adverse Events of MTX That Led to Suspension

The main EAs reported in our study were gastrointestinal (15.7%), mucocutaneus (3.0%) and hepatic (2.5%). We identified several studies in which Aes were associated with the main cause of MTX suspension. Alarcon G.S. et al. described that the most frequent AEs leading to discontinuation of MTX in North American RA patients (mean age: 61.2 ± 12.4 years) were gastrointestinal events (43.8%) followed by AEs related to skin involvements (22.8%) [9]. Nikiphorou E et al. reported in a cohort of UK RA patients (mean age of the patients was not specified) that side effects were the main reason for MTX withdrawal, of which, gastrointestinal events were the most frequent adverse effects (32.7%) [23]. In a more recent study, Nagafuchi H et al. reported in a retrospective cohort performed in Egyptian RA patients (with median age: 58.0 years) that the most frequent causes of withdrawals were infections (20.0%), malignancies (14.1%) and respiratory disorders (10.2%) [24]. In comparison, the rate of infections and respiratory disorders as causes for suspension were significantly lower (5.4% and 3.7%, respectively), and no malignancies were reported in our cohort. Instead, the main cause of suspension was gastrointestinal effects like the causes reported in cohorts from North American patients [9]. Other cohort studies have reported the incidence of AEs in RA patients treated with DMARDs. Singal V. et al. analyzed the AEs in young patients from India (mean age: 38 years) observing abnormal level of transaminases (29.1%) and excessive nausea along with vomiting (16.6%); however, this cohort did not focus on treatment suspension [25]. Sherbini A. A. et al., in a prospective cohort, analyzed the rates and baseline predictor of AEs observed in the first year of MTX treatment in RA patients from the UK (mean age: 59 years); at twelve months, 77.5% of their patients reported at least one adverse event, mainly gastrointestinal (42.0%), constitutional (39.6%), neurological (28.6%), mucocutaneus (26.0%) and pulmonary (20.9%). Nevertheless, they did not extend the time of follow-up in this interesting cohort [26]. Takahashi C et al. reported in a 76 week study, 34% of 79 Japanese patients with RA (mean age: 56.7) had AEs, mainly gastrointestinal symptoms and hepatotoxicity [27]. Cummins L et al. described in a prospective cohort of 181 Australian RA patients (mean age: 52 years) who received a combination of triple DMARDs including MTX + SSZ + HCQ, the tolerability, persistence and efficacy. Of them, MTX was withdrawn in 29% of their patients, in this cohort, the gastrointestinal intolerance (15.0%) and rash (11.0%) being the most frequent AEs [28]. All these results reflect the importance of surveilling gastrointestinal and cutaneous AEs in users of MTX and support our study findings.

4.3. Risk Factors Associated with MTX Suspension Due to AEs

We identified the risk factors associated with the suspension of MTX therapy due to adverse events. A MTX dose $\geq$ 15 mg/wk was found to increase 2.46-fold the risk of the suspension of MTX due to AEs. Two studies analyzed RA patients in which MTX withdrawal was associated with the use of lower doses of MTX compared to the doses observed in our patients. Ideguchi H et al., in Japanese RA patients (mean age: 57.6 $\pm$ 11.4 years), reported in their cohort study that MTX discontinuation is associated with lower MTX doses (>8 mg/wk), increasing the risk up to almost 3-fold [14]. Asai S et al., in a cross-sectional study in Japanese patients (Median age: 64), observed that MTX doses >8 mg/wk increased the risk of reflux and abdominal pain (OR: 1.62 and 1.62, respectively); however, association between these AEs and MTX suspension was not analyzed [29]. Shoda H. et al. performed a cohort in Japanese RA patients (mean age: 60.8), comparing the maintenance dose of MTX in patients who had AEs vs. RA patients without AEs, identifying a relation between higher doses and AEs (9.6 $\pm$ 4.2 mg/wk vs. 6.7 $\pm$ 3.0 mg/wk respectively, p = 0.03) [30]. These data support our results of a higher risk of withdrawals of this DMARD related to higher doses.

4.4. Folate Supplementation as Protective Factor for MTX Suspension Due to AEs

In our study, folic acid supplementation was observed as a protective factor associated with MTX persistence, reducing the probability of MTX suspension due to AEs by 0.28-fold. Two other studies also identified the supplementation of folic acid as a protective factor in MTX therapy. Ideguchi H et al., in Japanese RA patients (mean age: 57.6 $\pm$ 11.4 years), reported that a lack of folic acid supplementation increases the risk of MTX discontinuation (RR = 1.93, p = 0.029), although it is not directly associated with AE development [14]. Hoekstra M et al., in their cohort of Dutch RA patients (median age: 59.7), reported that folate supplementation was associated with MTX survival, acting as a protective factor (RR = 0.25, p < 0.001) [10].

4.5. Strengths and Limitations

The present study focused on MTX suspension due to AEs in elderly RA patients. There is limited information regarding suspension of MTX due to AEs in elderly RA patients. Our study shows that 19% to 35% of patients in our cohort of RA patients are aged $\geq$ 60 years old. Elderly RA patients represent a challenge for clinicians treating this subgroup of the population because they have an impairment in metabolism and excretion of several drugs, making them more susceptible to suffer adverse events linked to the drugs used for their treatments. The present study described the long-term incidence of suspension of MTX due to AEs. We identified that at 10 years, the rate of patients that suspended MTX was 35.6%, and at 15 years this increased up to 51.7%. The main AEs identified were gastrointestinal and mucocutaneous. Risk predictors were analyzed after using an adjusted multivariate analysis, the main risk factor being a higher dose of MTX and as a protective factor, the utilization of folic acid.

However, this study has several limitations; the main one of them is derived from the retrospective cohorts where we cannot exclude the possibility that some information regarding several other risk factors could be missing. Among them, we have no information regarding genetic variables, MTX and its metabolites serum levels, therapeutic adherence or other variables that may influence the development of AEs but are not usually registered in the clinical charts. Another limitation observed in long-term retrospective cohorts is the loss of patients during the follow-up; in this cohort, the number of patients who were censored during the study was increased by other causes different to AEs. We therefore used the density of incidence as the strategy to identify the rate of therapeutic suspension of MTX, whereas prospective cohort studies with lower follow-up could use cumulative incidence as a better measure of incidence. We adjusted the time for developing events using Kaplan–Meir curves and hazard ratio in the multivariable Cox regression analysis. One potential limitation in our study was the use of 1987 ACR criteria for the inclusion of patients with a diagnosis of RA; although these criteria have a good sensitivity (79%) and specificity (90%) in patients with established RA, these values can decrease in patients with early RA (sensitivity of 77% and specificity 77%) [31]. However, at the time of the cohort onset, this set of criteria were the most used in the clinical settings in our country. Another additional limitation of this cohort was the lack of data regarding the positivity of anti-CCP antibodies, these antibodies have been related to several outcomes including erosions [32] and some extraarticular manifestations (such as subcutaneous nodules and lung involvement) [33]. In this cohort, an assessment of anti-CCP antibodies at the onset and their relation with adverse events of MTX was not investigated. Finally, we excluded elderly RA patients treated with biologic DMARDs; although, nowadays, the use of biologic therapy is more prescribed in our institution, at the time of the cohort onset, only 10% of the patients had this type of therapy.

5. Conclusions

In elderly RA patients, the suspension of MTX usually occurs earlier in therapy, while as many as half of the patients tolerate it up to 15 years. The most frequent reason for suspending MTX is adverse events of a gastrointestinal and mucocutaneus nature. Higher doses of MTX were associated with an increased risk of suspension, while folate supplementation considerably improved MTX survival.

Author Contributions: Conceptualization, J.I.G.-N. and L.G.-L.; methodology, J.I.G.-N., C.A.N.-V., S.G.-V. and L.G.-L.; validation, M.F.A.-L., E.L.A.-C., R.A.-C., C.A.N.-V., F.G.-P., J.A.G.-A., J.M.P.-G., E.R.V.-T., M.A.M.-I., N.A.R.-J. and A.M.S.-C.; formal analysis, F.A.A.-S., C.A.N.-V., S.G.-V., J.A.G.-A. and E.G.C.-M.; investigation, A.P.S.-G., F.A.A.-S., M.F.A.-L., E.L.A.-C., M.A.M.-I., R.A.-C., C.A.N.-V., F.G.-P., J.A.G.-A., J.M.P.-G., N.A.R.-J. and A.M.S.-C.; resources, M.F.A.-L., R.A.-C., F.G.-P., J.M.P.-G., E.R.V.-T., N.A.R.-J., M.A.M.-I. and A.M.S.-C.; data curation, A.P.S.-G., F.A.A.-S., E.L.A.-C., C.A.N.-V., S.G.-V., J.A.G.-A. and E.G.C.-M.; writing—original draft, A.P.S.-G., F.A.A.-S., M.F.A.-L., E.L.A.-C., R.A.-C., C.A.N.-V., S.G.-V., J.A.G.-A. and E.G.C.-M.; writing—review and editing, A.P.S.-G., J.I.G.-N., F.A.A.-S., M.F.A.-L., E.R.V.-T., E.L.A.-C., R.A.-C., C.A.N.-V., S.G.-V., F.G.-P., J.A.G.-A., J.M.P.-G., N.A.R.-J., A.M.S.-C., E.G.C.-M. and L.G.-L.; supervision, J.I.G.-N. and L.G.-L.; project administration, E.G.C.-M. and L.G.-L.; funding acquisition, N.A.R.-J., A.M.S.-C. and E.G.C.-M. All authors have read and agreed to the published version of the manuscript.

Funding: This research received no external funding.

Institutional Review Board Statement: All study procedures were approved by the research and ethics committees of the University of Guadalajara (code of approval: CI-04021, date of approval 14 September 2024). This research protocol followed the Helsinki Declaration issued in Fortaleza, Brazil, in 2013 [19]. All the patients included in the study read and signed a voluntary consent form before participating.

Informed Consent Statement: Patient consent was waived due to this study being retrospective based on the review of clinical charts. This study did not involve confidential information and any possible identifiers, such as name, address, code, etc., of the patients were removed from the database before the analysis and interpretation.

Data Availability Statement: The dataset supporting the conclusions presented in this article is available on request from the corresponding author on reasonable request.

Acknowledgments: The authors would like to thank the Members of the Research Group for Factors Related to Therapeutic Outcomes in Autoimmune Diseases. Members: Senior researchers: Gamez-Nava Jorge Ivan, Gonzalez-Lopez Laura, Leaders of the group, Departamento de Fisiología, Programa de Doctorado en Farmacología and Programa de Doctorado en Salud Publica Centro Universitario de Ciencias de la Salud, Universidad de Guadalajara; Cardona-Muñoz Ernesto German, Centro Universitario de Ciencias de la Salud, Departamento de Fisiología, Universidad de Guadalajara. Associated Researchers: Research in Clinical and Laboratory Analysis: Avalos-Salgado Felipe Alexis, Centro Universitario de Ciencias de la Salud, Universidad de Guadalajara; Centro Universitario de Ciencias de la Salud, Universidad de Guadalajara; Fajardo-Robledo Nicte Selene, Centro Universitario de Ciencias Exactas e Ingenierías, Laboratorio de Investigación y Desarrollo Farmacéutico, Universidad de

Guadalajara; Saldaña-Cruz Ana Miriam, Rodriguez-Jimenez Norma Alejandra, Centro Universitario de Ciencias de la Salud, Departamento de Fisiología, Universidad de Guadalajara; Nava-Valdivia Cesar Arturo, Departamento de Microbiologia y Patologia, Centro Universitario de Ciencias de la Salud, Universidad de Guadalajara; Ponce-Guarneros Juan Manuel, Centro Universitario de Ciencias de la Salud, Departamento de Fisiología, Universidad de Guadalajara and Instituto Mexicano del Seguro Social, UMF 97, Guadalajara, Jalisco, Mexico; Alcaraz-Lopez Miriam Fabiola, Instituto Mexicano del Seguro Social, HGR 46, Guadalajara, Jalisco, Mexico. Statistical Team: Gamez-Nava Jorge Ivan, Departamento de Fisiología, Programa de Doctorado en Farmacología and Programa de Doctorado en Salud Publica Centro Universitario de Ciencias de la Salud, Universidad de Guadalajara; Alfredo Celis, Departamento de Salud Publica Centro Universitario de Ciencias de la Salud, Universidad de Guadalajara. Research Fellows: Santiago-Garcia Aline Priscilla, Jacobo-Cuevas Heriberto, OlivasFlores Eva, Gonzalez-Ponce Fabiola. Centro Universitario de Ciencias de la Salud, Programa de Doctorado en Farmacología, Universidad de Guadalajara.

Conflicts of Interest: The authors declare no conflict of interest.

References

1. Smolen, J.S.; Aletaha, D.; Barton, A.; Burmester, G.R.; Emery, P.; Firestein, G.S.; Kavanaugh, A.; McInnes, I.B.; Solomon, D.H.; Strand, V.; et al. Rheumatoid Arthritis. *Nat. Rev. Dis. Primers* **2018**, *4*, 18001. [CrossRef]
2. Silman, A.J.; Pearson, J.E. Epidemiology and genetics of rheumatoid arthritis. *Arthritis Res.* **2002**, *4* (Suppl. S3), S265–S272. [CrossRef]
3. NICE. Rheumatoid Arthritis in Adults: Management. 2018. Available online: www.nice.org.uk/guidance/ng100 (accessed on 15 February 2024).
4. Smolen, J.S.; Landewé, R.B.M.; Bergstra, S.A.; Kerschbaumer, A.; Sepriano, A.; Aletaha, D.; Caporali, R.; Edwards, C.J.; Hyrich, K.L.; Pope, J.E.; et al. EULAR recommendations for the management of rheumatoid arthritis with synthetic and biological disease-modifying antirheumatic drugs: 2022 update. *Ann. Rheum. Dis.* **2023**, *82*, 3–18. [CrossRef]
5. Zhao, Z.; Hua, Z.; Luo, X.; Li, Y.; Yu, L.; Li, M.; Lu, C.; Zhao, T.; Liu, Y. Application and pharmacological mechanism of methotrexate in rheumatoid arthritis. *Biomed. Pharmacother.* **2022**, *150*, 113074. [CrossRef]
6. Goycochea-Robles, M.V.; Arce-Salinas, C.A.; Guzmán-Vázquez, S.; Cardiel-Ríos, M.H. Prescription Rheumatology Practices Among Mexican Specialists. *Arch. Med Res.* **2007**, *38*, 354–359. [CrossRef]
7. Moura, C.S.; Schieir, O.; Valois, M.; Thorne, C.; Bartlett, S.J.; Pope, J.E.; Hitchon, C.A.; Boire, G.; Haraoui, B.; Hazlewood, G.S.; et al. Treatment Strategies in Early Rheumatoid Arthritis Methotrexate Management: Results from a Prospective Cohort. *Arthritis Care Res.* **2020**, *72*, 1104–1111. [CrossRef]
8. Alarcon, G.S.; Tracy, I.C.; Strand, G.M.; Singh, K.; Macaluso, M. Survival and drug discontinuation analyses in a large cohort of methotrexate treated rheumatoid arthritis patients. *Ann. Rheum. Dis.* **1995**, *54*, 708–712. [CrossRef] [PubMed]
9. Alarcóan, G.S.; Tracy, I.C.; Blackburn, W.D. Methotrexate in rheumatoid arthritis. Toxic effects as the major factor in limiting long-term treatment. *Arthritis Rheum.* **1989**, *32*, 671–676. [CrossRef] [PubMed]
10. Hoekstra, M.; Laar, M.A.F.J.V.D.; Moens, H.J.B.; Kruijsen, M.W.M.; Haagsma, C.J. Longterm observational study of methotrexate use in a Dutch cohort of 1022 patients with rheumatoid arthritis. *J. Rheumatol.* **2003**, *30*, 2325–2329. [PubMed]
11. Sevillano Gutierrez, J.; Capelusnik, D.; Schneeberger, E.; Citera, G. Tolerancia, sobrevida y adherencia al tratamiento con Metotrexato en pacientes con artritis reumatoidea. *Rev. Argent. De Reumatol.* **2019**, *30*, 13–17. [CrossRef]
12. Sherbini, A.A.; Sharma, S.D.; Gwinnutt, J.M.; Hyrich, K.L.; Verstappen, S.M.M. Prevalence and predictors of adverse events with methotrexate mono- and combination-therapy for rheumatoid arthritis: A systematic review. *Rheumatology* **2021**, *60*, 4001–4017. [CrossRef] [PubMed]
13. Verstappen, S.M.M.; Bakker, M.F.; Heurkens, A.H.M.; van der Veen, M.J.; A Kruize, A.; Geurts, M.A.W.; Bijlsma, J.W.J.; Jacobs, J.W.G. Adverse events and factors associated with toxicity in patients with early rheumatoid arthritis treated with methotrexate tight control therapy: The CAMERA study. *Ann. Rheum. Dis.* **2010**, *69*, 1044–1048. [CrossRef] [PubMed]
14. Ideguchi, H.; Ohno, S.; Ishigatsubo, Y. Risk Factors Associated with the Cumulative Survival of Low-Dose Methotrexate in 273 Japanese Patients with Rheumatoid Arthritis. *J. Clin. Rheumat.* **2007**, *13*, 73–78. [CrossRef] [PubMed]
15. Bliddal, H.; Eriksen, S.A.; Christensen, R.; Lorenzen, T.; Hansen, M.S.; Østergaard, M.; Dreyer, L.; Luta, G.; Vestergaard, P. Adherence to Methotrexate in Rheumatoid Arthritis: A Danish Nationwide Cohort Study. *Arthritis* **2015**, *2015*, 915142. [CrossRef] [PubMed]
16. World Health Organization. Ageing and Health. Available online: https://www.who.int/news-room/fact-sheets/detail/ageing-and-health#:~:text=By%202050,%20the%20world's%20population,2050%20to%20reach%20426%20million (accessed on 15 February 2024).
17. Morales-Romero, J.; Cázares-Méndez, J.M.; Gámez-Nava, J.I.; Triano-Páez, M.; Villa-Manzano, A.; López-Olivo, M.; Rodríguez-Arreola, B.; González-López, L. La atención médica en reumatología en un hospital de segundo nivel de atención [Patterns of health care in an out patient rheumatologic clinic]. *Reumatol. Clin.* **2005**, *1*, 87–94. [CrossRef] [PubMed]

18. Arnett, F.C.; Edworthy, S.M.; Bloch, D.A.; McShane, D.J.; Fries, J.F.; Cooper, N.S.; Healey, L.A.; Kaplan, S.R.; Liang, M.H.; Luthra, H.S.; et al. The American Rheumatism Association 1987 revised criteria for the classification of rheumatoid arthritis. *Arthritis. Rheum.* **1988**, *31*, 315–324. [CrossRef]
19. World Medical Association. World Medical Association Declaration of Helsinki: Ethical principles for medical research involving human subjects. *JAMA* **2013**, *310*, 2191–2194. [CrossRef]
20. Tutuncu, Z.; Reed, G.; Kremer, J.; Kavanaugh, A. Do patients with older-onset rheumatoid arthritis receive less aggressive treatment? *Ann. Rheum. Dis.* **2006**, *65*, 1226–1229. [CrossRef]
21. Mathieu, S.; Pereira, B.; Saraux, A.; Richez, C.; Combe, B.; Soubrier, M. Disease-modifying drug retention rate according to patient age in patients with early rheumatoid arthritis: Analysis of the ESPOIR cohort. *Rheumatol. Int.* **2021**, *41*, 879–885. [CrossRef]
22. Scully, C.J.; Anderson, C.J.; Cannon, G.W. Long-term methotrexate therapy for rheumatoid arthritis. *Semin. Arthritis Rheum.* **1991**, *20*, 317–331. [CrossRef]
23. Nikiphorou, E.; Negoescu, A.; Fitzpatrick, J.D.; Goudie, C.T.; Badcock, A.; Östör, A.J.K.; Malaviya, A.P. Indispensable or intolerable? Methotrexate in patients with rheumatoid and psoriatic arthritis: A retrospective review of discontinuation rates from a large UK cohort. *Clin. Rheumatol.* **2014**, *33*, 609–614. [CrossRef]
24. Nagafuchi, H.; Goto, Y.; Kiyokawa, T.; Kawahata, K. Reasons for discontinuation of methotrexate in the treatment of rheumatoid arthritis and challenges of methotrexate resumption: A single-center, retrospective study. *Egypt. Rheumatol. Rehabil.* **2022**, *49*, 63. [CrossRef]
25. Singal, V.; Chaturvedi, V.; Brar, K. Efficacy and Toxicity Profile of Methotrexate Chloroquine Combination in Treatment of Active Rheumatoid Arthritis. *Med. J. Armed Forces India* **2005**, *61*, 29–32. [CrossRef]
26. Sherbini, A.A.; Gwinnutt, J.M.; Hyrich, K.L.; RAMS Co-Investigators; Verstappen, S.M.M.; Adebajo, A.; Ahmed, K.; Al-Ansari, A.; Amarasena, R.; Bukhari, M.; et al. Rates and predictors of methotrexate-related adverse events in patients with early rheumatoid arthritis: Results from a nationwide UK study. *Rheumatology* **2022**, *61*, 3930–3938. [CrossRef] [PubMed]
27. Takahashi, C.; Kaneko, Y.; Okano, Y.; Taguchi, H.; Oshima, K.; Izumi, K.; Yamaoka, K.; Takeuchi, T. Association of erythrocyte methotrexate-polyglutamate levels with the efficacy and hepatotoxicity of methotrexate in patients with rheumatoid arthritis: A 76-week prospective study. *RMD Open* **2017**, *3*, e000363. [CrossRef] [PubMed]
28. Cummins, L.; Katikireddi, V.S.; Shankaranarayana, S.; Su, K.Y.C.; Duggan, E.; Videm, V.; Pahau, H.; Thomas, R. Safety and retention of combination triple disease-modifying anti-rheumatic drugs in new-onset rheumatoid arthritis. *Intern. Med. J.* **2015**, *45*, 1266–1273. [CrossRef]
29. Asai, S.; Nagai, K.; Takahashi, N.; Watanabe, T.; Matsumoto, T.; Asai, N.; Sobue, Y.; Ishiguro, N.; Kojima, T. Influence of methotrexate on gastrointestinal symptoms in patients with rheumatoid arthritis. *Int. J. Rheum. Dis.* **2019**, *22*, 207–213. [CrossRef] [PubMed]
30. Shoda, H.; Inokuma, S.; Yajima, N.; Tanaka, Y.; Oobayashi, T.; Setoguchi, K. Higher maximal serum concentration of methotrexate predicts the incidence of adverse reactions in Japanese rheumatoid arthritis patients. *Mod. Rheumatol.* **2007**, *17*, 311–316. [CrossRef]
31. Banal, F.; Dougados, M.; Combescure, C.; Gossec, L. Sensitivity and specificity of the American College of Rheumatology 1987 criteria for the diagnosis of rheumatoid arthritis according to disease duration: A systematic literature review and meta-analysis. *Ann. Rheum. Dis.* **2009**, *68*, 1184–1191. [CrossRef]
32. Sulaiman, F.N.; Wong, K.K.; Ahmad, W.A.W.; Ghazali, W.S.W. Anti-cyclic citrullinated peptide antibody is highly associated with rheumatoid factor and radiological defects in rheumatoid arthritis patients. *Medicine* **2019**, *98*, e14945. [CrossRef]
33. Korkmaz, C.; Us, T.; Kaşifoğlu, T.; Akgün, Y. Anti-cyclic citrullinated peptide (CCP) antibodies in patients with long-standing rheumatoid arthritis and their relationship with extra-articular manifestations. *Clin. Biochem.* **2006**, *39*, 961–965. [CrossRef] [PubMed]

Disclaimer/Publisher's Note: The statements, opinions and data contained in all publications are solely those of the individual author(s) and contributor(s) and not of MDPI and/or the editor(s). MDPI and/or the editor(s) disclaim responsibility for any injury to people or property resulting from any ideas, methods, instructions or products referred to in the content.

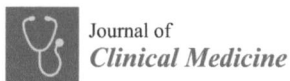

Review

Initial Treatment with Biological Therapy in Rheumatoid Arthritis

Jesús Tornero Molina [1,2,*], Blanca Hernández-Cruz [3] and Héctor Corominas [4,5]

1. Departamento de Reumatología, Hospital de Guadalajara, 19002 Guadalajara, Spain
2. Departamento de Medicina y Especialidades Médicas, Universidad de Alcalá, 28805 Madrid, Spain
3. Departamento de Reumatología, Hospital Universitario Virgen Macarena, 41009 Sevilla, Spain; blancahcruz@gmail.com
4. Departamento de Reumatología, Hospital Universitari de Sant Pau & Hospital Dos de Maig, 08025 Barcelona, Spain; vancor@yahoo.com
5. Medicine Faculty, Universitat Autònoma de Barcelona (UAB), 08193 Barcelona, Spain
* Correspondence: jtorneromolina@ser.es; Tel.: +34-949-20-92-00

Abstract: Background: We aimed to analyse the effectiveness, efficiency, and safety of initial treatment with biological therapies in rheumatoid arthritis (RA). Methods: Qualitative study. A group of RA experts was selected. A scoping review in Medline was conducted to analyse the evidence of initial RA treatment with biological therapies. Randomised clinical trials were selected. Two reviewers analysed the articles and compiled the data, whose quality was assessed using the Jadad scale. The experts discussed the review's findings and generated a series of general principles: Results: Seventeen studies were included. Most of the included patients were middle-aged women with early RA (1–7 months) and multiple poor prognostic factors. Initial treatment with TNF-alpha inhibitors combined with methotrexate (MTX) and an IL6R inhibitor (either in mono or combination therapy) is effective (activity, function, radiographic damage, quality of life), safe, and superior to MTX monotherapy in the short and medium term. In the long term, patients who received initial treatment with biologicals presented better results than those whose initial therapy was with MTX. Conclusions: Initial treatment of RA with biological therapies is effective, efficient, and safe in the short, medium, and long term, particularly for patients with poor prognostic factors.

Keywords: rheumatoid arthritis; biologic therapy; initial treatment; narrative review; experts' opinion

1. Introduction

Rheumatoid arthritis (RA) is a chronic inflammatory joint disease of autoimmune origin, with an estimated prevalence of around 1% [1]. The disease is associated with a major impact on the patient, their environment, and the healthcare system [2–4].

For many years, the pharmacological treatment of RA was essentially based on the use of corticosteroids and classical synthetic disease-modifying anti-rheumatic drugs (csDMARD) like methotrexate (MTX) [5]. However, the arrival of biologic DMARD (bDMARD) significantly changed treatment paradigms for RA patients [6].

Pivotal studies on bDMARD showed their efficacy and safety for patients with RA refractory to csDMARD [5,7], which led regulatory agencies to approve the use of these drugs for this group of RA patients. Subsequent publications have presented the results of *post hoc* analyses and studies specifically designed to analyse bDMARD as the initial treatment for RA (csDMARD-naïve patients) [8,9]. This is why the summaries of products for some bDMARD contemplate the drug's use in patients with severe, active, progressive RA not previously treated with MTX or other csDMARD. However, the guidelines of national and international scientific societies still recommend using csDMARD, particularly MTX, as the initial treatment for RA [6,10]. These guidelines highlight the high cost of many bDMARDs as a limitation to their wider use [11,12].

On the other hand, the approval of biosimilar medicines has ushered in more competitive pricing, bringing a considerable reduction in bDMARD costs [13]. A report by BioSim (the Spanish Association of Biosimilar Medicines) estimates savings derived from the introduction of biosimilars for the 2009–2019 period to be 2306 million euros in Spain [14]. It also highlights adalimumab (ADA) as the drug that generates the most savings [14]. There are currently over 60 biosimilar medicines corresponding to 17 drugs, 4 of which are for immune-mediated diseases: infliximab (IFX), ADA, etanercept (ETN), tocilizumab (recently approved by the European Medicines Agency), and rituximab, which are widely used [15]. The guidelines of scientific societies acknowledge that biosimilar medicines have contributed to a substantial reduction in the cost of medicines, following a policy of rational prescribing based on the principle that if two medicines are equally effective and safe for a specific patient, the least expensive should be used [6].

In light of this, we can consider the use of bDMARD as the initial treatment for RA, at least for some subgroups of patients. The design of this project aimed to address this topic, with the objectives of analysing the existing evidence on initial treatment with bDMARD and issuing a series of positions for better stratification of RA patients. Bearing in mind that many countries recommend biosimilar TNF-alpha inhibitors as the first choice for bDMARD and, among patients with intolerance to/contraindications for MTX, an interleukin 6 receptor (IL6R) inhibitor, this document focuses on these pharmacological groups. Abatacept and rituximab are currently reserved for special situations, and in clinical practice, Janus kinase inhibitors are used in later lines of treatment.

We believe that this document will help rheumatologists in their therapeutic decision-making for RA patients.

2. Materials and Methods

This qualitative study is based on a scoping review of the literature and on expert opinion. The project was conducted in full compliance with the principles established in the Declaration of Helsinki for medical research involving human subjects in its latest version [16] and in accordance with applicable regulations on Good Clinical Practice.

Participant selection and the first nominal group meeting. A group of three rheumatologists with extensive experience and knowledge of RA management were selected. In a first meeting, they analysed the current status of RA management and defined the objectives, scope, and literature review to be undertaken.

Scoping review of the literature. The objective was to assess the efficacy, effectiveness, and safety of the initial treatment of RA with bDMARD.

With the help of an expert documentalist, different search strategies were designed for Medline (up to January 2023) that combined both MeSH and free-text terms. Examples of terms used are "rheumatoid arthritis" or "disease-modifying anti-rheumatic drugs". Searches were also made using PubMed's Clinical Queries tool (see Supplementary Table S1).

Studies that met the following inclusion and exclusion criteria were selected: The population included patients with RA (according to international criteria [17]), adults (>18 years), regardless of disease duration or severity (P); RA patients receiving initial treatment with bDMARD, i.e., naïve for any csDMARD such as oral (po), subcutaneous (sc), or other MTX. No restrictions were imposed regarding dose, treatment duration, use as monotherapy or in combination (I), a control, or either a placebo or with an active ingredient (C). We also included studies that analysed any variable related with efficacy/effectiveness, such as RA activity including DAS28 (disease activity score), CDAI (clinical disease activity index), SDAI (simplified disease activity index), disease remission, function assessed with the HAQ (Health Assessment Questionnaire), structural damage viewed in a simple radiography or magnetic resonance imaging (MRI), PRO (patient-reported outcomes), acute phase reactants such as erythrocyte sedimentation rate (ESR) or C-reactive protein (CRP), quality of life assessed with RAQoL (Rheumatoid Arthritis Quality of Life) Questionnaire or others, cost-effectiveness and safety variables (serious adverse events, infection rate, etc.). The types of studies accepted were randomised clinical trials (RCT) with their corresponding extension studies and post hoc analyses. Figure 1 shows the study flow chart.

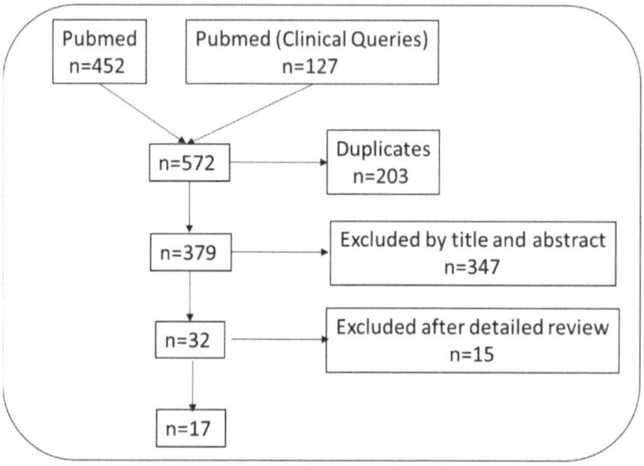

Figure 1. Studies flow chart.

All of the citations found using the different search strategies were downloaded to the EndNote® reference management software package (Version number 20). Two reviewers (EL, TO) independently analysed the citations in duplicate. The search results were first refined by title and abstract, with another purge after a detailed reading of the resulting citations. The two reviewers compiled data from the included studies. To assess the methodological quality of the studies included, a Jadad scale was used (from 1 to 5, with "quality" defined as an RCT with a score of ≥ 3). A descriptive-qualitative analysis was performed. Meta-analysis was only performed in cases of homogeneity.

Finally, as part of the secondary search, the bibliographic references of the included articles and the abstracts of international conferences were reviewed.

Second meeting of the nominal group. The nominal group discussed the review results at the second meeting, during which the experts reached a consensus on a series of points related to the use of bDMARD as an initial treatment for RA.

Preparation of the final document. The final text took into account both the narrative review and the nominal group's decisions. For each of the expert points, we assessed the strength of the recommendation (very low, low, moderate, or high). The resulting document was given to the experts for their final evaluation and comments.

3. Results

A total of 17 articles [18–34] were included, whereas 15 were excluded (see Supplementary Material, Table S2) [8,9,35–47]. A summary of the main outcomes is depicted in Table 1, while the supplementary material provides the evidence tables (Tables S3 and S4).

Here we present the expert opinions along with the literature search results.

General indications on initial treatment with bDMARD.

1. Based on the body of evidence and the current context of daily practice, it is possible to consider the use of bDMARD as an initial treatment for RA. Strengths of the recommendation: Moderate

With regard to TNF-alpha inhibitors, one RCT found that the combination IFX + MTX po was significantly superior to MTX po in improving synovitis and bone marrow oedema (measured by MRI), both at weeks 18 and 52 [19]. The combination was also superior in ACR20/50/70 responses at week 22, with a similar (non-significant) trend observed at week 52 [19].

Data from the *BeSt* study show that the triple therapy of csDMARD with prednisone and the combination IFX + MTX (po and sc) improved HAQ faster (3rd month) than the other treatment groups analysed, an improvement that was sustained until month 12 ($p < 0.05$). Moreover, these strategies were also significantly superior in improving structural damage (<0.001), although this effect disappeared in the second year [20–22]. Long-term (10-year) follow-up showed that the different combination therapies produced similar global outcomes (non-significant differences), although patients treated with IFX + MTX showed less radiographic progression and better physical functioning than the other strategies [23].

Table 1. Main conclusions of the included studies [18–34]. The study's primary outcomes are highlighted.

1	The use of initial treatment with IFX + MTX is significantly superior to MTX (in the short and long term) to MTX regarding RA activity (DAS28, DAS28 remission, imaging techniques, etc.), HAQ, radiographic progression, and quality of life (RAQoL)
2	Initial treatment with IFX + MTX is superior to other strategies: sequential csDMARD monotherapy and stepped combination treatment with csDMARDs regarding the previously mentioned variables
3	Initial use of ADA + MTX during the first year is significantly superior (in the short and long term) to MTX regarding RA activity (DAS28, DAS28/CDAI/SDAI/ACR-EULAR remission, low disease activity, joint counts, etc.). HAQ, quality of life (SF-36-physical component), and probably regarding radiographic progression
4	Current evidence on initial treatment with ETN + MTX is based on a single study and is inconclusive
5	Initial use of CZP + MTX is significantly superior (in the short and long term) to MTX regarding RA activity (DAS28, DAS28 remission, CDAI, CDAI remission, SDAI, acute phase reactants, etc.), HAQ, and radiographic progression. However, the CZP + MTX combination has not been shown to be superior to the combination of MTX with prednisone or to the combination of SSZ + HCQ + intra-articular corticosteroids
6	Initial use of ABT + MTX achieves remission rates of 52% at 24 weeks, higher than those obtained with the combination of MTX + corticosteroids or SSZ + HCQ+ intra-articular corticosteroids
7	Initial use of TCZ + MTX or TCZ in monotherapy is significantly superior (in the short and long term) to MTX regarding RA activity (DAS28, DAS28 remission, CDAI, CDAI remission, EULAR and ACR responses, etc.), HAQ, radiographic progression, and quality of life

Abbreviations: IFX = infliximab; ADA = adalimumab; ETN = etanercept; CZP = certolizumab pegol; TCZ = tocilizumab; SSZ = sulphasalazine; HCQ = hydroxychloroquine; MTX = methotrexate; csDMARDs = classical synthetic disease-modifying anti-rheumatic drugs; RA = rheumatoid arthritis; SF-36 = 36-item short-form health survey; ACR = American College of Rheumatology; DAS28 = disease activity score of 28 joints; CEDAI = clinical disease activity index; SDAI = simplified disease activity index; HAQ = health assessment questionnaire; EULAR = European Alliance of Associations for Rheumatology; RAQoL = rheumatoid arthritis quality of life scale.

In the IDEA RCT, the combination of initial therapy with IFX + MTX po or MTX + intravenous methylprednisolone achieved similar DAS28 remission rates at week 78: 50% vs. 48% ($p = 0.795$); however, DAS28 remission was reached more quickly with IFX + MTX. Although both groups obtained a high proportion of patients without radiographic progression, no differences were detected [24].

The HIT-HARD [26], GUEPAR [27], and OPERA [28] RCTs evaluated ADA as the initial treatment for RA. The outcomes of the HIT HARD study at week 24 showed that ADA + MTX sc was significantly superior to MTX sc in terms of DAS28, HAQ, and DAS28 remission (47.9% vs. 29.5%; $p = 0.021$), as well as in ACR 50 and ACR 70 responses [26]. From week 24, all patients received MTX sc monotherapy. Radiographic progression at week 48 was significantly greater in patients who had received MTX sc monotherapy as the initial treatment [26]. The OPERA study compared ADA po + MTX vs. MTX po [28]. At one year of treatment, the combination ADA + MTX was significantly superior to MTX in terms of DAS28-CRP, CDAI, SDAI, HAQ, ACR/EULAR28 and ACR/EULAR40, ACR50 and ACR70 responses, and in remission, defined with DAS28, CDAI, SDAI, and ACR/EULAR. The SF-12 questionnaire revealed a significant improvement in quality of life for physical but not mental health, which was echoed in the EQ-5D ($p = 0.015$) [28]. Finally, the GUEPAR study reported that initial treatment with ADA + MTX po was significantly superior at 3 months to MTX po in improving rigidity, ACR 20/50/70 response, good EULAR response (63% vs. 25%), and DAS28 remission (36% vs. 12%). No differences existed between the groups for pain, fatigue, or ESR [27].

For ETN, the EMPIRE study [29] included 110 patients with early-onset synovitis (41% met RA criteria according to 1987 ACR criteria and 94% according to 2010 ACR-EULAR criteria). At week 52 of treatment, 32.5% of patients with ETN + MTX po did not present painful or swollen joints vs. 28.1% with MTX po (no statistically significant differences).

Nor were any differences found in ACR remission, SDAI remission, DAS44-CRP, HAQ-DI, SF-36, EQ5D-3L, radiographic progression, or in the variables assessed at week 72 [29].

There are 3 published good-quality RCTs on the initial treatment of RA with certolizumab pegol (CZP) [30–32]. The outcomes of *C-EARLY* show that the combination CZP + MTX po is significantly superior to MTX po in controlling disease activity, sustaining clinical response, functional improvement, and inhibiting radiographic progression. In week 52, 28.9% of patients in the CZP + MTX group reached DAS28 remission: 28.9% vs. 15% for MTX ($p < 0.001$) [30]. The study also revealed significant differences in favour of CZP + MTX in sustained low disease activity (DAS28 $\leq$ 3.2), ACR 50 response, functioning, inhibition of radiographic progression, and both CDAI and SDAI remission. The study went on to assess whether, for patients who had achieved sustained low disease activity after 1 year of treatment with standard doses of CZP (200 mg/2 weeks) + MTX po, continuing with a standard or optimised dose of CZP (200 mg/4 weeks) was superior to interrupting CZP (and continuing with MTX po) for an additional period of 1 year (a total of 104 weeks). At week 104, the proportion of patients with sustained low disease activity was higher in the CZP-treated group, both at standard and optimised doses (48.8% and 53.2%) than in patients who continued with MTX (39.2%), although the differences were only significant for the comparison of optimised dose vs. MTX ($p = 0.041$). The trend was similar for inhibition of radiographic progression and physical functioning [32].

There are 3 articles available for TCZ, based on 2 studies. One good quality study, *U-Act-Early* [33,34], and another moderate quality study [31]. TCZ as monotherapy or in combination with MTX po were superior to MTX po in different outcome measures. At week 24, almost double the number of patients receiving TCZ achieved DAS28 and CDAI remission compared with MTX (86% and 83% with TCZ + MTX and TCZ, respectively, vs. 44% with MTX, $p < 0.0001$). The therapies with TCZ were also significantly superior to MTX in terms of good EULAR response (89% vs. 87% vs. 49%), ACR (20/50/70/90 responses), and HAQ. In week 104, little progression was observed in all groups, but it was significantly lower in both TCZ arms than in the MTX po arm [34]. Patients in this study underwent an additional follow-up of 3 years in real life. The data for effectiveness were sustained, with no differences between the groups. During 5 years of follow-up, the accumulated time of sustained remission was significantly higher in the groups that began therapy with TCZ (median 216 and 190 days for the TCZ + MTX combination and TCZ, respectively) than for MTX (median 172). However, no differences were observed in radiographic progression between the groups [33].

2. Initial treatment with bDMARD should be considered, particularly for RA patients with a high inflammatory load and/or other poor prognostic factors. Strengths of the recommendation: High

Although RA is a heterogeneous, dynamic disease, different studies have shown that the baseline presence of certain factors is associated with a worse prognosis in terms of activity (e.g., remission) and radiographic damage [48]. Among these factors, we highlight a positive rheumatoid factor (RF) and/or anti–citrullinated protein antibodies, high counts of acute phase reactants, high disease activity (multiple inflamed joints, high activity index, etc.), significant functional limitation, or the presence of erosion in imaging tests [48].

Most patients included in the RCT analysed presented poor prognostic factors at baseline (see Table 2). The mean age of patients included was between 45 and 55 years, RF positivity was occasionally even higher than 90%, the mean DAS28 in most cases was higher than 5, and many patients presented structural damage in radiographic imaging [18–34].

Table 2. Basal characteristics of RA patients in the included studies [18–34].

	Age (Years)	Women	RA Duration	RF+	ACPA+	RA Activity	Structural Damage
IFX	45–55	60–71%	5–7.4 months	61–67%	Hasta 90%	DAS28 > 5	70%
ADA	46–56	63–79%	3–4.4 months	69–74%	-	DAS28 5.5–6.3	SHS 6.3–7.5
ETN	48	76%	7 months	53%	77%	DAS28-CRP 4.17	mTTS 6.69–8.01
CZP	50–52	69–76%	3–7 months	72–97%	-	DAS28 6.7	77.3%
TCZ	53–55	61–76%	1 month	75%	-	DAS28 5.2	SHS 0

Abbreviations: RA = rheumatoid arthritis; RF = rheumatoid factor; ACPA = anti-citrullinated peptide antibodies; IFX = infliximab; ADA = adalimumab; ETN = etanercept; CZP = certolizumab pegol; TCZ = tocilizumab; DAS28 = disease activity score of 28 joints; CRP = C reactive protein; SHS = Sharp-van der Heijde index; mTTS = modified Sharp-van der Heijde index.

On the other hand, early, aggressive treatment has been shown to improve the long-term prognosis of this disease [49]. This therapy is associated with higher clinical response rates, lower disability, and less structural damage [50,51]. Although a larger body of specific evidence is necessary, in the BeSt study's 10-year follow-up, patients who received IFX + MTX showed less radiographic progression and better physical functioning than patients following other strategies [23]. The data at 5 years for TCZ are similar [33], as are the 10-year extension data for ADA of the PREMIER study (almost 30% of whose patients had previously received csDMARD) [52]. However, it is important to consider each case individually. The decision to use bDMARD as initial treatment should be discussed with the patient, evaluating the potential risks and benefits of these drugs on a case-by-case basis.

3. If considering a TNF-alpha inhibitor as an initial treatment for RA, its use is recommended in combination with MTX, whereas if considering an IL6R inhibitor, monotherapy is possible. Strength of the recommendation: Moderate

Most of the RCTs analysed included patients with MTX po either combined with a TNF-alpha inhibitor or as monotherapy [18–25,27–32]. The studies used different doses and regimens of MTX po, but the majority began with a dose of 7.5–10 mg/week, progressively increasing each 2–4 weeks to a maximum of 30 mg/week; however, most studies used a maximum dose of MTX between 15 and 20 mg/week.

As we have described, the use of MTX in combination with a TNF-alpha inhibitor is an effective and safe initial treatment for RA [18–25,27–32]. Although we have not found comparative evidence between TNF-alpha inhibitors for initial treatment as monotherapy and in combination with MTX, based on publications referring to patients with refractory RA, experts recommend the use of TNF-alpha inhibitors with MTX as the initial therapy [7]. In this context, as well as being more effective, MTX can prevent immunogenicity or reduce the use of corticosteroids [53]. On the other hand, MTX po might be recommended because it is the drug for which most evidence is available due to its lower price (cost-effectiveness). However, it is important to remember that the bioavailability of parenteral MTX is higher than that of MTX po, particularly at doses of $\geq$15 mg/week [54,55], and that in patients with an inadequate response to orally administered MTX (15 mg/week), dose scaling using parenteral MTX is more clinically effective [55,56]. Likewise, we should always consider patient opinion and preference when making therapeutic decisions. So, in some cases, we may consider the use of parenteral MTX with TNF-alpha inhibitors as the initial treatment.

On the other hand, there are considerable variations in the use of MTX in clinical practice, including the initial dose, dose scaling, maximum dose, etc. [57,58]. A sub-analysis of the AR Excellence study [59] highlighted these variations, finding that MTX scaling to its full dose did not occur as quickly as it should and that there was not correct use of parenteral MTX administration.

The outcomes reported for the use of IL6R as initial treatment [33,34] are similar to those reported for patients with RA refractory to csDMARD, so its use can be considered a monotherapy.

4. Initial treatment of RA with bDMARD in monotherapy or in combination therapy is safe. Strength of the recommendation: Moderate

Data on the safety of bDMARD as an initial treatment are similar to those reported in studies on RA refractory to csDMARD [18–34]. It should be noted that the data analysed is for RCTs with different follow-up periods and even changes in treatment within the same study.

Infections are still the most frequent adverse event with the use of bDMARD as the initial treatment for RA, although the percentage of severe infections is generally low and similar to existing reports [18–34]. No new signs related to the active infection by hepatitis or tuberculosis viruses were detected. Haematological adverse events are not very frequent, and when they do occur, they are mild and reversible. An increase in liver enzymes is a relatively frequent adverse event, but in most cases, it is mild [18–34]. There are exceptional reports of severe cases but no clearly established causal relationship. Based on the data from the included studies, the use of bDMARD as an initial treatment cannot be associated with the development of any type of cancer [18–34]. A larger number of specific, long-term studies on patients in real life are necessary to analyse this issue in greater depth.

On the other hand, the global percentage of adverse events of combinations of bDMARD with MTX in some studies is superior to that of MTX monotherapy, specifically for certain types of adverse events such as infections [33], but combination has not been associated with a higher risk of serious adverse events of any type.

5. Initial treatment of RA with biosimilars of TNF-alpha inhibitor biological drugs is cost-effective and this specific variable should be included in treatment stratification. Strength of the recommendation: Moderate

Clinical variables, along with patient opinion and preferences, are essential elements in RA therapy decision-making. However, we must not forget the current healthcare context and its sustainability. This is why the experts consider that the cost-effectiveness of bDMARD is another important variable to take into account.

Different reports at international conferences have informed us about studies into the cost-effectiveness of biological therapy treatment in Spain [60–62]. As no effectiveness difference was seen, a cost minimization analysis was performed that showed that currently the most cost-effective option for immune-mediated diseases such as Crohn's or RA is ADA [60,61]. Specifically in the case of RA, it represents the cheapest biological therapy, with an estimated annual cost of 4650 euros vs. the 4650–10,000 euros for other treatments [60].

In line with these data, a study on cost-effectiveness in Norway [63], where the healthcare system promotes the use of biosimilars to reduce costs, found that since the introduction of biosimilars, the number of RA patients receiving treatment with bDMARD and small molecule inhibitors has increased from 39% in 2010 to 45% in 2019. The proportion of patients who reached DAS28 also increased from 42% to 67%. However, the annual cost of treating a patient with these therapies decreased by 47% [63].

Another pharmacoeconomic study from the perspective of the Italian national health system found that for psoriasis patients, there is a high similarity in cost per responder with two ADA biosimilars (MSB1102 and ABP 501) compared with MTX sc, with cost-effectiveness closest at 52 weeks between MSB1102 (799 euros) and MTX sc (625 euros) [64].

Finally, a cost-effectiveness study on the efficiency of early treatment with biologicals [65] found that for RA patients refractory to csDMARD, adding a biosimilar TNF-alpha inhibitor to MTX at 6 months increased the total treatment cost by only £70, compared to continuing MTX monotherapy and waiting until 12 months (price in pounds sterling for 2017) [65].

4. Discussion

This project shows that the initial RA treatments of TNF-alpha inhibitors combined with MTX and of IL6R (as monotherapy or in combination) are effective, efficient, and safe, with data for effectiveness that in some cases surpasses csDMARD results [18–34].

For several reasons, including effectiveness, safety, cost-effectiveness, type of health care system, etc., the current strategy consists of starting treatment with csDMARD, habitually as a monotherapy. This review highlights that, in many cases, patients who began an initial treatment with bDMARD presented better outcomes (considering activity, physical functioning, PROs, quality of life, and image) than those who had done so with csDMARD [18–34]. This suggests that the option should be considered in clinical practice.

It should be noted that most of the studies we excluded had a significantly high percentage (between 20 and 30%) of patients included who had previously used csDMARD [37–40]. This population may have characteristics and/or responses that are different from those of csDMARD-naïve patients. The patients included in this review were experiencing early-stage RA and had more than one variable for poor prognosis, and it is particularly for this subset of patients that initial treatment with bDMARD should be considered [18–34] or at the very least they should follow the current T2T strategy, changing stage in a short period of time (a maximum of 3 months) to more effective therapeutic options. To the best of our knowledge, there have been no similar initiatives in this field, and we consider that our results may be of interest in clinical practise to manage the initial treatment of RA patients.

It is striking that national and international consensus documents do not consider the use of bDMARD as an initial treatment for RA, citing various reasons, the foremost of which is cost [10]. Bearing in mind the current context, in which the arrival of biosimilars has brought a considerable reduction in the net cost of bDMARD [13], this position should be reconsidered. But taking into account the risks with the use of bDMARDs, we consider it very important to individualise the use of bDMARD as an initial treatment, trying to select patients that might benefit most. In our opinion, this treatment strategy might be particularly effective for RA patients with poor prognostic factors.

The evidence for initial treatment with ETN deserves particular comment, although we can only draw conclusions based on one study, EMPIRE [29], which limits the robustness of our conclusions. The study did not find differences between the combination ETN + MTX and MTX monotherapy that were as consistent as those found in studies of other biologicals. There are different factors that could explain these results. The study included 110 patients, which is probably a small sample size (the calculation of the sample size was based on radiographic criteria, not on RA activity, as in other RCTs). The patients presented early-onset synovitis (some did not meet RA criteria), with data on activity and other severity factors that were lower than the other studies included. This RCT also allowed the use of MTX at comparatively higher doses than in other RCTs. All of these factors could cause the study not to have reached statistical significance in many of the outcome variables.

Another point to note is that recommendations include the use of MTX po (vs. MTX sc) in combination with bDMARD, both because more evidence is available and due to cost. However, the option of MTX sc should be evaluated case by case since its bioavailability is greater and the patient may prefer this route of administration [54,55].

Among the limitations of our work, we note that some of the studies included are post-hoc analyses or exploratory studies, so their outcomes should be interpreted with caution. Likewise, the inclusion of RCT means that the population consists of patients who are not 100% representative of the general RA population seen in conventional clinical practice. Finally, the lack of robust comparative data between combination therapy and monotherapy of biologicals could weaken our findings.

5. Conclusions and Future Directions

Initial treatment with bDMARD in RA patients is effective, has an acceptable safety profile, and, in our current context, should be considered, particularly for patients with poor prognostic factors. The final decision on RA treatment should be made on a case-by-case basis and in consensus with patients.

On the other hand, more research is needed in order to expedite and optimise treatment stratification by using advanced integrative modelling of complex health data (genetics, biomarkers, clinical data, etc.).

Supplementary Materials: The following supporting information can be downloaded at: https://www.mdpi.com/article/10.3390/jcm13010048/s1. Table S1: Excluded studies and reasons for exclusion; Table S2: Evidence table. Main characteristics of included studies; Table S3: Main results of included studies [66]. Table S4: Main results of included studies.

Author Contributions: Conceptualization, J.T.M., B.H.-C. and H.C.; Formal analysis, J.T.M., B.H.-C. and H.C.; Investigation, J.T.M., B.H.-C. and H.C.; Methodology, J.T.M.; Project administration, J.T.M.; Supervision, J.T.M.; Visualization, J.T.M.; Writing—original draft, J.T.M.; Writing—review and editing, J.T.M., B.H.-C. and H.C. All authors have read and agreed to the published version of the manuscript.

Funding: This project was funded by an unrestricted grant from Fresenius Kabi, Spain.

Acknowledgments: We would like to thank Estíbaliz Loza for her help with the methodological tasks, review of this study, and writing of this manuscript.

Conflicts of Interest: The authors received honoraria from Fresenius Kabi Spain for participating in this project.

References

1. Almutairi, K.B.; Nossent, J.C.; Preen, D.B.; Keen, H.I.; Inderjeeth, C.A. The Prevalence of Rheumatoid Arthritis: A Systematic Review of Population-based Studies. *J. Rheumatol.* **2021**, *48*, 669–676. [CrossRef] [PubMed]
2. Alcaide, L.; Torralba, A.I.; Eusamio Serre, J.; García Cotarelo, C.; Loza, E.; Sivera, F. Current state, control, impact and management of rheumatoid arthritis according to patient: AR 2020 national survey. *Reumatol. Clin. (Engl. Ed.)* **2022**, *18*, 177–183. [CrossRef] [PubMed]
3. Gil-Conesa, M.; Del-Moral-Luque, J.A.; Gil-Prieto, R.; Gil-de-Miguel, Á.; Mazzuccheli-Esteban, R.; Rodríguez-Caravaca, G. Hospitalization burden and comorbidities of patients with rheumatoid arthritis in Spain during the period 2002–2017. *BMC Health Serv. Res.* **2020**, *20*, 374. [CrossRef] [PubMed]
4. Leon, L.; Abasolo, L.; Fernandez-Gutierrez, B.; Jover, J.A.; Hernandez-Garcia, C. Direct medical costs and their predictors in the EMAR-II cohort: "Variability in the management of rheumatoid arthritis and spondyloarthritis in Spain". *Reumatol. Clin. (Engl. Ed.)* **2018**, *14*, 4–8. [CrossRef] [PubMed]
5. Kerschbaumer, A.; Sepriano, A.; Smolen, J.S.; van der Heijde, D.; Dougados, M.; van Vollenhoven, R.; McInnes, I.B.; Bijlsma, J.W.J.; Burmester, G.R.; de Wit, M.; et al. Efficacy of pharmacological treatment in rheumatoid arthritis: A systematic literature research informing the 2019 update of the EULAR recommendations for management of rheumatoid arthritis. *Ann. Rheum. Dis.* **2020**, *79*, 744–759. [CrossRef] [PubMed]
6. Smolen, J.S.; Landewé, R.B.M.; Bergstra, S.A.; Kerschbaumer, A.; Sepriano, A.; Aletaha, D.; Caporali, R.; Edwards, C.J.; Hyrich, K.L.; Pope, J.E.; et al. EULAR recommendations for the management of rheumatoid arthritis with synthetic and biological disease-modifying antirheumatic drugs: 2022 update. *Ann. Rheum. Dis.* **2023**, *82*, 3–18. [CrossRef] [PubMed]
7. Singh, J.A.; Hossain, A.; Tanjong Ghogomu, E.; Kotb, A.; Christensen, R.; Mudano, A.S.; Maxwell, L.J.; Shah, N.P.; Tugwell, P.; Wells, G.A. Biologics or tofacitinib for rheumatoid arthritis in incomplete responders to methotrexate or other traditional disease-modifying anti-rheumatic drugs: A systematic review and network meta-analysis. *Cochrane Database Syst. Rev.* **2016**, *2016*, Cd012183. [CrossRef] [PubMed]
8. Singh, J.A.; Hossain, A.; Mudano, A.S.; Tanjong Ghogomu, E.; Suarez-Almazor, M.E.; Buchbinder, R.; Maxwell, L.J.; Tugwell, P.; Wells, G.A. Biologics or tofacitinib for people with rheumatoid arthritis naive to methotrexate: A systematic review and network meta-analysis. *Cochrane Database Syst. Rev.* **2017**, *5*, Cd012657. [CrossRef]
9. Simpson, E.L.; Ren, S.; Hock, E.S.; Stevens, J.W.; Binard, A.; Pers, Y.M.; Archer, R.; Paisley, S.; Stevenson, M.D.; Herpin, C.; et al. Rheumatoid arthritis treated with 6-months of first-line biologic or biosimilar therapy: An updated systematic review and network meta-analysis. *Int. J. Technol. Assess. Health Care* **2019**, *35*, 36–44. [CrossRef]
10. Fraenkel, L.; Bathon, J.M.; England, B.R.; St Clair, E.W.; Arayssi, T.; Carandang, K.; Deane, K.D.; Genovese, M.; Huston, K.K.; Kerr, G.; et al. 2021 American College of Rheumatology Guideline for the Treatment of Rheumatoid Arthritis. *Arthritis Care Res.* **2021**, *73*, 924–939. [CrossRef]
11. Putrik, P.; Ramiro, S.; Kvien, T.K.; Sokka, T.; Pavlova, M.; Uhlig, T.; Boonen, A. Inequities in access to biologic and synthetic DMARDs across 46 European countries. *Ann. Rheum. Dis.* **2014**, *73*, 198–206. [CrossRef] [PubMed]

12. Bergstra, S.A.; Branco, J.C.; Vega-Morales, D.; Salomon-Escoto, K.; Govind, N.; Allaart, C.F.; Landewé, R.B.M. Inequity in access to bDMARD care and how it influences disease outcomes across countries worldwide: Results from the METEOR-registry. *Ann. Rheum. Dis.* **2018**, *77*, 1413–1420. [CrossRef] [PubMed]
13. Kay, J.; Schoels, M.M.; Dörner, T.; Emery, P.; Kvien, T.K.; Smolen, J.S.; Breedveld, F.C. Consensus-based recommendations for the use of biosimilars to treat rheumatological diseases. *Ann. Rheum. Dis.* **2018**, *77*, 165–174. [CrossRef] [PubMed]
14. Asociación Española de Medicamentos Biosimilares. Análisis de Impacto Presupuestario de los Medicamentos Biosimilares en el Sistema Nacional de Salud de España (2009–2022). Available online: https://www.biosim.es/documentos/AIP_biosimilares_Hygeia_UCM_BioSim_nov2020.pdf (accessed on 1 June 2023).
15. Cornejo Uixeda, S.; Quintana Vergara, B.; Sánchez Alcaraz, A. Análisis de la utilización de medicamentos biosimilares. *Rev. De La OFIL* **2020**, *30*, 80–81.
16. Association, W.M. World Medical Association Declaration of Helsinki: Ethical principles for medical research involving human subjects. *JAMA* **2013**, *310*, 2191–2194. [CrossRef]
17. Aletaha, D.; Neogi, T.; Silman, A.J.; Funovits, J.; Felson, D.T.; Bingham, C.O., III; Birnbaum, N.S.; Burmester, G.R.; Bykerk, V.P.; Cohen, M.D.; et al. 2010 Rheumatoid arthritis classification criteria: An American College of Rheumatology/European League Against Rheumatism collaborative initiative. *Arthritis Rheum.* **2010**, *62*, 2569–2581. [CrossRef] [PubMed]
18. Bejarano, V.; Conaghan, P.G.; Quinn, M.A.; Saleem, B.; Emery, P. Benefits 8 years after a remission induction regime with an infliximab and methotrexate combination in early rheumatoid arthritis. *Rheumatology* **2010**, *49*, 1971–1974. [CrossRef] [PubMed]
19. Durez, P.; Malghem, J.; Nzeusseu Toukap, A.; Depresseux, G.; Lauwerys, B.R.; Westhovens, R.; Luyten, F.P.; Corluy, L.; Houssiau, F.A.; Verschueren, P. Treatment of early rheumatoid arthritis: A randomized magnetic resonance imaging study comparing the effects of methotrexate alone, methotrexate in combination with infliximab, and methotrexate in combination with intravenous pulse methylprednisolone. *Arthritis Rheum.* **2007**, *56*, 3919–3927. [CrossRef]
20. Goekoop-Ruiterman, Y.P.; de Vries-Bouwstra, J.K.; Allaart, C.F.; van Zeben, D.; Kerstens, P.J.; Hazes, J.M.; Zwinderman, A.H.; Peeters, A.J.; de Jonge-Bok, J.M.; Mallée, C.; et al. Comparison of treatment strategies in early rheumatoid arthritis: A randomized trial. *Ann. Intern. Med.* **2007**, *146*, 406–415. [CrossRef]
21. Goekoop-Ruiterman, Y.P.; de Vries-Bouwstra, J.K.; Allaart, C.F.; van Zeben, D.; Kerstens, P.J.; Hazes, J.M.; Zwinderman, A.H.; Ronday, H.K.; Han, K.H.; Westedt, M.L.; et al. Clinical and radiographic outcomes of four different treatment strategies in patients with early rheumatoid arthritis (the BeSt study): A randomized, controlled trial. *Arthritis Rheum.* **2005**, *52*, 3381–3390. [CrossRef]
22. Goekoop-Ruiterman, Y.P.; de Vries-Bouwstra, J.K.; Allaart, C.F.; van Zeben, D.; Kerstens, P.J.; Hazes, J.M.; Zwinderman, A.H.; Ronday, H.K.; Han, K.H.; Westedt, M.L.; et al. Clinical and radiographic outcomes of four different treatment strategies in patients with early rheumatoid arthritis (the BeSt study): A randomized, controlled trial. *Arthritis Rheum.* **2008**, *58*, S126–S135. [CrossRef] [PubMed]
23. Markusse, I.M.; Akdemir, G.; Dirven, L.; Goekoop-Ruiterman, Y.P.; van Groenendael, J.H.; Han, K.H.; Molenaar, T.H.; Le Cessie, S.; Lems, W.F.; van der Lubbe, P.A.; et al. Long-Term Outcomes of Patients With Recent-Onset Rheumatoid Arthritis After 10 Years of Tight Controlled Treatment: A Randomized Trial. *Ann. Intern. Med.* **2016**, *164*, 523–531. [CrossRef] [PubMed]
24. Nam, J.L.; Villeneuve, E.; Hensor, E.M.; Conaghan, P.G.; Keen, H.I.; Buch, M.H.; Gough, A.K.; Green, M.J.; Helliwell, P.S.; Keenan, A.M.; et al. Remission induction comparing infliximab and high-dose intravenous steroid, followed by treat-to-target: A double-blind, randomised, controlled trial in new-onset, treatment-naive, rheumatoid arthritis (the IDEA study). *Ann. Rheum. Dis.* **2014**, *73*, 75–85. [CrossRef] [PubMed]
25. Quinn, M.A.; Conaghan, P.G.; O'Connor, P.J.; Karim, Z.; Greenstein, A.; Brown, A.; Brown, C.; Fraser, A.; Jarret, S.; Emery, P. Very early treatment with infliximab in addition to methotrexate in early, poor-prognosis rheumatoid arthritis reduces magnetic resonance imaging evidence of synovitis and damage, with sustained benefit after infliximab withdrawal: Results from a twelve-month randomized, double-blind, placebo-controlled trial. *Arthritis Rheum.* **2005**, *52*, 27–35. [CrossRef] [PubMed]
26. Detert, J.; Bastian, H.; Listing, J.; Weiß, A.; Wassenberg, S.; Liebhaber, A.; Rockwitz, K.; Alten, R.; Krüger, K.; Rau, R.; et al. Induction therapy with adalimumab plus methotrexate for 24 weeks followed by methotrexate monotherapy up to week 48 versus methotrexate therapy alone for DMARD-naive patients with early rheumatoid arthritis: HIT HARD, an investigator-initiated study. *Ann. Rheum. Dis.* **2013**, *72*, 844–850. [CrossRef] [PubMed]
27. Soubrier, M.; Puéchal, X.; Sibilia, J.; Mariette, X.; Meyer, O.; Combe, B.; Flipo, R.M.; Mulleman, D.; Berenbaum, F.; Zarnitsky, C.; et al. Evaluation of two strategies (initial methotrexate monotherapy vs its combination with adalimumab) in management of early active rheumatoid arthritis: Data from the GUEPARD trial. *Rheumatology* **2009**, *48*, 1429–1434. [CrossRef]
28. Hørslev-Petersen, K.; Hetland, M.L.; Junker, P.; Pødenphant, J.; Ellingsen, T.; Ahlquist, P.; Lindegaard, H.; Linauskas, A.; Schlemmer, A.; Dam, M.Y.; et al. Adalimumab added to a treat-to-target strategy with methotrexate and intra-articular triamcinolone in early rheumatoid arthritis increased remission rates, function and quality of life. The OPERA Study: An investigator-initiated, randomised, double-blind, parallel-group, placebo-controlled trial. *Ann. Rheum. Dis.* **2014**, *73*, 654–661. [CrossRef]
29. Nam, J.L.; Villeneuve, E.; Hensor, E.M.; Wakefield, R.J.; Conaghan, P.G.; Green, M.J.; Gough, A.; Quinn, M.; Reece, R.; Cox, S.R.; et al. A randomised controlled trial of etanercept and methotrexate to induce remission in early inflammatory arthritis: The EMPIRE trial. *Ann. Rheum. Dis.* **2014**, *73*, 1027–1036. [CrossRef]
30. Emery, P.; Bingham, C.O., III; Burmester, G.R.; Bykerk, V.P.; Furst, D.E.; Mariette, X.; van der Heijde, D.; van Vollenhoven, R.; Arendt, C.; Mountian, I.; et al. Certolizumab pegol in combination with dose-optimised methotrexate in DMARD-naïve patients with early, active rheumatoid arthritis with poor prognostic factors: 1-year results from C-EARLY, a randomised, double-blind, placebo-controlled phase III study. *Ann. Rheum. Dis.* **2017**, *76*, 96–104. [CrossRef]

31. Hetland, M.L.; Haavardsholm, E.A.; Rudin, A.; Nordström, D.; Nurmohamed, M.; Gudbjornsson, B.; Lampa, J.; Hørslev-Petersen, K.; Uhlig, T.; Grondal, G.; et al. Active conventional treatment and three different biological treatments in early rheumatoid arthritis: Phase IV investigator initiated, randomised, observer blinded clinical trial. *BMJ* **2020**, *371*, m4328. [CrossRef]
32. Weinblatt, M.E.; Bingham, C.O., III; Burmester, G.R.; Bykerk, V.P.; Furst, D.E.; Mariette, X.; van der Heijde, D.; van Vollenhoven, R.; VanLunen, B.; Ecoffet, C.; et al. A Phase III Study Evaluating Continuation, Tapering, and Withdrawal of Certolizumab Pegol After One Year of Therapy in Patients With Early Rheumatoid Arthritis. *Arthritis Rheumatol.* **2017**, *69*, 1937–1948. [CrossRef] [PubMed]
33. Verhoeven, M.M.A.; Tekstra, J.; Welsing, P.M.J.; Pethö-Schramm, A.; Borm, M.E.A.; Bruyn, G.A.W.; Bos, R.; Griep, E.N.; Klaasen, R.; van Laar, J.M.; et al. Effectiveness and safety over 3 years after the 2-year U-Act-Early trial of the strategies initiating tocilizumab and/or methotrexate. *Rheumatology* **2020**, *59*, 2325–2333. [CrossRef] [PubMed]
34. Bijlsma, J.W.J.; Welsing, P.M.J.; Woodworth, T.G.; Middelink, L.M.; Pethö-Schramm, A.; Bernasconi, C.; Borm, M.E.A.; Wortel, C.H.; Ter Borg, E.J.; Jahangier, Z.N.; et al. Early rheumatoid arthritis treated with tocilizumab, methotrexate, or their combination (U-Act-Early): A multicentre, randomised, double-blind, double-dummy, strategy trial. *Lancet* **2016**, *388*, 343–355. [CrossRef] [PubMed]
35. Breedveld, F.C.; Weisman, M.H.; Kavanaugh, A.F.; Cohen, S.B.; Pavelka, K.; van Vollenhoven, R.; Sharp, J.; Perez, J.L.; Spencer-Green, G.T. The PREMIER study: A multicenter, randomized, double-blind clinical trial of combination therapy with adalimumab plus methotrexate versus methotrexate alone or adalimumab alone in patients with early, aggressive rheumatoid arthritis who had not had previous methotrexate treatment. *Arthritis Rheum.* **2006**, *54*, 26–37. [CrossRef] [PubMed]
36. Kavanaugh, A.; Fleischmann, R.M.; Emery, P.; Kupper, H.; Redden, L.; Guerette, B.; Santra, S.; Smolen, J.S. Clinical, functional and radiographic consequences of achieving stable low disease activity and remission with adalimumab plus methotrexate or methotrexate alone in early rheumatoid arthritis: 26-week results from the randomised, controlled OPTIMA study. *Ann. Rheum. Dis.* **2013**, *72*, 64–71. [CrossRef]
37. Bathon, J.M.; Martin, R.W.; Fleischmann, R.M.; Tesser, J.R.; Schiff, M.H.; Keystone, E.C.; Genovese, M.C.; Wasko, M.C.; Moreland, L.W.; Weaver, A.L.; et al. A comparison of etanercept and methotrexate in patients with early rheumatoid arthritis. *N. Engl. J. Med.* **2000**, *343*, 1586–1593. [CrossRef]
38. Emery, P.; Breedveld, F.C.; Hall, S.; Durez, P.; Chang, D.J.; Robertson, D.; Singh, A.; Pedersen, R.D.; Koenig, A.S.; Freundlich, B. Comparison of methotrexate monotherapy with a combination of methotrexate and etanercept in active, early, moderate to severe rheumatoid arthritis (COMET): A randomised, double-blind, parallel treatment trial. *Lancet* **2008**, *372*, 375–382. [CrossRef]
39. Emery, P.; Breedveld, F.; van der Heijde, D.; Ferraccioli, G.; Dougados, M.; Robertson, D.; Pedersen, R.; Koenig, A.S.; Freundlich, B. Two-year clinical and radiographic results with combination etanercept-methotrexate therapy versus monotherapy in early rheumatoid arthritis: A two-year, double-blind, randomized study. *Arthritis Rheum.* **2010**, *62*, 674–682. [CrossRef]
40. Kekow, J.; Moots, R.J.; Emery, P.; Durez, P.; Koenig, A.; Singh, A.; Pedersen, R.; Robertson, D.; Freundlich, B.; Sato, R. Patient-reported outcomes improve with etanercept plus methotrexate in active early rheumatoid arthritis and the improvement is strongly associated with remission: The COMET trial. *Ann. Rheum. Dis.* **2010**, *69*, 222–225. [CrossRef]
41. Rantalaiho, V.; Kautiainen, H.; Korpela, M.; Hannonen, P.; Kaipiainen-Seppänen, O.; Möttönen, T.; Kauppi, M.; Karjalainen, A.; Laiho, K.; Laasonen, L.; et al. Targeted treatment with a combination of traditional DMARDs produces excellent clinical and radiographic long-term outcomes in early rheumatoid arthritis regardless of initial infliximab. The 5-year follow-up results of a randomised clinical trial, the NEO-RACo trial. *Ann. Rheum. Dis.* **2014**, *73*, 1954–1961. [CrossRef]
42. St Clair, E.W.; van der Heijde, D.M.; Smolen, J.S.; Maini, R.N.; Bathon, J.M.; Emery, P.; Keystone, E.; Schiff, M.; Kalden, J.R.; Wang, B.; et al. Combination of infliximab and methotrexate therapy for early rheumatoid arthritis: A randomized, controlled trial. *Arthritis Rheum.* **2004**, *50*, 3432–3443. [CrossRef] [PubMed]
43. Tam, L.S.; Shang, Q.; Li, E.K.; Wang, S.; Li, R.J.; Lee, K.L.; Leung, Y.Y.; Ying, K.Y.; Yim, C.W.; Kun, E.W.; et al. Infliximab is associated with improvement in arterial stiffness in patients with early rheumatoid arthritis -- a randomized trial. *J. Rheumatol.* **2012**, *39*, 2267–2275. [CrossRef] [PubMed]
44. Burmester, G.R.; Rigby, W.F.; van Vollenhoven, R.F.; Kay, J.; Rubbert-Roth, A.; Kelman, A.; Dimonaco, S.; Mitchell, N. Tocilizumab in early progressive rheumatoid arthritis: FUNCTION, a randomised controlled trial. *Ann. Rheum. Dis.* **2016**, *75*, 1081–1091. [CrossRef] [PubMed]
45. Jones, G.; Sebba, A.; Gu, J.; Lowenstein, M.B.; Calvo, A.; Gomez-Reino, J.J.; Siri, D.A.; Tomsic, M.; Alecock, E.; Woodworth, T.; et al. Comparison of tocilizumab monotherapy versus methotrexate monotherapy in patients with moderate to severe rheumatoid arthritis: The AMBITION study. *Ann. Rheum. Dis.* **2010**, *69*, 88–96. [CrossRef] [PubMed]
46. Kume, K.; Amano, K.; Yamada, S.; Hatta, K.; Ohta, H.; Kuwaba, N. Tocilizumab monotherapy reduces arterial stiffness as effectively as etanercept or adalimumab monotherapy in rheumatoid arthritis: An open-label randomized controlled trial. *J. Rheumatol.* **2011**, *38*, 2169–2171. [CrossRef] [PubMed]
47. Stevenson, M.; Archer, R.; Tosh, J.; Simpson, E.; Everson-Hock, E.; Stevens, J.; Hernandez-Alava, M.; Paisley, S.; Dickinson, K.; Scott, D.; et al. Adalimumab, etanercept, infliximab, certolizumab pegol, golimumab, tocilizumab and abatacept for the treatment of rheumatoid arthritis not previously treated with disease-modifying antirheumatic drugs and after the failure of conventional disease-modifying antirheumatic drugs only: Systematic review and economic evaluation. *Health Technol. Assess.* **2016**, *20*, 1–610. [CrossRef]

48. Archer, R.; Hock, E.; Hamilton, J.; Stevens, J.; Essat, M.; Poku, E.; Clowes, M.; Pandor, A.; Stevenson, M. Assessing prognosis and prediction of treatment response in early rheumatoid arthritis: Systematic reviews. *Health Technol. Assess.* **2018**, *22*, 1–294. [CrossRef]
49. Burgers, L.E.; Raza, K.; van der Helm-van Mil, A.H. Window of opportunity in rheumatoid arthritis—Definitions and supporting evidence: From old to new perspectives. *RMD Open* **2019**, *5*, e000870. [CrossRef]
50. John, J.C. Early rheumatoid arthritis—Is there a window of opportunity? *J. Rheumatol.* **2007**, *80*, 1.
51. Breedveld, F. The value of early intervention in RA—A window of opportunity. *Clin. Rheumatol.* **2011**, *30*, 33–39. [CrossRef]
52. Keystone, E.C.; Breedveld, F.C.; van der Heijde, D.; Landewé, R.; Florentinus, S.; Arulmani, U.; Liu, S.; Kupper, H.; Kavanaugh, A. Longterm effect of delaying combination therapy with tumor necrosis factor inhibitor in patients with aggressive early rheumatoid arthritis: 10-year efficacy and safety of adalimumab from the randomized controlled PREMIER trial with open-label extension. *J. Rheumatol.* **2014**, *41*, 5–14. [CrossRef] [PubMed]
53. Garcês, S.; Demengeot, J.; Benito-Garcia, E. The immunogenicity of anti-TNF therapy in immune-mediated inflammatory diseases: A systematic review of the literature with a meta-analysis. *Ann. Rheum. Dis.* **2013**, *72*, 1947–1955. [CrossRef] [PubMed]
54. Braun, J.; Kastner, P.; Flaxenberg, P.; Wahrisch, J.; Hanke, P.; Demary, W.; von Hinuber, U.; Rockwitz, K.; Heitz, W.; Pichlmeier, U.; et al. Comparison of the clinical efficacy and safety of subcutaneous versus oral administration of methotrexate in patients with active rheumatoid arthritis: Results of a six-month, multicenter, randomized, double-blind, controlled, phase IV trial. *Arthritis Rheum.* **2008**, *58*, 73–81. [CrossRef] [PubMed]
55. Tornero Molina, J.; Calvo Alen, J.; Ballina, J.; Belmonte, M.; Blanco, F.J.; Caracuel, M.; Carbonell, J.; Corominas, H.; Chamizo, E.; Hidalgo, C.; et al. Recommendations for the use of parenteral methotrexate in rheumatic diseases. *Reumatol. Clin. (Engl. Ed.)* **2018**, *14*, 142–149. [CrossRef] [PubMed]
56. Islam, M.S.; Haq, S.A.; Islam, M.N.; Azad, A.K.; Islam, M.A.; Barua, R.; Hasan, M.M.; Mahmood, M.; Safiuddin, M.; Rahman, M.M.; et al. Comparative efficacy of subcutaneous versus oral methotrexate in active rheumatoid arthritis. *Mymensingh Med. J. MMJ* **2013**, *22*, 483–488. [PubMed]
57. Harris, J.A.; Bykerk, V.P.; Hitchon, C.A.; Keystone, E.C.; Thorne, J.C.; Boire, G.; Haraoui, B.; Hazlewood, G.; Bonner, A.J.; Pope, J.E.; et al. Determining best practices in early rheumatoid arthritis by comparing differences in treatment at sites in the Canadian Early Arthritis Cohort. *J. Rheumatol.* **2013**, *40*, 1823–1830. [CrossRef] [PubMed]
58. Ferraz-Amaro, I.; Seoane-Mato, D.; Sanchez-Alonso, F.; Martin-Martinez, M.A.; emAR II Study Group. Synthetic disease-modifying antirheumatic drug prescribing variability in rheumatoid arthritis: A multilevel analysis of a cross-sectional national study. *Rheumatol. Int.* **2015**, *35*, 1825–1836. [CrossRef] [PubMed]
59. Tornero-Molina, J.; Andreu, J.L.; Martín-Martínez, M.-A.; Corominas, H.; Pérez Venegas, J.J.; Román-Ivorra, J.A.; Sánchez-Alonso, F. Metotrexato en pacientes con artritis reumatoide en España: Subanálisis del proyecto AR Excellence. *Reumatol. Clínica* **2019**, *15*, 338–342. [CrossRef]
60. Martínez-Sesmero, J.M.; Schoenenberger-Arnaiz, J.A.; Crespo-Diz, C.; Cerezales, M. AB1389 Cost-Minimization Analysis in Rheumatoid Arthritis in Spain. *Ann. Rheum. Dis.* **2022**, *81*, 1799–1800. [CrossRef]
61. Schoenenberger Arnaiz, J.; Crespo Diz, C.; Martínez Sesmero, J.; Cerezales, M. 4CPS-083 Cost-effectiveness analysis of adalimumab and its clinical alternatives in immune-mediated inflammatory diseases in Spain. *Eur. J. Hosp. Pharm.* **2022**, *29*, A55–A56. [CrossRef]
62. Schoenenberger-Arnaiz, J.A.; Martínez-Sesmero, J.M.; Crespo-Diz, C.; Cerezales, M.; Guigini, M. Adalimumab and its clinical alternatives in Crohn's disease and ulcerative colitis in Spain. *United Eur. Gastroenterol. J.* **2022**, *10* (Suppl. 8), 1064.
63. Brkic, A.; Diamantopoulos, A.P.; Haavardsholm, E.A.; Fevang, B.T.S.; Brekke, L.K.; Loli, L.; Zettel, C.; Rødevand, E.; Bakland, G.; Mielnik, P.; et al. Exploring drug cost and disease outcome in rheumatoid arthritis patients treated with biologic and targeted synthetic DMARDs in Norway in 2010–2019—A country with a national tender system for prescription of costly drugs. *BMC Health Serv. Res.* **2022**, *22*, 48. [CrossRef] [PubMed]
64. Maurelli, M.; Girolomoni, G.; Gisondi, P. Cost per responder of adalimumab biosimilars versus methotrexate in patients with psoriasis: A real-life experience. *J. Dermatolog. Treat.* **2023**, *34*, 2218504. [CrossRef] [PubMed]
65. Patel, D.; Shelbaya, A.; Cheung, R.; Aggarwal, J.; Park, S.H.; Coindreau, J. Cost-Effectiveness of Early Treatment with Originator Biologics or Their Biosimilars After Methotrexate Failure in Patients with Established Rheumatoid Arthritis. *Adv. Ther.* **2019**, *36*, 2086–2095. [CrossRef]
66. Atsumi, T.; Tanaka, Y.; Yamamoto, K.; Takeuchi, T.; Yamanaka, H.; Ishiguro, N.; Eguchi, K.; Watanabe, A.; Origasa, H.; Yasuda, S.; et al. Clinical benefit of 1-year certolizumab pegol (CZP) add-on therapy to methotrexate treatment in patients with early rheumatoid arthritis was observed following CZP discontinuation: 2-year results of the C-OPERA study, a phase III randomised trial. *Ann. Rheum. Dis.* **2017**, *76*, 1348–1356. [CrossRef]

Disclaimer/Publisher's Note: The statements, opinions and data contained in all publications are solely those of the individual author(s) and contributor(s) and not of MDPI and/or the editor(s). MDPI and/or the editor(s) disclaim responsibility for any injury to people or property resulting from any ideas, methods, instructions or products referred to in the content.

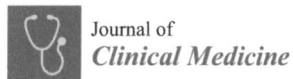

Article

The Real-World Effectiveness, Persistence, Adherence, and Safety of Janus Kinase Inhibitor Baricitinib in Rheumatoid Arthritis: A Long-Term Study

Alberto Calvo-Garcia [1], Esther Ramírez Herráiz [1], Irene María Llorente Cubas [2], Blanca Varas De Dios [3], Juana Benedí González [4], Alberto Morell Baladrón [1] and Rosario García-Vicuña [2,5,*]

[1] Pharmacy Service, Hospital Universitario La Princesa, IIS-Princesa, 28006 Madrid, Spain; alberto.calvo@salud.madrid.org (A.C.-G.); eramirezh@salud.madrid.org (E.R.H.); alberto.morell@salud.madrid.org (A.M.B.)
[2] Rheumatology Service, Hospital Universitario La Princesa, IIS-Princesa, 28006 Madrid, Spain; irenemaria.llorente@salud.madrid.org
[3] Rheumatology Service, Hospital Universitario Santa Cristina, 28006 Madrid, Spain; blanca.varas@salud.madrid.org
[4] Pharmacology, Pharmacognosy and Botany Department, Pharmacy Faculty, Complutense University of Madrid, 28040 Madrid, Spain; jbenedi@farm.ucm.es
[5] Department of Medicine, Faculty of Medicine, Autonomous University of Madrid, 28049 Madrid, Spain
* Correspondence: mariadelrosario.garcia@salud.madrid.org

Abstract: Background/Aim: Baricitinib (BAR) is the first oral selective Janus kinase inhibitor approved in Europe for rheumatoid arthritis (RA). Real-world data are still needed to clarify its long-term benefits/risk profile. This study aimed to evaluate the effectiveness, persistence, adherence, and safety of BAR in a real-world setting. **Methods**: An ambispective study was conducted between October 2017 and December 2021 in RA patients starting BAR. The effectiveness was evaluated, assessing changes from the baseline of the Disease Activity Score using 28-joint counts-C reactive protein (DAS28CRP), and the achievement of low disease activity/remission. Drug persistence was evaluated using Kaplan–Meier analysis. Adherence was estimated using the medication possession ratio (MPR) and the 5-item Compliance Questionnaire for Rheumatology. Safety was assessed determining global incidence proportion and adverse event adjusted incidence rates. **Results**: In total, 61/64 recruited patients were finally analyzed, 83.6% were female, 78.7% were seropositive, the mean age was 58.1 (15.4) years, and the disease duration was 13.9 (8.3) years. A total of 32.8% of patients were naïve to biologics and 16.4% received BAR as monotherapy. The median exposure to BAR was 12.4 (6.6–31.2) months (range 3.1–51.4). A significant change in DAS28CRP was observed after treatment (difference -1.2, $p = 0.000$). 70.5% and 60.7% of patients achieved low disease activity or remission, respectively, and 50.8% (31/61) remained on BAR throughout the follow-up, with a median persistence of 31.2 (9.3–53.1) months. The average MPR was 0.96 (0.08) and all patients exhibited "good adherence" according to the questionnaire. In total, 21.3% of patients discontinued baricitinib due to toxicity. **Conclusions**: In our real-world practice, BAR demonstrated effectiveness, large persistence, high adherence to treatment, and an acceptable safety profile.

Keywords: JAK-inhibitor; baricitinib; rheumatoid arthritis; real-word data; persistence; adherence; safety; unmet needs

1. Introduction

Rheumatoid arthritis (RA) is a chronic autoimmune disease, typically characterized by polyarticular joint inflammation, with potential extra-articular involvement and frequent comorbidities. The persistent inflammation produces a decrease in the patients' functional capacity and in their quality of life [1].

The physiopathology of RA includes chronic synovial membrane inflammation with the subsequent destruction of the joint cartilage and bone [2]. The current pathogenic model proposes autoimmunity as the main disease trigger in genetically predisposed individuals, resulting in the early presence of circulating auto-antibodies to environmental-induced neoepitopes (anti-citrullinated protein antibodies [ACPAs] and antibodies against immunoglobulin G, such as the rheumatoid factor [RF]) [2].

The main goal of RA treatment is to achieve remission or, at least, low disease activity (LDA) through a "treat to target" strategy [1]. Briefly, disease activity target goals are defined at disease onset, and this activity is tightly monitored, aiming to adjust treatment until the predefined goals are achieved. Disease activity can be assessed using composite indices, such as the Disease Activity Score, using 28-joint counts (DAS28), the Clinical Disease Activity Index (CDAI), and the Simplified Disease Activity Index (SDAI) [1].

Current treatment guidelines for RA recommend conventional synthetic disease-modifying anti-rheumatic drugs (csDMARDs) as the first step in treatment, and when the treatment goals are not met, they endorse adding or switching to either a biologic DMARD (bDMARD), or a targeted synthetic DMARD (tsDMARD) [3]. tsDMARDs inhibit intracellular signaling pathways, specifically the Janus kinase/signal transducer and the activator of the transcription (JAK-STAT) pathway. Baricitinib (BAR), which predominantly inhibits JAK1 and JAK2 isoenzymes, was one of the first JAK inhibitors (JAKi) available for RA treatment [4].

In randomized clinical trials (RCT), BAR demonstrated efficacy in patients naïve to bDMARDs and in those with an inadequate response to csDMARDs or Tumor Necrosis Factor inhibitors (TNFi) [5–7]. Furthermore, BAR, in combination with methotrexate (MTX), achieved better results in some early disease activity outcomes than the combination of MTX with adalimumab (ADA) [8].

The increasing incorporation of JAKi into RA therapy, as well as emerging safety issues regarding tofacitinib [9] and even BAR [10], warrant more real-world data (RWD) on effectiveness, safety, and persistence of BAR, in order to consolidate this drug as one of the alternatives for RA treatment. In addition, since the complexity and chronicity of anti-rheumatic treatment may influence adherence, monitoring adherence is mandatory to identify adherence problems and tailor the interventions to solve them [11]. The lack of medication compliance may lead to early treatment failure and the switch to more intensive treatments. Therefore, this study was designed to evaluate the effectiveness, persistence, adherence, and safety of BAR in a real-world setting.

2. Materials and Methods

2.1. Study Design and Population

This was a longitudinal ambispective chart review conducted between October 2017 and December 2021 in La Princesa University Hospital in Madrid, Spain (See Figure 1 for study design). Patients eligible for inclusion were aged ≥18 years, diagnosed with RA according to the American College of Rheumatology (ACR)/European League against Rheumatism (EULAR) 2010 classification criteria [12], and had initiated BAR treatment between October 2017 and June 2021. All consecutive patients whose BAR prescription started within in this inclusion period were recruited for the study. The index date was defined as the first BAR prescription date, and the follow-up was defined as the period between the index date and death, loss to follow-up, or last chart review data, whichever came first. The patient recruitment period lasted from September 2019 to June 2021 and the chart review covered data collection from October 2017 to December 2021. For patients who initiated BAR before September 2019, data were collected retrospectively until that date; subsequently, these patients were followed together with the rest of the patients until December 2021, to ensure that patients initiating BAR in June 2021 had a minimum follow-up of 6 months. The population sample size was calculated based on data from our hospital pharmacy electronic prescription records, where an average of 75 RA patients per year were eligible to start on or switch to bDMARDs or JAK inhibitors (JAKi). Employing a confidence level of 95% and a margin of error of 5%, along with an expected loss of 10–15% during the follow-up period, we determined that a sample size of 64–67 would adequately represent our population.

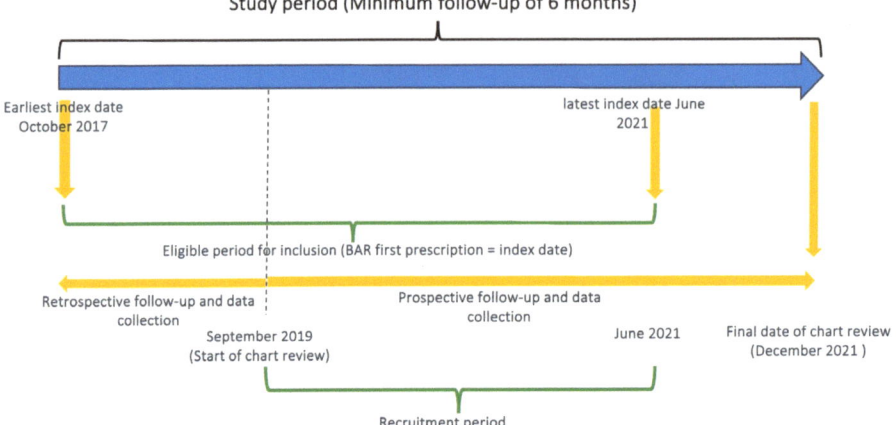

Figure 1. Overall study design. The index date is defined as the first baricitinib prescription date. The follow-up period is defined as the interval from the index date until the date of the final chart review, or any event resulting in the early end of follow-up, treatment withdrawal, or loss to follow-up, whichever comes first.

The indication for BAR did not include the recent recommendations from The Pharmacovigilance Risk Assessment Committee (PRAC), endorsed by the European Medicines Agency, to minimize the risk of serious side effects of JAKi, because they were published after the end of the observation period [13].

2.2. Outcomes

The pre-defined primary endpoints for effectiveness were changes from the baseline in DAS28-C reactive protein (CRP), and rates of low disease activity (LDA) (2.6 < DAS28-erytrocyte sedimentation rate [ESR] $\leq$ 3.2), and disease remission (DAS28CRP < 2.6) [14] at months 6, 12, 24, and at the end of follow-up. As the secondary endpoint, rates of EULAR response at the end of the follow-up were also assessed. The DAS28CRP score was chosen to evaluate effectiveness, based on EULAR/ACR recommendations for defining RA activity in studies with patients and its widespread use in clinical practice [15].

The primary endpoints for treatment persistence were the number of days on BAR treatment until discontinuation or the end of follow-up period (compiled from electronic prescribing and dispensing records) [16] and the rate of patients who maintained BAR at 6, 12, 24, 36, and 48 months and at the end of follow-up period. In addition to overall persistence, the median persistence was differentially assessed in patients who discontinued treatment due to a loss of effectiveness or to toxicity. Adherence was calculated using two methods. The first method was the assessment of the medication possession ratio (MPR), defined as the sum of the days' supply for all fills of the drug in a given time period divided by the number of days in this period (compiled from electronic prescribing and dispensing records). Patients were considered adherent when their MPR was $\geq$0.8 [17]. The second method was the 5-item Compliance Questionnaire for Rheumatology (CQR5), a simplified and validated Spanish version of the 19-item CQR [18–20]. This questionnaire was only applied to patients with a prospective follow-up.

To evaluate safety, the global incidence proportion (IP) and adjusted incidence rate (IR) per 100 patient years (PY) of adverse events (AEs) were calculated. Deviations in laboratory values were defined according to the specifications in the BAR summary of product characteristics [21]. AEs were classified according to the Common Terminology Criteria for Adverse Events (CTCAE) Version 5.0 [22].

2.3. Statistical Analysis

Summary statistics are expressed as means (standard deviation) or medians (25–75 interquartile range [IQR]) for quantitative variables, or n (percentage) for qualitative variables. Paired analyses of DAS28CRP and laboratory values were performed using the Wilcoxon signed-rank test. Stratified analyses for disease activity and persistence were performed using the Pearson's chi-squared test in different subgroups according to: the presence/absence of RF and/or ACPAs, previous exposure to bDMARDs or JAKi, and combination treatment with csDMARDs or BAR monotherapy. Kaplan–Meier curves were plotted for the evaluation of BAR persistence. SPSS version 22.0 was used.

3. Results

3.1. Baseline Population Demographics and Treatments Patterns

In total, 64 patients started treatment with BAR during the inclusion period, although only 61 fulfilled the inclusion criteria and were included in the statistical analysis. A total of 15 patients initiated BAR before the prospective study started and 13 discontinued treatment until that date. Therefore, those data were collected retrospectively.

Baseline demographics and clinical characteristics are shown in Table 1. Most patients were female, 51/61 (83.6%), with a mean (SD) age at initiation of BAR of 58.1 (15.4) years and a mean RA disease duration of 13.9 (8.3) years. In total, 48 (78.7%) patients were positive for RF and/or ACPA, and more than a half, 34/61 (55.7%), had erosive disease. In total, 30 (49.1%) patients were under glucocorticoid treatment when BAR treatment started.

Table 1. Baseline characteristics of the study population (n = 61).

Gender (n, % female)	51 (83.6)
Age at initiation of BAR (years, mean, SD)	58.1 (15.4)
Disease duration (years, mean, SD)	13.9 (8.3)
RF positive (n, %)	47 (77.0)
ACPAs positive (n, %)	43 (70.5)
Erosive disease (n, %)	34 (55.7)
Extra-articular disease (n, %)	26 (42.6)
Rheumatic nodules	10 (16.4)
Sjögren syndrome	7 (11.5)
Interstitial pneumonitis	4 (6.6)
Neuropathies	2 (3.3)
Peripheral ulcerative keratitis	1 (1.6)
Raynaud syndrome	1 (1.6)
Felty syndrome	1 (1.6)
Glucocorticoid treatment (n, %)	30 (49.1)
Naïve to bDMARDs or JAKi treatment (n, %)	20 (32.8)
Previous exposure to bDMARDs or JAKi (n, %)	41 (67.2)
Number or previous bDMARDs	
One previous bDMARD	6 (9.8)
Two previous bDMARDs	14 (23.0)
Three previous bDMARDs	8 (13.1)
Four previous bDMARDs	7 (11.5)
Five previous bDMARDs	2 (3.3)
Six previous bDMARDs	2 (3.3)
Seven previous bDMARDs	1 (1.6)
Eight previous bDMARD	1 (1.6)

Table 1. *Cont.*

Type of previous bDMARDs	
TNFi	41 (67.2)
IL-6Ri	18 (29.1)
CTLA4-Ig	19 (31.1)
Anti-CD20 B cell depletion	21 (34.4)
Previous exposure to one JAKi (tofacitinib) (n, %)	7 (11.5)
BAR monotherapy (n, %)	10 (16.4)
BAR in combination with csDMARDs	51 (83.6)
Methotrexate	31 (50.8)
Leflunomide	14 (23.0)
Hydroxychloroquine	3 (4.9)
Sulfasalazine	2 (3.3)
Methotrexate plus leflunomide	1 (1.6)
Baseline DAS28CRP (mean, SD)	3.9 (0.9)
Baseline ESR (mml/h, mean, SD)	27.8 (23.2)
Baseline CRP (mg/dL, mean, SD)	2.0 (4.8)

ACPAs: Anti-citrullinated protein antibodies; BAR: baricitinib; bDMARDs: biologic disease-modifying antirheumatic drugs; csDMARDs: conventional synthetic disease-modifying anti-rheumatic drugs; DAS28CRP: Disease activity score using 28-joint counts-C reactive protein; ESR: Erythrocyte sedimentation rate; IL-6Ri: IL6 receptor inhibitors; RF: Rheumatoid factor; SD: Standard deviation; TNFi: TNF inhibitors.

Regarding previous exposure to bDMARDs, 20 (32.8%) patients were naïve to bDMARDs or JAKi, and the median (25–75 IQR) number of previous bDMARDs or JAKi was 2 (0–4). Among patients with previous exposure to b/sdDMARDs (41/61), all patients had been treated with TNFi, while approximately one third of the overall population was first exposed to different non-TNF biologic targeted therapies (Table 1). A total of 7 (11.5%) patients had experienced previous failure to one JAKi, tofacitinib. Regarding combination treatment, 51 (83.6%) patients had used BAR in combination with csDMARDs. The mean follow-up time of the study population was 19.1 (1.4) months with a range of 3.1–51.4 months.

3.2. Effectiveness

A significant change in DAS28CRP was observed at the end of the follow-up period (difference of 1.2, $p = 0.000$) (Table 2). The median exposure to BAR was 12.4 (6.6–31.2) months.

Table 2. Variation in disease activity and laboratory parameters under baricitinib treatment.

	Baseline	Final	p
DAS28CRP (average, SD)	3.9 (0.9)	2.7 (1.3)	0.000
CRP (mg/dL, average, SD)	2.0 (4.8)	1.1 (1.7)	0.105
ESR (mml/h, average, SD)	29.0 (23,2)	25.7 (22.9)	0.604
Lymphocyte count (cells/mm^3, mean, SD)	2641 (1501)	2482.6 (1505)	0.154
Neutrophil count (cells/mm^3, mean, SD)	4198 (2126)	4157 (2132)	0.865
Hemoglobin (g/dL, mean, SD)	13.5 (1.5)	12.9 (1.4)	0.000

DAS28CRP: Disease activity score using 28-joint counts-C reactive protein; SD: Standard deviation; ESR: Erythrocyte sedimentation rate.

According to DAS28CRP, 37/61 (60.7%) patients achieved disease remission, whereas 43/61 (70.5%) achieved LDA along the follow-up period. The evolution of DAS28CRP along the follow-up period and the proportion of patients who achieved disease remission or LDA at months 6, 12, and 24 are shown in Figure 2.

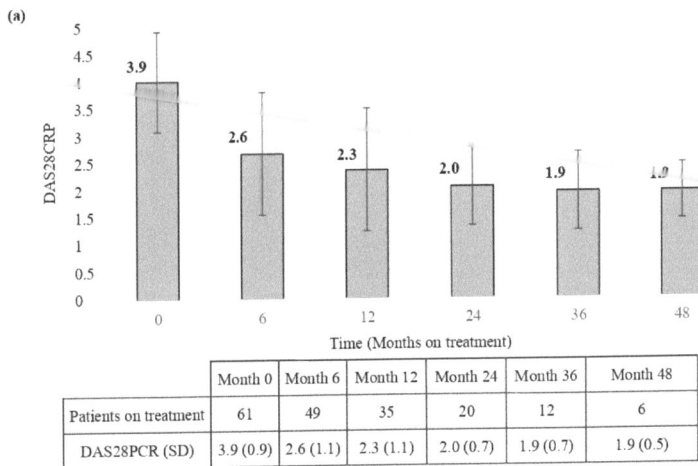

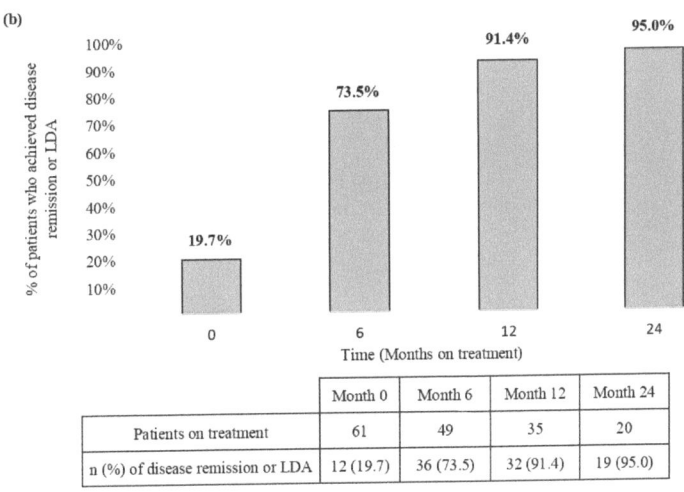

Figure 2. Baricitinib effectiveness. Change in disease activity from the baseline, assessed by the disease activity score using 28-joint counts-C reactive protein (**a**) and the proportion of patients who achieved disease remission or low disease activity at months 6, 12, and 24 (**b**). DAS28CRP: Disease activity score using 28-joint counts-C reactive protein; SD: standard deviation; LDA: low disease activity.

At the end of the follow-up period, 33/61 (54.1%) patients exhibited good response, 10/61 (16.4%) moderate response, and 18/61 (29.5%) no response according to EULAR criteria.

Combined LDA/remission rates under BAR treatment were similar in patients with RF and/or ACPA positive status and in those with a negative status, (70.8% [34/48] vs. 69.2% [9/13] [$p = 0.911$]). Notably, LDA/remission rates were significantly higher in bDMARDs/JAKi-naïve patients compared to previously exposed patients, (95.0% [19/20] vs. 58.5% [24/41], respectively [$p = 0.014$]). According to the number of previous bDMARDs/JAKi, global LDA/remission rates varied from 95.0% (19/20) in bDMARDs/JAKi-naïve patients to 66.7% (4/6) in patients with one previous bDMARDs/JAKi, and 57.1% (20/35) in patients with two or more previous drugs ($p = 0.040$). Finally, no significant differences were found between patients on monotherapy with BAR and patients on combination regimen with csDMARDs, 70.0% (7/10) vs. 70.6% (36/51), respectively ($p = 0.970$).

3.3. Persistence

In total, 31 (31/61, 50.8%) patients remained on treatment with BAR at the end of the follow-up period, with a mean time on treatment of 12.4 (6.6–31.2) months and a median persistence of 31.2 (9.3–53.1) months. The Kaplan–Meier curves for the global population and those stratified according to the cause of BAR discontinuation are shown in Figure 3.

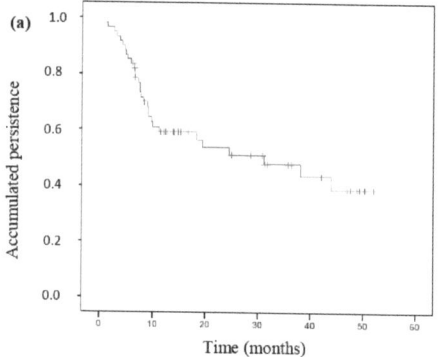

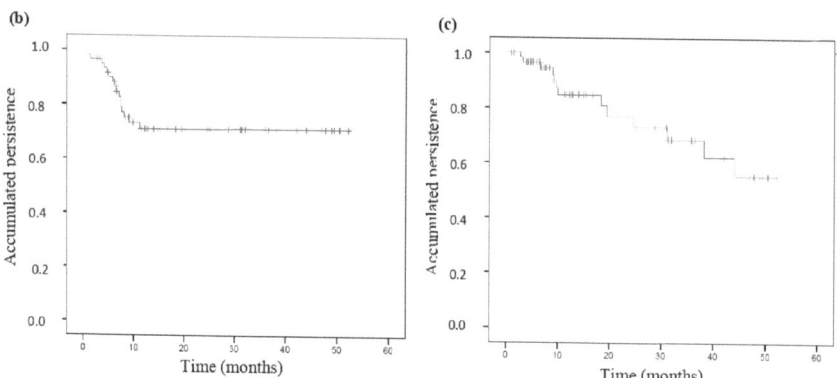

Figure 3. Baricitinib persistence. Drug retention in the global population (n = 61) (**a**); in patients who discontinued treatment due to loss of effectiveness (n = 16) (**b**), or due to intolerance/safety issues (n = 10) (**c**). CI: confidence interval.

During follow-up, BAR treatment was discontinued in 16/61 (26.2%) patients due to the lack of effectiveness, and in 13/61 (21.3%) patients due to intolerance/safety issues. Finally, 1/61 (1.6%) patient ended BAR treatment by their own decision. The retention rates at different time points are shown in Figure 4.

The stratified analysis of persistence according to the presence/absence of RF and/or ACPAs, previous exposure to bDMARDs or JAKi, and in combination treatment with csDMARDs or BAR monotherapy is shown in Figure 5. The log-rank test indicated a significant difference only in the stratified analysis by previous exposure to bDMARDs/JAKi: median persistence was not obtained in naïve patients (the median could not be calculated as it did not reach a 0.5 probability) vs. 11.2 (0.1–25.4) months in the group of patients with prior exposure ($p = 0.039$).

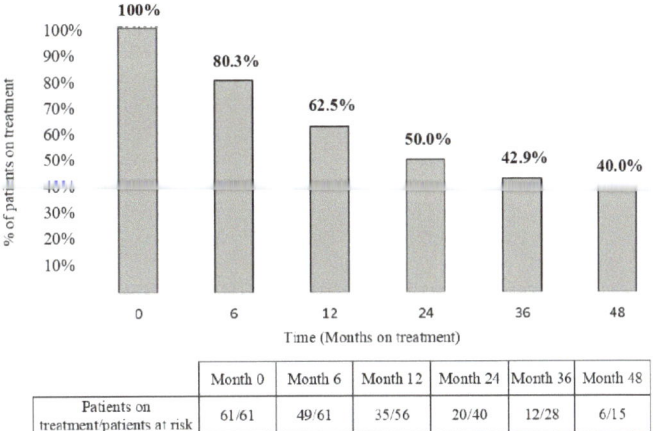

	Month 0	Month 6	Month 12	Month 24	Month 36	Month 48
Patients on treatment/patients at risk	61/61	49/61	35/56	20/40	12/28	6/15

Figure 4. Retention rates of baricitinib treatment at different time points.

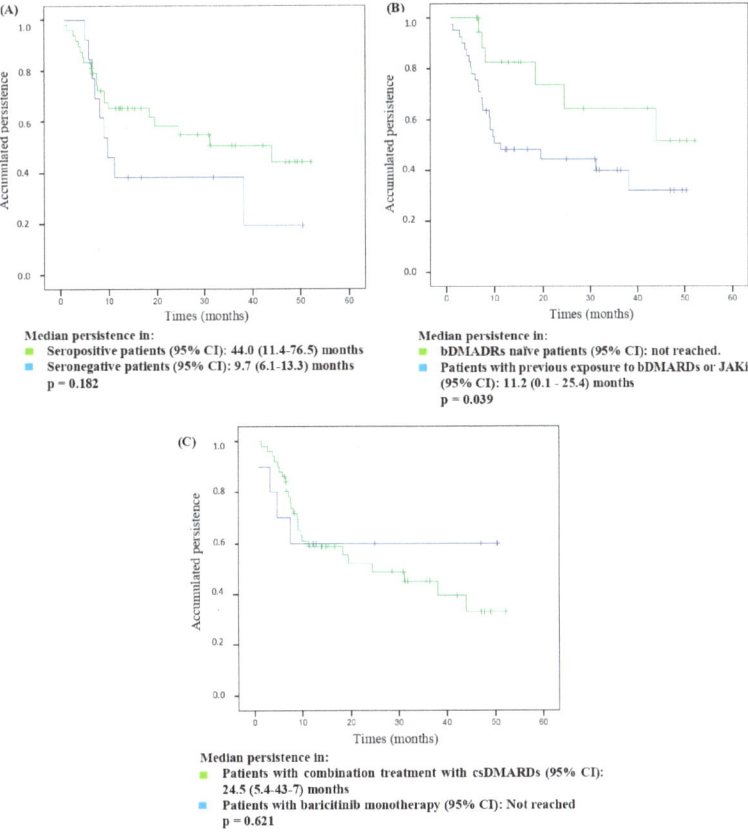

Figure 5. Baricitinib persistence in different subgroups according to: (**A**) the presence/absence of the rheumatoid factor and/or anti-citrullinated protein antibodies; (**B**) previous exposure to bDMARDs or JAKi; (**C**) and combination treatment with csDMARDs or baricitinib monotherapy. The log-rank test was used to compare Kaplan–Meier curves. CI: confidence interval; csDMARDs: conventional synthetic disease-modifying anti-rheumatic drugs, bDMARDs: biological disease-modifying anti-rheumatic drugs; JAKi: Janus Kinase inhibitors.

3.4. Adherence

The average MPR of all patients was 0.96 (0.08). According to this parameter, all patients but one were adherent to treatment. In total, 46 patients in the prospective study completed the CQR5 questionnaire, and all of them were considered "good adherents".

3.5. Safety

AEs occurred in 40/61 (65.6%) patients, with an IR per 100 PY of 15.2 (95% CI 15.4–15.1), while severe AEs (SAEs) occurred in 9/61 (14.8%) patients, with an IR per 100 PY of 3.5 (3.3–3.7) (Table 3).

Table 3. Adverse events during baricitinib exposure.

	IP (n, %)	IR per 100 PY (95% CI)
Patients with any AE (Total AEs = 104)	40/61 (65.6)	15.2 (15.1–15.3)
Anemia	24/61 (39.3)	9.1 (9.0–9.2)
Any infection	22/61 (36.1)	8.4 (8.2–8.6)
Herpes Zoster	7/61 (11.5)	2.7 (2.4–3.0)
URTI	7/61 (11.5)	2.7 (2.4–3.0)
Skin and soft tissue infection	5/61 (8.2)	1.9 (1.7–2.1)
Bacterial pneumonia	3/61 (4.9)	1.1 (0.8–1.4)
Influenza A	2/61 (3.3)	0.8 (0.6–1.0)
Oral herpes simple	2/61 (3.3)	0.8 (0.6–1.0)
Hypercholesterolemia	20/61 (32.8)	7.6 (7.4–7.8)
Abnormal liver enzymes (ALT or AST)	19/61 (31.1)	7.2 (6.9–7.5)
Nausea and vomiting	4/61 (6.6)	1.5 (1.3–1.7)
Cancer	3/61 (4.9)	1.1 (0.8–1.4)
Alopecia	2/61 (3.3)	0.8 (0.6–1.0)
Skin disorders	2/61 (3.3)	0.8 (0.6–1.0)
Asthenia	2/61 (3.3)	0.8 (0.6–1.0)
Weight gain	1/61 (1.6)	0.4 (0.2–0.6)
Venous thrombotic event	1/61 (1.6)	0.4 (0.2–0.6)
Hypertriglyceridemia	1/61 (1.6)	0.4 (0.2–0.6)
Rhabdomyolysis	1/61 (1.6)	0.4 (0.2–0.6)
Platelet increase	1/61 (1.6)	0.4 (0.2–0.6)
Patients with SAEs (Grade 3–4) (Total SAEs = 11)	9/61 (14.8)	3.5 (3.3–3.7)
Bacterial pneumonia with intravenous treatment	3/61 (4.9)	1.1 (0.8–1.4)
Cancer	3/61 (4.9)	1.1 (0.8–1.4)
Abnormal liver enzymes (ALT or AST)	1/61 (1.6)	0.4 (0.2–0.6)
Venous thrombotic event	1/61 (1.6)	0.4 (0.2–0.6)
Hypertriglyceridemia	1/61 (1.6)	0.4 (0.2–0.6)
Skin disorders (Urticaria)	1/61 (1.6)	0.4 (0.2–0.6)
Platelet increase	1/61 (1.6)	0.4 (0.2–0.6)

IP: incidence proportion; IR: incidence rate; PY: patient-year; CI: Confidence interval; AEs: adverse events; SAEs: severe AEs; URTI: upper respiratory tract infection; ALT: alanine transaminase; AST: aspartate transaminase.

The most prevalent AEs were anemia in 24/61 (39.3%) patients, infection in 22/61 (36.1%), hypercholesterolemia in 20/61 (32.8%), and abnormal liver enzymes in 19/61 (31.1%). Herpes Zoster (HZ) infection occurred in 7/61 (11.5%) patients (Table 3). Regarding laboratory parameters during BAR treatment, significant changes from the baseline values were only found in mean hemoglobin concentration (13.5 [1.5] g/dL vs. 12.9 [1.4] g/dL, $p = 0.000$) (Table 2).

A total of 13 out of 61 (21.3%) patients discontinued BAR treatment due to toxicity. Three of them discontinued treatment due to HZ infection; three due to cancer (two lung carcinoma and one breast carcinoma), two due to grade 2 anemia; two due to grade 2 abnormal liver enzymes; one patient due to grade 4 hypertriglyceridemia, grade 4 abnormal liver enzymes, and grade 3 urticaria; one patient due to increased platelet count (>1,000,000 cells/mm^3); and one patient due to central retinal vein occlusion. No deaths were recorded.

4. Discussion

The main findings in our study were the high rates of effectiveness, persistence, and adherence of BAR in a long-standing and mostly bDMARD experienced population with a significant proportion of seropositivity and erosive disease; nonetheless, biologic-naïve patients achieved a better response to BAR treatment.

BAR has recently been incorporated into RA therapy after favorable efficacy results in randomized clinical trials [5–8]. In clinical practice, BAR has been postulated as one of the alternatives for unmet therapeutic needs in RA patients; in addition, recent safety concerns with tofacitinib [9] have led regulatory agencies to endorse measures to minimize risks in all JAKi treatments for chronic inflammatory diseases [13,23]. Accordingly, a repurposing of these drugs in the RA armamentarium, at least in some subpopulations, has emerged. Our safety data from a population not selected following current recommendations may provide additional information to that on published RWD on BAR treatment [4,24,25]. Unlike most real-world studies, we provide long-term safety data as adjusted incidence rates (IR) per 100 patient years, demonstrating an acceptable safety profile of BAR.

The characteristics of our patients (age around 60 years, long-standing RA with poor prognostic factors and few patients naïve to biologics or JAKi) are in line with most of the compiled real-world evidence [4,25]. In contrast, our use of BAR in monotherapy is less frequent than that of most published studies, which also show wide geographical heterogeneity [4].

Regarding effectiveness, a recent systematic review of BAR RWD reveals that most of the studies report LDA/disease remission rates after a six-month follow-up [25]. Herein we report high rates of LDA/disease remission in extended timeframes, in accordance with the results of a long-term study [26], as well as EULAR response at the end of follow-up. The rapid decrease in DAS28CRP was detected in the first six months, which led to sustained remission, i.e., more than 70% of patients in remission at 6 months of follow-up and more than 90% at 12 or successive months. These findings corroborate the effectiveness of BAR observed in other real-world studies [27–36].

BAR treatment effectiveness was not significantly affected by the presence of RF and/or ACPAs, nor by combination treatment with csDMARDs, in accordance with studies by Takahasi et al. [27] and Guidelli et al. [37], but contrary to results from Iwamoto et al. [28], in which patients on combination treatment with MTX achieved a better response. In our study, patients naïve to bDMARDs or JAKi treatment had higher LDA and disease remission rates than patients with previous exposure to bDMARDs, in line with previous studies [27,28,36,37]. Therefore, this result supports that bDMARD- naïve patients may benefit more from BAR treatment.

In our population, persistence at four years of follow-up was large; median time to BAR discontinuation was 31 months, and half of the patients remained on treatment at the end of follow-up. Retention rates at 6, 12, and 24 months were 80, 62.5, and 50%, respectively, similar to those described in other observational studies [27,29–32,36,38–41], while Japanese [42] and two Italian cohorts [43,44] showed BAR´ survival rates at 2 years higher than 70%. Beyond this time point, available RWD are limited [26,43,44]. In our study, about 40% of the refractory patients who completed the 36- or 48-month follow-up were still on treatment. In improving these results, a recent retrospective multicenter Italian study with 478 patients observed a persistence rate of 53.4% at 48 months [44]. However, compared to our population, this cohort had a lower disease duration (78 months (32–163)), lower seropositivity for RF and ACPA (60.1% and 55.2%, respectively), and fewer patients were exposed to TNFi (34%) or biologics with other mechanisms of action (1.7–17.6% for different drugs) [44]. All this data pointed to a more severe or multidrug-resistant population in our study. In this regard, a long-term extension study from Smolen et al. [26]

described a lower discontinuation rate of BAR at 36 months, although in this study the patients were recruited in RCTs and were naïve to ts/b or even csDMARDs, reflecting a selected population far from the context of RWD studies.

The Kaplan–Meier curve of persistence in patients who discontinued BAR treatment due to a lack of effectiveness showed a rapid initial decrease followed by a stabilization in the following months. This pattern indicates that most discontinuations due to lack of effectiveness were due to primary failure, as they occurred in the first months of treatment, in accordance with results of other studies [27,30,40]. Treatment discontinuations due to toxicity were more gradual over time. Our discontinuation rates related with a lack of effectiveness or adverse events match those in other studies [36,42–44] and are also consistent with descriptions across different JAKi [29,42,45].

The median persistence was much bigger in bDMARD- or JAKi-naïve patients than in those with prior exposure to bDMARDs or JAKi, in accordance with previous data reported in larger Spanish [31] and Italian cohorts [44] and with the conclusions of an exhaustive review of real-world studies [4]. In contrast, in the retrospective Japanese ANSWER cohort [42], the number of prior bDMARDs or JAKi did not affect JAKi (BAR and tofacitinib) retention, in accordance with other studies analyzing overall persistence of several JAKi [42,45]. However, concerning the type of prior biologic therapy, the use of IL-6Ri has been postulated as a potential risk factor for the early discontinuation of JAKi due to inefficacy [42,45].

In our study, statistical significance was not reached in the stratified analysis according to presence/absence of RF/ACPA, and we cannot rule out that the population size was behind these results. Indeed, the median persistence was much bigger in patients with seropositive status than in those with seronegative status (44.0 vs. 9.7 months). Interestingly, a similar trend in persistence associated with seropositive status was also described in a Spanish multicenter cohort [31], which reached statistical significance in a multicenter Italian study [37]. However, this finding was not corroborated in a recent single-center study [43] and, therefore, further research is warranted to clarify this discrepancy. Finally, no difference in persistence was found in the stratified analysis in patients with BAR monotherapy or combination treatment with csDMARDs, also in accordance with previous reports [28,31,42].

The adherence to treatment, assessed by RMP and CQR5, was high, close to 100%. These results are in contrast with a recent US experience [46] reporting only 31.8% of patients with good adherence to BAR (defined as proportion of days covered [PDC] $\geq$ 80%) and the poor adherence to oral RA treatment determined in a study conducted in Spain with csDMARDs [47]. In accordance with our findings, a high adherence to both JAKi (BAR and tofacitinib) was demonstrated in the study of Codes-Mendez et al. [48], suggesting that a good tolerance and rapid abrogation of symptoms can improve patient compliance with treatment. Nonetheless, due to the high adherence rates, no comparison between effectiveness and adherence was performed in our population.

Concerning safety, more than half of our patients reported AEs. However, most of them were moderate, leading to BAR discontinuation in thirteen patients and SAE occurrence in nine patients. To adjust for population size and exposure time, our safety data are shown as incidence rate per 100 PY. Comparison with similar published real-world studies is challenging as they are cohorts with limited sample sizes or shorter follow-up periods than ours and do not estimate incidence rates per PY [25]. Therefore, for SAEs we must use publications of national databases or registries, bearing in mind that our values reflect crude and not standardized IRs. In our study, the AE with the highest IR per 100 PY was anemia. In contrast to findings by Takahashi et al. [27], and Deprez et al. [38], which reported the normalization of hemoglobin values after a decrease in the first months of treatment, we observed a significant decrease in hemoglobin values along the follow-up that never led to BAR discontinuation. Regarding infections, HZ was the most common reported infection and one of the main causes of BAR discontinuation, similarly to other publications [8,27,28,49–52], although none of these infections were considered SAE. It should be noted that all but one patient with HZ were under glucocorticoid treatment at the time of infection. Indeed, glucocorticoid treatment and older age have been described as risk factors for HZ and other infections [53]. Vaccination against HZ is currently recommended for all patients prior to the initiation of JAKi treatment and could be considered for those already on treatment [54]. Only bacterial pneumonia was considered a serious infection with an IR per 100 PY of 1.1 (0.8–1.4), which ranges within the lowest SAE rates for BAR reported by Salinas et.al in a meta-analysis of multi-databases using disease registries and claims [55], although we used crude and not standardized adjusted IRs.

Regarding cardiovascular SAEs, in addition to findings with tofacitinib in the oral surveillance trial for RA [9], several RWD studies with JAKi have observed an increased risk of major adverse cardiovascular events (MACE) or thromboembolism in elderly patients with certain cardiovascular risk factors [55–57]. No MACE was recorded in our cohort and only one venous thrombotic event was observed in line with standardized incidence rates described by Uchida et al. [53] or in the meta-analysis published by Salinas et al. [55].

Three patients discontinued BAR due to a new diagnosis of cancer, with a crude IR per 100 PY of 1.1 (0.8–1.4), consistent with known data from RWD studies [35,50,52,53,55,58]. The two patients with lung carcinoma were ≥65 years old and smokers, two conditions in which treatment with BAR would not have been initiated following current recommendations.

To conclude, despite the severity of RA in our population, we have not found any increase in SAEs compared to the safety profile reported in RWD studies. However, given recent recommendations, it is necessary to assess inter-individual risk/benefit ratio at the initiation of BAR treatment.

This study has some limitations. First, those related to the non-interventional, ambispective design. Second, the limited sample size; we cannot rule out that a larger population could have provided significant differences in some outcomes of the stratified group analysis. Third, the single center population can limit the generalization of the results, although our findings are consistent with those reported in multicenter experiences in our country [31]. Finally, we did not collect information on the smoking status, body mass index, or other confounding variables that could interfere with the therapeutic response [59] or interpretation of safety data.

5. Conclusions

In this real-world study, BAR was mainly used in patients with moderate, erosive, seropositive, long-standing RA, previously exposed to more than one b/tsDMARDs. These characteristics have been associated with more severe disease and a greater difficulty in reaching the therapeutic target. Despite this, BAR can provide significant benefits in several outcomes in RA patients, even in those with long-standing, severe, and refractory disease. However, patients without previous exposure to biologics appear to benefit more from the drug. A good adherence and the acceptable safety profile of BAR contribute to a high persistence. Together with considering safety concerns, which are mandatory in the selection of treatment candidates, all previous data support a good risk/benefit ratio of BAR in daily clinical practice. Additional prospective studies with a greater sample size are needed to confirm these findings.

Author Contributions: Conceptualization, E.R.H., A.M.B. and R.G.-V.; Data curation, A.C.-G. and E.R.H.; Formal analysis, A.C.-G and E.R.H.; Funding acquisition, A.M.B.; Investigation, A.C.-G., E.R.H., I.M.L.C., B.V.D.D. and R.G.-V.; Methodology, E.R.H. and R.G.-V.; Project administration, E.R.H.; Resources, E.R.H., I.M.L.C., B.V.D.D., A.M.B. and R.G.-V.; Supervision, E.R.H., J.B.G. and R.G.-V.; Validation, E.R.H. and R.G.-V.; Writing—original draft, A.C.-G.; Writing—review and editing, E.R.H. and R.G.-V. All authors have read and agreed to the published version of the manuscript.

Funding: This research received no external funding. The APC was funded by a grant to A.M.B. through the Biomedical Research Foundation (FIB) of the Hospital Universitario la Princesa.

Institutional Review Board Statement: This study was conducted according to the guidelines of the Declaration of Helsinki and approved by the Institutional Review Board of Hospital Universitario de La Princesa (IRB 25 April 2019, approval number 3742).

Informed Consent Statement: Informed consent was obtained from all subjects involved in the study.

Data Availability Statement: The datasets generated during and/or analyzed during the current study are available from the corresponding author on reasonable request.

Acknowledgments: The authors send their thanks to Manuel Gómez-Gutierrez, from the Methodology Unit, Hospital Universitario la Princesa, for his help in translation and editing.

Conflicts of Interest: A.C.-G. and I.M.L.C. declare personal fees for participating in research from Lilly, outside of the submitted work. R.G.-V. reports research or educational support to her institution from Abbvie, BMS, MSD, Janssen, Lilly, Novartis, and Sanofi; have received personal fees for participating on advisory boards or delivering presentations sponsored by Abbvie, Biogen, BMS, Lilly, Pfizer, Sandoz and Sanofi; all outside of the submitted work. E.R.H., B.V.D.D., J.B.G. and A.M.B. declare that they have no conflicts of interest.

References

1. Aletaha, D.; Smolen, J. Diagnosis and Management of Rheumatoid Arthritis: A Review. *JAMA* **2018**, *320*, 1360–1372. [CrossRef]
2. Firestein, G.; McInnes, I.B. Immunopathogenesis of rheumatoid arthritis. *Immunity* **2017**, *46*, 183–196. [CrossRef] [PubMed]
3. Smolen, J.S.; Landewé, R.B.M.; Bergstra, S.A.; Kerschbaumer, A.; Sepriano, A.; Aletaha, D.; Caporali, R.; Edwards, C.J.; Hyrich, K.L.; Pope, J.E.; et al. EULAR recommendations for the management of rheumatoid arthritis with synthetic and biological disease-modifying antirheumatic drugs: 2022 update. *Ann. Rheum. Dis.* **2023**, *82*, 3–18. [CrossRef]
4. Taylor, P.C.; Laedermann, C.; Alten, R.; Feist, E.; Choy, E.; Haladyj, E.; De La Torre, I.; Richette, P.; Finckh, A.; Tanaka, Y. A JAK Inhibitor for Treatment of Rheumatoid Arthritis: The Baricitinib Experience. *J. Clin. Med.* **2023**, *12*, 4527. [CrossRef]
5. Fleischmann, R.; Schiff, M.; van der Heijde, D.; Ramos-Remus, C.; Spindler, A.; Stanislav, M.; Zerbini, C.A.; Gurbuz, S.; Dickson, C.; de Bono, S.; et al. Baricitinib, Methotrexate, or Combination in Patients with RA and No or Limited Prior DMARDs Treatment. *Arthritis Rheumatol.* **2017**, *69*, 506–517. [CrossRef]
6. Dougados, M.; van der Heijde, D.; Chen, Y.C.; Greenwald, M.; Drescher, E.; Liu, J.; Beattie, S.; Witt, S.; de la Torre, I.; Gaich, C.; et al. Baricitinib in patients with inadequate response or intolerance to conventional synthetic DMARDs: Results from the RA-BUILD study. *Ann. Rheum. Dis.* **2017**, *76*, 88–95. [CrossRef]
7. Genovese, M.C.; Kremer, J.; Zamani, O.; Ludivico, C.; Krogulec, M.; Xie, L.; Beattie, S.D.; Koch, A.E.; Cardillo, T.E.; Rooney, T.P.; et al. Baricitinib in Patients with Refractory Rheumatoid Arthritis. *N. Engl. J. Med.* **2016**, *374*, 1243–1252. [CrossRef] [PubMed]
8. Taylor, P.C.; Keystone, E.C.; van der Heijde, D.; Weinblatt, M.E.; Del Carmen Morales, L.; Reyes Gonzaga, J.; Yakushin, S.; Ishii, T.; Emoto, K.; Beattie, S.; et al. Baricitinib versus Placebo or Adalimumab in Rheumatoid Arthritis. *N. Engl. J. Med.* **2017**, *376*, 652–662. [CrossRef]
9. Ytterberg, S.R.; Bhatt, D.L.; Mikuls, T.R.; Koch, G.G.; Fleischmann, R.; Rivas, J.L.; Germino, R.; Menon, S.; Sun, Y.; Wang, C.; et al. Cardiovascular and Cancer Risk with Tofacitinib in Rheumatoid Arthritis. *N. Engl. J. Med.* **2022**, *386*, 316–326. [CrossRef]
10. Taylor, P.C.; Bieber, T.; Alten, R.; Witte, T.; Galloway, J.; Deberdt, W.; Issa, M.; Haladyj, E.; De La Torre, I.; Grond, S.; et al. Baricitinib Safety for Events of Special Interest in Populations at Risk: Analysis from Randomised Trial Data Across Rheumatologic and Dermatologic Indications. *Adv. Ther.* **2023**, *40*, 1867–1883. [CrossRef]
11. Sabaté, E. Adherence to Long-Term Therapies: Evidence for Action. 2003. Available online: http://www.who.int/chronic_conditions/adherencereport/en/ (accessed on 15 July 2023).
12. Aletaha, D.; Neogi, T.; Silman, A.J.; Funovits, J.; Felson, D.T.; Bingham, C.O., 3rd; Birnbaum, N.S.; Burmester, G.R.; Bykerk, V.P.; Cohen, M.D.; et al. American College of Rheumatology/European League Against Rheumatism collaborative initiative. *Arthritis Rheum.* **2010**, *62*, 2569–2581. [CrossRef]
13. Europen Medicine Agency. EMA Confirms Measures to Minimise Risk of Serious Side Effects with Janus Kinase Inhibitors for Chronic Inflammatory Disorders. Available online: https://www.ema.europa.eu/en/medicines/human/referrals/janus-kinase-inhibitors-jaki (accessed on 6 March 2023).
14. Fransen, J.; van Riel, P.L. The Disease Activity Score and the EULAR response criteria. *Rheum. Dis. Clin. N. Am.* **2009**, *35*, 745–757. [CrossRef]
15. Aletaha, D.; Landewe, R.; Karonitsch, T.; Bathon, J.; Boers, M.; Bombardier, C.; Bombardieri, S.; Choi, H.; Combe, B.; Dougados, M.; et al. Reporting disease activity in clinical trials of patients with rheumatoid arthritis: EULAR/ACR collaborative recommendations. *Ann. Rheum. Dis.* **2008**, *67*, 1360–1364. [CrossRef]
16. Raebel, M.A.; Schmittdiel, J.; Karter, A.J.; Konieczny, J.L.; Steiner, J.F. Standardizing terminology and definitions of medication adherence and persistence in research employing electronic databases. *Med. Care* **2013**, *51*, S11–S21. [CrossRef]
17. Martínez-López de Castro, N.; Álvarez-Payero, M.; Samartín-Ucha, M.; Martín-Vila, A.; Piñeiro-Corrales, G.; Pego Reigosa, J.M.; Rodríguez-Rodríguez, M.; Melero-González, R.B.; Maceiras-Pan, F.J. Adherence to biological therapies in patients with chronic inflammatory arthropathies. *Farm. Hosp.* **2019**, *43*, 134–139. [CrossRef]

18. de Klerk, E.; van der Heijde, D.; Landewé, R.; van der Tempel, H.; van der Linden, S. The compliance-questionnaire-rheumatology compared with electronic medication event monitoring: A validation study. *J. Rheumatol.* **2003**, *30*, 2469–2475.
19. Hughes, L.D.; Done, J.; Young, A. A 5 item version of the Compliance Questionnaire for Rheumatology (CQR5) successfully identifies low adherence to DMARDs. *BMC Musculoskelet Disord.* **2013**, *14*, 286. [CrossRef]
20. Fernández-Avila, D.G.; Accini, M.; Tobón, M.; Moreno, S.; Rodriguez, V.; Matín Gutierrez, J. Validación y calibración al español del cuestionario CQR para la medición de adherencia a la terapia antirreumática en un grupo de pacientes colombianos con artritis reumatoide. *Clin. Exp. Rheumatol.* **2019**, *26*, 105–110. [CrossRef]
21. Agencia Española de Medicamentos y Productos Sanitarios. Ficha Técnica Olumiant (Baricitinib). Available online: https://cima.aemps.es/cima/pdfs/ft/1161170010/FT_1161170010.pdf (accessed on 15 July 2022).
22. United Stated Deparment of Health and Human Service. Common Terminology Criteria for Adverse Events (CTCAE). Available online: https://ctep.cancer.gov/protocoldevelopment/electronic_applications/docs/ctcae_v5_quick_reference_5x7.pdf (accessed on 15 July 2022).
23. US Food and Drug Administration. FDA Requires Warnings about Increased Risk of Serious Heart-Related Events, Cancer, Blood Clots, and Death for JAK Inhibitors That Treat Certain Chronic Inflammatory Conditions. Available online: https://www.fda.gov/drugs/drug-safety-and-availability/fda-requires-warnings-about-increased-risk-serious-heart-related-events-cancer-blood-clots-and-death (accessed on 6 March 2023).
24. Kearsley-Fleet, L.; Davies, R.; De Cock, D.; Watson, K.D.; Lunt, M.; Buch, M.H.; Isaacs, J.D.; Hyrich, K.L. Biologic refractory disease in rheumatoid arthritis: Results from the British Society for Rheumatology Biologics Register for Rheumatoid Arthritis. *Ann. Rheum. Dis.* **2018**, *77*, 1405–1412. [CrossRef]
25. Hernández-Cruz, B.; Kiltz, U.; Avouac, J.; Treuer, T.; Haladyj, E.; Gerwien, J.; Gupta, C.D.; Conti, F. Evidence on Baricitinib for the Treatment of Rheumatoid Arthritis. *Rheumatol. Ther.* **2023**, *10*, 1417–1457. [CrossRef]
26. Smolen, J.S.; Xie, L.; Jia, B.; Taylor, P.C.; Burmester, G.; Tanaka, Y.; Elias, A.; Cardoso, A.; Ortmann, R.; Walls, C.; et al. Efficacy of baricitinib in patients with moderate-to-severe rheumatoid arthritis with 3 years of treatment: Results from a long-term study. *Rheumatology* **2021**, *60*, 2256–2266. [CrossRef] [PubMed]
27. Takahashi, N.; Asai, S.; Kobayakawa, T.; Kaneko, A.; Watanabe, T.; Kato, T.; Nishiume, T.; Ishikawa, H.; Yoshioka, Y.; Kanayama, Y.; et al. Predictors for clinical effectiveness of baricitinib in rheumatoid arthritis patients in routine clinical practice: Data from a Japanese multicenter registry. *Sci. Rep.* **2020**, *10*, 21907. [CrossRef] [PubMed]
28. Iwamoto, N.; Sato, S.; Kurushima, S.; Michitsuji, T.; Nishihata, S.; Okamoto, M.; Tsuji, Y.; Endo, Y.; Shimizu, T.; Sumiyoshi, R.; et al. Real-world comparative effectiveness and safety of tofacitinib and baricitinib in patients with rheumatoid arthritis. *Arthritis Res. Ther.* **2021**, *23*, 197. [CrossRef] [PubMed]
29. Fitton, J.; Melville, A.R.; Emery, P.; Nam, J.L.; Buch, M.H. Real-world single centre use of JAK inhibitors across the rheumatoid arthritis pathway. *Rheumatology* **2021**, *60*, 4048–4054. [CrossRef] [PubMed]
30. Barbulescu, A.; Askling, J.; Chatzidionysiou, K.; Forsblad-d'Elia, H.; Kastbom, A.; Lindström, U.; Turesson, C.; Frisell, T. Effectiveness of baricitinib and tofacitinib compared with bDMARDs in RA: Results from a cohort study using nationwide Swedish register data. *Rheumatology* **2022**, *61*, 3952–3962. [CrossRef]
31. Hernández-Cruz, B.; Rosas, J.; Díaz-Torné, C.; Belzunegui, J.; García-Vicuña, R.; Inciarte-Mundo, J.; Pons, A.; Millán, A.M.; Jeria-Navarro, S.; Valero, J.A.; et al. Real-World Treatment Patterns and Clinical Outcomes of Baricitinib in Rheumatoid Arthritis Patients in Spain: Results of a Multicenter, Observational Study iRoutine Clinical Practice (The ORBIT-RA Study). *Rheumatol. Ther.* **2022**, *9*, 589–608. [CrossRef] [PubMed]
32. Spinelli, F.R.; Ceccarelli, F.; Garufi, C.; Duca, L.; Mancuso, S.; Cipriano, E.; Dell'Unto, E.; Alessandri, C.; Di Franco, M.; Perricone, C.; et al. Effectiveness and safety of baricitinib in rheumatoid arthritis: A monocentric, longitudinal, real-life experience. *Clin. Exp. Rheumatol.* **2021**, *39*, 525–531. [CrossRef]
33. González-Freire, L.; Giménez-Candela, R.M.; Castro-Luaces, S.; Veiga-Villaverde, A.B.; Crespo-Diz, C. Baricitinib and tofacitinib in patients with rheumatoid arthritis: Results of regular clinical practice. *Farm. Hosp.* **2021**, *45*, 165–169.
34. González Mazarío, R.; Fragío Gil, J.J.; Ivorra Cortés, J.; Grau García, E.; Cañada Martínez, A.J.; González Puig, L.; Negueroles Albuixech, R.M.; Román Ivorra, J.A. Efectividad y seguridad en el mundo real de los inhibidores de JAK en la artritis reumatoide: Estudio unicéntrico. *Reumatol. Clin.* **2022**, *18*, 523–530. [CrossRef]
35. Takagi, M.; Atsumi, T.; Matsuno, H.; Tamura, N.; Fujii, T.; Okamoto, N.; Takahashi, N.; Nakajima, A.; Nakajima, A.; Tsujimoto, N.; et al. Safety and Effectiveness of Baricitinib for Rheumatoid Arthritis in Japanese Clinical Practice: 24-Week Results of All-Case Post-Marketing Surveillance. *Mod. Rheumatol.* **2023**, *4*, 647–656. [CrossRef]
36. Alten, R.; Burmester, G.R.; Matucci-Cerinic, M.; Salmon, J.H.; Lopez-Romero, P.; Fakhouri, W.; de la Torre, I.; Zaremba-Pechmann, L.; Holzkämper, T.; Fautrel, B. The RA-BE-REAL Multinational, Prospective, Observational Study in Patients with Rheumatoid Arthritis Receiving Baricitinib, Targeted Synthetic, or Biologic Disease-Modifying Therapies: A 6-Month Interim Analysis. *Rheumatol. Ther.* **2023**, *10*, 73–93. [CrossRef]
37. Guidelli, G.M.; Viapiana, O.; Luciano, N.; De Santis, M.; Boffini, N.; Quartuccio, L.; Birra, D.; Conticini, E.; Chimenti, M.S.; Bazzani, C.; et al. Efficacy and safety of baricitinib in 446 patients with rheumatoid arthritis: A real-life multicentre study. *Clin. Exp. Rheumatol.* **2021**, *39*, 868–873. [CrossRef]
38. Deprez, V.; Le Monnier, L.; Sobhy-Danial, J.M.; Grados, F.; Henry-Desailly, I.; Salomon-Goëb, S.; Rabin, T.; Ristic, S.; Fumery, M.; Fardellone, P.; et al. Therapeutic Maintenance of Baricitinib and Tofacitinib in Real Life. *J. Clin. Med.* **2020**, *9*, 3319. [CrossRef]

39. Scheepers, L.; Yang, Y.; Chen, Y.L.; Jones, G. Persistence of Janus-kinase (JAK) inhibitors in rheumatoid arthritis: Australia wide study. *Semin. Arthritis Rheum.* **2024**, *64*, 152314. [CrossRef]
40. Rosas, J.; Senabre-Gallego, J.M.; Santos-Soler, G.; Antonio Bernal, J.; Pons Bas, A. Efficacy and Safety of Baricitinib in Patients with Rheumatoid Arthritis and Inadequate Response to Conventional Synthetic DMARDs and/or Biological DMARDs: Data from a Local Registry. *Reumatol. Clin.* **2022**, *18*, 188–189. [CrossRef]
41. Retuerto, M.; Trujillo, E.; Valero, C.; Fernandez-Espartero, C.; Soleto, C.Y.; Garcia-Valle, A.; Aurrecoechea, E.; Garijo, M.; Lopez, A.; Loricera, J.; et al. Efficacy and safety of switching Jak inhibitors in rheumatoid arthritis: An observational study. *Clin. Exp. Rheumatol.* **2021**, *39*, 453–455. [CrossRef]
42. Ebina, K.; Hirano, T.; Maeda, Y.; Yamamoto, W.; Hashimoto, M.; Murata, K.; Onishi, A.; Jinno, S.; Hara, R.; Son, Y.; et al. Drug retention of sarilumab, baricitinib, and tofacitinib in patients with rheumatoid arthritis: The ANSWER cohort study. *Clin. Rheumatol.* **2021**, *40*, 2673–2680. [CrossRef]
43. Baldi, C.; Berlengiero, V.; Falsetti, P.; Cartocci, A.; Conticini, E.; D'Alessandro, R.; D'Ignazio, E.; Bardelli, M.; Fabbroni, M.; Cantarini, L.; et al. Baricitinib retention rate: 'real-life' data from a mono-centric cohort of patients affected by rheumatoid arthritis. *Front. Med.* **2023**, *10*, 1176613. [CrossRef]
44. Parisi, S.; Andrea, B.; Chiara, D.M.; Alberto, L.G.; Maddalena, L.; Palma, S.; Olga, A.; Massimo, R.; Marino, P.; Rosalba, C.; et al. Analysis of survival rate and persistence predictors of baricitinib in real-world data from a large cohort of rheumatoid arthritis patients. *Curr. Res. Pharmacol. Drug Discov.* **2024**, *6*, 100178. [CrossRef]
45. Martinez-Molina, C.; Gich, I.; Diaz-Torné, C.; Park, H.S.; Feliu, A.; Vidal, S.; Corominas, H. Patient-related factors influencing the effectiveness and safety of Janus Kinase inhibitors in rheumatoid arthritis: A real-world study. *Sci. Rep.* **2024**, *14*, 172. [CrossRef]
46. Bergman, M.; Chen, N.; Thielen, R.; Zueger, P. One-Year Medication Adherence and Persistence in Rheumatoid Arthritis in Clinical Practice: A Retrospective Analysis of Upadacitinib, Adalimumab, Baricitinib, and Tofacitinib. *Adv. Ther.* **2023**, *40*, 4493–4503. [CrossRef] [PubMed]
47. Marras, C.; Monteagudo, I.; Salvador, G.; de Toro, F.J.; Escudero, A.; Alegre-Sancho, J.J.; Raya, E.; Ortiz, A.; Carmona, L.; Mestre, Y.; et al. Identification of patients at risk of non-adherence to oral antirheumatic drugs in rheumatoid arthritis using the Compliance Questionnaire in Rheumatology: An ARCO sub-study. *Rheumatol. Int.* **2017**, *37*, 1195–1202. [CrossRef] [PubMed]
48. Codes-Mendez, H.; Martinez-Molina, C.; Masip, M.; Riera, P.; Pagès Puigdemont, N.; Riera Magallón, A.; Lobo Prat, D.; Sainz Comas, L.; Corominas, H.; Díaz-Torné, C. Therapeutic adherence and persistence of tofacitinib and baricitinib in rheumatoid arthritis patients in daily clinical practice. *Ann. Rheum. Dis.* **2022**, *81*, 1330. [CrossRef]
49. Peng, L.; Xiao, K.; Ottaviani, S.; Stebbing, J.; Wang, Y.J. A real-world disproportionality analysis of FDA Adverse Event Reporting System (FAERS) events for baricitinib. *Expert. Opin. Drug Saf.* **2020**, *19*, 1505–1511. [CrossRef] [PubMed]
50. Taylor, P.C.; Takeuchi, T.; Burmester, G.R.; Durez, P.; Smolen, J.S.; Deberdt, W.; Issa, M.; Terres, J.R.; Bello, N.; Winthrop, K.L. Safety of baricitinib for the treatment of rheumatoid arthritis over a median of 4.6 and up to 9.3 years of treatment: Final results from long-term extension study and integrated database. *Ann. Rheum. Dis.* **2022**, *81*, 335–343. [CrossRef] [PubMed]
51. Choi, W.; Ahn, S.M.; Kim, Y.G.; Lee, C.K.; Yoo, B.; Hong, S. Safety of JAK inhibitor use in patients with rheumatoid arthritis who developed herpes zoster after receiving JAK inhibitors. *Clin. Rheumatol.* **2022**, *41*, 1659–1663. [CrossRef] [PubMed]
52. Frisell, T.; Bower, H.; Morin, M.; Baecklund, E.; Di Giuseppe, D.; Delcoigne, B.; Feltelius, N.; Forsblad-d'Elia, H.; Lindqvist, E.; Lindström, U.; et al. Safety of biological and targeted synthetic disease-modifying antirheumatic drugs for rheumatoid arthritis as used in clinical practice: Results from the ARTIS programme. *Ann. Rheum. Dis.* **2023**, *82*, 601–610. [CrossRef] [PubMed]
53. Uchida, T.; Iwamoto, N.; Fukui, S.; Morimoto, S.; Aramaki, T.; Shomura, F.; Aratake, K.; Eguchi, K.; Ueki, Y.; Kawakami, A. Comparison of risks of cancer, infection, and MACEs associated with JAK inhibitor and TNF inhibitor treatment: A multicenter cohort study. *Rheumatology* **2023**, *62*, 3358–3365. [CrossRef] [PubMed]
54. Waldman, R.A.; Sharp, K.L.; Adalsteinsson, J.A.; Grant-Kels, J.M. Herpes zoster subunit vaccine for patients initiating a Janus kinase inhibitor. *J. Am. Acad. Dermatol.* **2022**, *88*, 697–698. [CrossRef]
55. Salinas, C.A.; Louder, A.; Polinski, J.; Zhang, T.C.; Bower, H.; Phillips, S.; Song, Y.; Rashidi, E.; Bosan, R.; Chang, H.C.; et al. Evaluation of VTE, MACE, and Serious Infections among Patients with RA Treated with Baricitinib Compared to TNFi: A Multi-Database Study of Patients in Routine Care Using Disease Registries and Claims Databases. *Rheumatol. Ther.* **2023**, *10*, 201–223. [CrossRef]
56. Gouverneur, A.; Avouac, J.; Prati, C.; Cracowski, J.L.; Schaeverbeke, T.; Pariente, A.; Truchetet, M.E. JAK inhibitors and risk of major cardiovascular events or venous thromboembolism: A self-controlled case series study. *Eur. J. Clin. Pharmacol.* **2022**, *78*, 1981–1990. [CrossRef] [PubMed]
57. Hoisnard, L.; Pina Vegas, L.; Dray-Spira, R.; Weill, A.; Zureik, M.; Sbidian, E. Risk of major adverse cardiovascular and venous thromboembolism events in patients with rheumatoid arthritis exposed to JAK inhibitors versus adalimumab: A nationwide cohort study. *Ann. Rheum. Dis.* **2023**, *82*, 182–188. [CrossRef] [PubMed]
58. Qian, J.; Xue, X.; Shannon, J. Characteristics of adverse event reporting of Xeljanz/Xeljanz XR, Olumiant, and Rinvoq to the US Food and Drug Administration. *J. Manag. Care Spec. Pharm.* **2022**, *28*, 1046–1052. [CrossRef] [PubMed]
59. Kiely, P.D. Biologic efficacy optimization—A step towards personalized medicine. *Rheumatology* **2016**, *55*, 780–788. [CrossRef]

Disclaimer/Publisher's Note: The statements, opinions and data contained in all publications are solely those of the individual author(s) and contributor(s) and not of MDPI and/or the editor(s). MDPI and/or the editor(s) disclaim responsibility for any injury to people or property resulting from any ideas, methods, instructions or products referred to in the content.

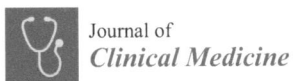

Article

Are There Sex-Related Differences in the Effectiveness of Janus Kinase Inhibitors in Rheumatoid Arthritis Patients?

Cristina Martinez-Molina [1,2,*], Anna Feliu [1], Hye S. Park [2,3], Ana Juanes [1], Cesar Diaz-Torne [2,3], Silvia Vidal [2,4,†] and Hèctor Corominas [2,3,*,†]

1. Department of Pharmacy, Hospital de la Santa Creu i Sant Pau, Sant Antoni Maria Claret 167, 08025 Barcelona, Spain
2. Department of Medicine, Universitat Autònoma de Barcelona (UAB), Av. Can Domènech 737, 08193 Bellaterra, Spain
3. Department of Rheumatology and Systemic Autoimmune Diseases, Hospital de la Santa Creu i Sant Pau, Sant Antoni Maria Claret 167, 08025 Barcelona, Spain
4. Group of Immunology-Inflammatory Diseases, Institut de Recerca Sant Pau (IR SANT PAU), Sant Quintí 77-79, 08041 Barcelona, Spain
* Correspondence: cmartinezmo@santpau.cat (C.M.-M.); hcorominas@santpau.cat (H.C.)
† These authors contributed equally to this work.

Citation: Martinez-Molina, C.; Feliu, A.; Park, H.S.; Juanes, A.; Diaz-Torne, C.; Vidal, S.; Corominas, H. Are There Sex-Related Differences in the Effectiveness of Janus Kinase Inhibitors in Rheumatoid Arthritis Patients? *J. Clin. Med.* **2024**, *13*, 2355. https://doi.org/10.3390/jcm13082355

Academic Editors: Eugen Feist and Jürgen Rech

Received: 17 March 2024
Revised: 8 April 2024
Accepted: 16 April 2024
Published: 18 April 2024

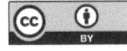

Copyright: © 2024 by the authors. Licensee MDPI, Basel, Switzerland. This article is an open access article distributed under the terms and conditions of the Creative Commons Attribution (CC BY) license (https://creativecommons.org/licenses/by/4.0/).

Abstract: Background: There is evidence suggesting the existence of sex differences in the effectiveness of specific drug classes for rheumatoid arthritis (RA). Our study stands as the first to elucidate sex-related differences in the effectiveness of Janus kinase (JAK) inhibitors. **Methods**: The study involved 150 RA patients treated with tofacitinib, baricitinib, upadacitinib, or filgotinib between September 2017 and October 2023. Sex differences in achieving remission and low disease activity (LDA) were identified through logistic regression analyses. Sex disparities in treatment effectiveness survival were evaluated through the Kaplan–Meier estimate, employing the log-rank test for comparison. The Cox model was applied to analyze the variable sex as a potential factor that could influence the maintenance of the JAK inhibitor treatment effectiveness. **Results**: Concerning the achievement of remission and LDA, no differences were observed between sexes in terms of the 28-joint Disease Activity Score (DAS28) C-reactive protein (CRP), the Clinical Disease Activity Index (CDAI), and the Simplified Disease Activity Index (SDAI). With respect to the DAS28-erythrocyte sedimentation rate (ESR), female patients, compared to males, possessed 70% lower odds of achieving remission ($p = 0.018$) and 66% lower odds of achieving LDA ($p = 0.023$). No differences were observed in treatment effectiveness survival between sexes ($p = 0.703$). Sex was not found to influence the survival of JAK inhibitor treatment effectiveness ($p = 0.704$). **Conclusions**: Being a female or male patient does not entail differences in the effectiveness of the JAK inhibitor treatment. Our findings encourage the consideration of a global pool of composite indices (DAS28-ESR/CRP, CDAI, SDAI) to measure RA disease activity, thus individualizing the target value as advocated by the treat-to-target strategy.

Keywords: rheumatoid arthritis; Janus kinase inhibitor; tofacitinib; baricitinib; upadacitinib; filgotinib; treat-to-target; treatment effectiveness; sex-related differences

1. Introduction

Rheumatoid arthritis is a chronic inflammatory autoimmune disease that predominantly affects female more than male patients, typically represented in a 3:1 sex ratio [1]. Although the reason for this sexual disparity is not fully understood, multiple elements could potentially play a pathogenic role in rheumatoid arthritis.

According to the treat-to-target (T2T) strategy, the assessment of disease activity is required in routine clinical practice to guide treatment decisions [2,3]. To date, four validated composite measures are all applicable for this purpose. In 1995, the 28-joint Disease

Activity Score (DAS28) was validated as a composite measure, using the erythrocyte sedimentation rate (ESR) as an inflammatory marker [4]. In 2004, the C-reactive protein (CRP) was included in the DAS28-CRP [5]. Finally, the Clinical Disease Activity Index (CDAI) and the Simplified Disease Activity Index (SDAI) emerged as the two other simplified validated measures, widely accepted in clinical practice [6]. Achieving clinical remission, or at least low disease activity, constitutes the primary target for rheumatoid arthritis treatment, as defined by the T2T recommendations [2,3] and advocated by several rheumatoid arthritis guidelines [7–9].

In light of these shared treatment targets between sexes, it has been suggested that female patients with rheumatoid arthritis tend to exhibit worse responses to biologic Disease-Modifying Antirheumatic Drugs (bDMARDs) compared to males [10–12]. Previous studies have considered being male as a predictive factor for achieving remission in the bDMARD treatment [13,14]. However, the magnitude of these sex disparities could differ depending on the specific drug class. Biological mechanisms related to sex, including immune profiles, could contribute to diverse treatment responses across the different rheumatoid arthritis drug classes.

The therapeutic arsenal for moderate to severe active rheumatoid arthritis has recently evolved to the regular use of targeted synthetic (ts) DMARDs (tsDMARDs), i.e., the Janus kinase (JAK) inhibitors, such as tofacitinib, baricitinib, upadacitinib, or filgotinib. Due to the fact that JAK inhibitors are the most recent drug class for rheumatoid arthritis treatment (Figure 1), it is notable how little published literature exists addressing sex disparities. The goal of the present study was to assess sex-related differences in the effectiveness of JAK inhibitor treatment in rheumatoid arthritis patients. The results may enhance the understanding of how sex, as a patient-related factor, might influence the JAK inhibitor treatment in rheumatoid arthritis.

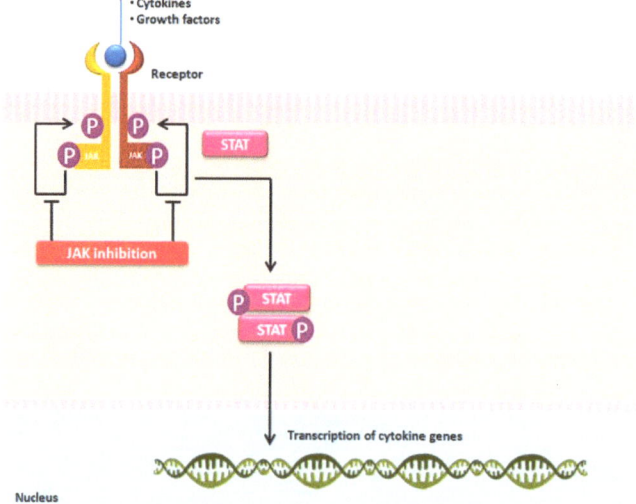

Figure 1. The mechanism of action of Janus kinase (JAK) inhibitors: tofacitinib, baricitinib, upadacitinib, and filgotinib. An extracellular recognition of cytokines and growth factors by their receptors leads to the intracellular phosphorylation of JAK enzymes. The involvement of specific JAKs (JAK1, JAK2, JAK3, and tyrosine kinase 2, TYK2) depends on their selective interactions with cytokine-receptor families. Activated JAKs phosphorylate the receptors, facilitating the recruitment and activation of signal transducer and activator of transcription (STAT) factors. Intracellular signals are transmitted through JAKs and seven STAT family members (STAT1-4, STAT5A, STAT5B, and STAT6) that promote transcription. JAK inhibitors mitigate cytokine effects by inhibiting the JAK-STAT signaling pathway.

2. Materials and Methods

2.1. Study Design and Patient Population

An observational retrospective study was conducted in a university hospital, which included real-world patients (aged ≥ 18 years) diagnosed according to the 2010 American College of Rheumatology (ACR)—European League Against Rheumatism (EULAR) classification criteria for rheumatoid arthritis [15]. All patients included were individually informed about the study protocol and were given the option to decline the extraction of data. Clinical data were collected from electronic medical records in October 2023. All patients were treated with either tofacitinib, baricitinib, upadacitinib, or filgotinib between September 2017 and October 2023.

2.2. Assessments

The exposure of interest of the study was focused on the sex of patients, categorized as female and male. The primary outcome was to assess sex differences in achieving both remission and low disease activity at the first 6 months of the JAK inhibitor treatment. This specific time frame, up to the first 6 months of treatment, was deemed appropriate for evaluating the primary outcome. According to the ACR-EULAR recommendations [7–9], if the T2T goal is not achieved within the first 6 months, a change in the treatment strategy should be considered. The secondary outcome was to determine sex disparities in the survival of the JAK inhibitor treatment effectiveness by analyzing the treatment retention. The retention of treatment was described as the time period from the treatment initiation and the definitive treatment discontinuation. With respect to disease activity, it was categorized based on the updated recommendations from the ACR [16], into remission, low disease activity, moderate disease activity, and high disease activity. Remission was determined by DAS28-ESR < 2.6, DAS28-CRP < 2.4, CDAI ≤ 2.8, and SDAI ≤ 3.3. Low disease activity was defined as DAS28-ESR < 3.2, DAS28-CRP < 2.9, and CDAI ≤ 10, SDAI ≤ 11.

2.3. Statistical Analyses

Demographic and clinical patient characteristics were separately detailed by sex. Differences between female and male patients were evaluated using the Mann–Whitney test (for ordinal or quantitative variables) and Fisher's exact test (for categorical variables). Ordinal and quantitative variables are presented using the median and the interquartile range (IQR). Categorical variables are described as absolute number (n) and percentage (%).

The percentages of female and male patients achieving remission and low disease activity were determined at the first 6 months of the JAK inhibitor treatment. In order to evaluate the probability of attaining the study outcomes in female patients compared to males (control group), logistic regression analyses were conducted. Both crude and adjusted analyses for JAK inhibitor type, concomitant GC use, and concomitant csDMARD use were performed. All covariates that were statistically significant ($p < 0.05$) or exhibited borderline significance ($p < 0.1$ and >0.05) in the crude analyses were included in the adjusted analyses.

The JAK inhibitor retention due to the lack of treatment effectiveness was examined through the Kaplan–Meier estimate and the Cox proportional hazard regression model. The Kaplan–Meier estimate, for the discontinuation reason of lack of treatment effectiveness, was employed to evaluate the survival curves of female and male patients, with the log-rank test used for comparison. The bivariate Cox model was applied to analyze the variable sex as a potential factor that could influence that retention of the JAK inhibitor treatment.

The statistical analyses were performed utilizing STATA software version 12. A *p*-value of <0.05 was considered statistically significant.

2.4. Ethics Approval and Consent to Participate

Approval was obtained from the ethics committee of a hospital (IIBSP-JAG-2023-168). This study involving human participants was in accordance with the 1964 Helsinki declaration and its later amendments or comparable ethical standards.

3. Results

A total of 150 rheumatoid arthritis patients who received JAK inhibitor treatment were identified between September 2017 and October 2023. Their demographic and clinical characteristics are summarized in Table 1. No differences were observed in the JAK inhibitor type distribution between sexes. At JAK inhibitor treatment initiation, female and male patients presented comparable years of age, body mass index (BMI), years of disease duration, rheumatoid arthritis seropositivity considering rheumatoid factor (RF) and anti-cyclic citrullinated peptide (anti-CCP), prior conventional synthetic (cs) DMARD (csDMARD) use, and prior bDMARD use. Both sexes showed similar use of concomitant glucocorticoids (GC) and concomitant csDMARDs at the JAK inhibitor treatment initiation. In terms of disease activity, similar scores were noted between female and male patients, with the exception of the DAS28-ESR, which was higher in female patients, both at baseline ($p = 0.043$) and at the first 6 months of treatment ($p = 0.014$).

Table 1. Demographic and clinical patient characteristics.

Parameters	Female (n = 128)	Male (n = 22)	p-Value
Age (years), median [IQR]	65 [52–71]	61 [53–75]	0.855
BMI [weight(kg)/height(m^2)], median [IQR]	27.0 [24.0–30.3]	27.9 [25.4–30.7]	0.407
RA disease duration (years), median [IQR]	14.0 [5.0–24.5]	9.5 [5.0–19.0]	0.126
RA seropositivity, n (%)			
RF	77 (60.2)	15 (68.2)	0.636
Anti-CCP	96 (75.0)	17 (77.3)	1.000
Previous csDMARDs, n (%)			
Methotrexate	127 (99.2)	22 (100)	1.000
Leflunomide	62 (48.5)	8 (36.4)	0.358
Sulfasalazine	32 (25.0)	5 (22.7)	1.000
Other csDMARDs	50 (39.1)	5 (22.7)	0.159
Previous bDMARDs, n (%)			
Adalimumab	63 (49.2)	10 (45.5)	0.820
Certolizumab	41 (32.0)	7 (31.8)	1.000
Etanercept	51 (39.9)	10 (45.5)	0.645
Golimumab	27 (21.1)	4 (18.2)	1.000
Infliximab	22 (17.2)	1 (4.6)	0.200
Tocilizumab	65 (50.8)	7 (31.8)	0.112
Sarilumab	26 (20.3)	2 (9.1)	0.372
Abatacept	56 (43.8)	7 (31.8)	0.355
Rituximab	32 (25.0)	2 (9.1)	0.165
JAK inhibitor type, n (%)			0.198
Tofacitinib	40 (31.3)	11 (50.0)	
Baricitinib	69 (53.9)	7 (31.8)	
Upadacitinib	9 (7.0)	2 (9.1)	
Filgotinib	10 (7.8)	2 (9.1)	
Concomitant GC use, n (%)	79 (61.7)	14 (63.6)	1.000
PDN dose (mg/day), median [IQR]	5.0 [0.0–5.0]	5.0 [0.0–5.0]	0.671
Concomitant csDMARD use, n (%)	35 (27.3)	8 (36.4)	0.446
Methotrexate	24 (18.8)	5 (22.7)	0.770
Leflunomide	1 (0.8)	2 (9.1)	0.056
Sulfasalazine	5 (3.9)	0 (0.0)	1.000
Other csDMARD	5 (3.9)	1 (4.6)	1.000
RA disease activity at baseline, median [IQR]			
DAS28-ESR	5.4 [4.8–6.1]	5.0 [4.0–5.5]	0.043
DAS28-CRP	4.7 [4.1–5.3]	4.6 [4.1–5.1]	0.572
CDAI	25.5 [19.5–32.0]	19.0 [16.0–26.0]	0.098
SDAI	25.6 [18.0–31.5]	20.3 [16.2–26.2]	0.288

Table 1. Cont.

Parameters	Female (n = 128)	Male (n = 22)	p-Value
RA disease activity at 6 months, median [IQR]			
DAS28-ESR	3.7 [2.9–5.2]	3 [1.7–4.4]	0.014
DAS28-CRP	2.9 [1.9–4.3]	2.3 [1.6–4.2]	0.232
CDAI	10 [5.0–23.5]	6.5 [4.0–17.0]	0.093
SDAI	10.2 [5.2–23.2]	5.7 [3.1–18.6]	0.091

IQR—interquartile range [P25-P75], BMI—body mass index, RA—rheumatoid arthritis, RF—rheumatoid factor, anti-CCP—anti-cyclic citrullinated peptide, csDMARD—conventional synthetic Disease Modifying Anti-Rheumatic Drug, bDMARD—biologic Disease Modifying Anti-Rheumatic Drug, JAK—Janus kinase, GC—glucocorticoid, PDN—prednisone, DAS28-ESR—Disease Activity Score 28-joint count using Erythrocyte Sedimentation Rate, DAS28-CRP—Disease Activity Score 28-joint count using C-Reactive Protein, CDAI—Clinical Disease Activity Index, SDAI—Simplified Disease Activity Index.

The main findings from the logistic regression analyses are shown in Table 2. Compared to males, female patients were less likely to achieve the DAS28-ESR remission [unadjusted odds ratio (OR): 0.32; 95% confidence interval (CI): 0.12–0.83; p = 0.019] or the DAS28-ESR low disease activity (OR: 0.34; 95% CI: 0.13–0.85; p = 0.022), at the first 6 months of the JAK inhibitor treatment. The multivariate model showed similar results, with adjusted odds ratio (ORadj) of 0.30 (95% CI: 0.11–0.81; p = 0.018) and 0.34 (95% CI: 0.13–0.86; p = 0.023), respectively. There were no significant differences between sexes in the achievement of remission and low disease activity for the DAS28-CRP, the CDAI, and the SDAI.

Table 2. Logistic remission analyses examining the effect of sex on the study outcomes.

Outcomes at 6 Months	Female, n (%)	Male, n (%)	OR for Female [95% CI]	p-Value	ORadj for Female [95% CI]	p-Value
DAS28-ESR remission	23 (18.0)	9 (40.9)	0.32 [0.12–0.83]	0.019	0.30 [0.11–0.81]	0.018
DAS28-ESR LDA	42 (32.8)	13 (59.1)	0.34 [0.13–0.85]	0.022	0.34 [0.13–0.86]	0.023
DAS28-CRP remission	44 (34.4)	11 (50.0)	0.52 [0.21–1.30]	0.165	0.52 [0.20–1.32]	0.169
DAS28-CRP LDA	61 (47.7)	13 (59.1)	0.63 [0.25–1.58]	0.324	0.61 [0.24–1.58]	0.309
CDAI remission	9 (7.0)	3 (13.6)	0.48 [0.12–1.93]	0.301	0.47 [0.11–1.98]	0.305
CDAI LDA	67 (52.3)	14 (63.6)	0.63 [0.25–1.60]	0.329	0.58 [0.22–1.58]	0.289
SDAI remission	20 (15.6)	6 (27.3)	0.49 [0.17–1.41]	0.189	0.54 [0.18–1.62]	0.273
SDAI LDA	68 (53.1)	13 (59.1)	0.78 [0.31–1.97]	0.605	0.74 [0.28–1.95]	0.546

OR—odds ratio, CI—confidence interval, ORadj—odds ratio adjusted, DAS28-ESR—Disease Activity Score 28-joint count using Erythrocyte Sedimentation Rate, LDA—low disease activity, DAS28-CRP—Disease Activity Score 28-joint count using C-Reactive Protein, CDAI—Clinical Disease Activity Index, SDAI—Simplified Disease Activity Index.

JAK inhibitor retention, for the discontinuation reason of lack of treatment effectiveness, is depicted in Figure 2. No differences were observed in retention rates between female and male patients (p = 0.703). Sex was not found to influence the survival of the JAK inhibitor treatment effectiveness [hazard ratio (HR) for female patients: 1.16; 95% CI: 0.55–2.45; p = 0.704].

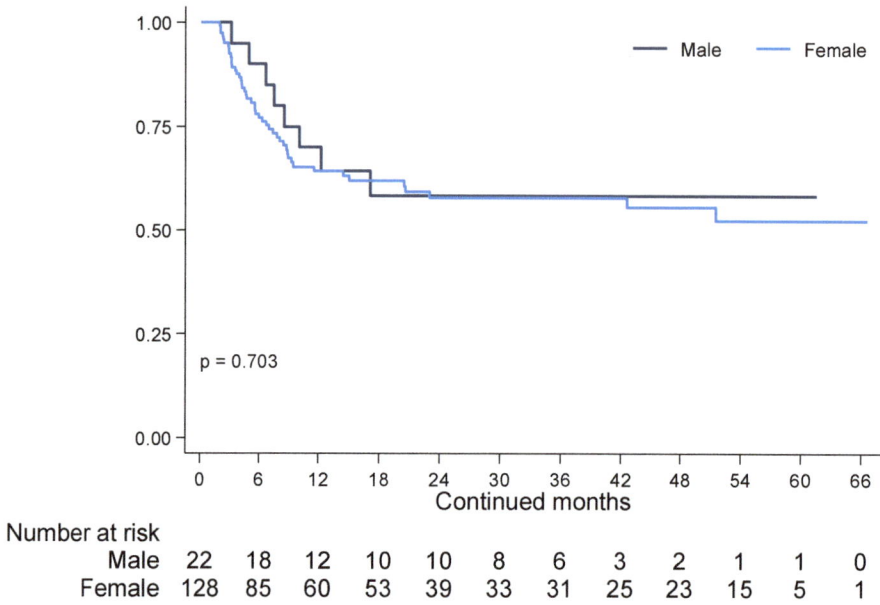

Figure 2. JAK inhibitor retention due to the lack of treatment effectiveness. Similar JAK inhibitor retentions due to the lack of treatment effectiveness were observed between female and male patients ($p = 0.703$) during the follow-up period from September 2017 to October 2023.

4. Discussion

This study assessed sex-related differences in the effectiveness of tofacitinib, baricitinib, upadacitinib, and filgotinib in the clinical context of rheumatoid arthritis treatment. Taking into account the available literature, there are currently limited published real-world studies addressing this concern. Indirectly, previous studies have suggested that being either a female or male patient does not influence the survival of the JAK inhibitor treatment effectiveness [17–19]. To the best of our knowledge, this study stands as the first to elucidate sex-related disparities in the achievement of JAK inhibitor treatment effectiveness, while also shedding light on the survival of the effectiveness of these small molecules.

In terms of achieving remission and low disease activity at the first 6 months of the JAK inhibitor treatment, no significant differences between sexes were observed concerning the DAS28-CRP, the CDAI, or the SDAI. With respect to the DAS28-ESR, female patients, compared to males, possessed 70% lower odds of achieving remission (ORadj for female: 0.30; 95% CI: 0.11–0.81; $p = 0.018$) and, similarly, 66% lower odds of achieving low disease activity (ORadj for female: 0.34; 95% CI: 0.13–0.86; $p = 0.023$). ESR and CRP are acute-phase reactants commonly used in routine clinical practice as inflammation biomarkers, with ESR levels typically being higher in female than in male patients [20–22]. In this manner, sex disparities in ESR levels were reflected in the DAS28-ESR values both at baseline (female: 5.4 [4.8–6.1]; male: 5 [4–5.5]; $p = 0.043$) and at 6 months of the JAK inhibitor treatment (female: 3.7 [2.9–5.2]; male: 3 [1.7–4.4]; $p = 0.014$), leading to the misclassification in female patients of both the DAS28-ESR remission and the DAS28-ESR low disease activity. In accordance with the foregoing, our study findings suggest that, specifically for JAK inhibitor treatment, being a female or male patient does not influence the achievement of remission or low disease activity.

In terms of the survival of the JAK inhibitor treatment effectiveness, Figure 2 illustrates the treatment strategy selected based on the clinical judgment of our clinical rheumatologists in response to the lack of treatment effectiveness. According to both the T2T strategy [2,3] and the rheumatoid arthritis guidelines [7–9], if substantial improvement in disease activity is not plausible within the first 3 months of treatment, or if the primary target remains unattained by 6 months, treatment adjustment or modification of the therapy is recommended. The unobserved significant differences between female and male patients in the JAK inhibitor treatment retention rates ($p = 0.703$), as well as the non-determination of sex as a potential factor that could influence the maintenance of the treatment effectiveness (HR: 1.16; 95% CI: 0.55–2.45; $p = 0.704$), suggest that being a female or male patient does not influence the maintenance of the effectiveness of these small molecules.

The present study had some inherent limitations. The first of these was the population size and that it was exclusively conducted at a single healthcare center. However, the results obtained align with previous indirect data regarding discrepancies in the survival of the JAK inhibitor treatment effectiveness between female and male patients. Second was the disparity in sex distribution, reflecting real-world clinical data of a disease that predominantly affects females over males. Third, due to the retrospective nature of this study, despite adjusting for potential confounders, there remains the possibility that treatment retention may have been influenced by unmeasured cofounders not accounted for in our adjusted models. Fourth, JAK inhibitors other than tofacitinib, baricitinib, upadacitinib, or filgotinib —the four small molecules currently approved in Europe for the treatment of rheumatoid arthritis—were not considered in our study, i.e., peficitinib. Fifth, adjustments in dosage or frequency of drug treatment were not monitored in our study. JAK inhibitors are approved at specific dosages, with certain treatment adjustments recommended based on specific patient characteristics and concomitant treatments. We assumed that all patients received their required dosage and frequency in accordance with the approved recommendations for JAK inhibitor treatment. Sixth, it would be interesting to precisely understand the influence of sex on the components of the four validated disease activity measures; however, data regarding this aspect were lacking in the present study.

The main strength of our study lies in the inclusion of rheumatoid arthritis patients undergoing treatment in real-world clinical settings, with the primary aim of elucidating whether sex-related disparities exist that could influence the achievement and survival of the JAK inhibitor treatment effectiveness, thereby establishing the initial findings on this matter within the published literature.

5. Conclusions

To sum up, the findings of our study suggest that being a female or male patient does not entail differences in the effectiveness of the JAK inhibitor treatment, taking into account the potential misclassification in female patients for both the DAS28-ESR remission and the DAS28-ESR low disease activity, attributable to sex disparities in the ESR levels. This study encourages the consideration of a global pool of validated composite indices (DAS28-ESR, DAS28-CRP, CDAI, and SDAI) to measure rheumatoid arthritis disease activity, thus individualizing the target value based on patient-related factors, as advocated by the T2T strategy [2,3].

Author Contributions: Conceptualization, C.M.-M., H.C. and S.V.; resources, A.F., A.J., C.D.-T., C.M.-M., H.C., H.S.P. and S.V.; investigation, C.M.-M.; formal analysis, C.M.-M.; visualization, C.M.-M.; writing—original draft preparation, C.M.-M.; writing—review and editing, H.C. and S.V.; supervision, H.C. and S.V. All authors have read and agreed to the published version of the manuscript.

Funding: This research received no external funding.

Institutional Review Board Statement: The study was conducted in accordance with the Declaration of Helsinki, and approved by the Ethics Committee of Hospital de la Santa Creu i Sant Pau (IIBSP-JAG-2023-168, 29 December 2023).

Informed Consent Statement: Informed consent was obtained from all subjects involved in the study.

Data Availability Statement: The datasets used and/or analyzed during the current study are available from the corresponding author on reasonable request.

Conflicts of Interest: The authors declare no conflicts of interest.

References

1. Scott, D.L.; Wolfe, F.; Huizinga, T.W. Rheumatoid arthritis. *Lancet* **2010**, *376*, 1094–1108. [CrossRef]
2. Smolen, J.S.; Aletaha, D.; Bijlsma, J.W.; Breedveld, F.C.; Boumpas, D.; Burmester, G.; Combe, B.; Cutolo, M.; de Wit, M.; Dougados, M.; et al. Treating rheumatoid arthritis to target: Recommendations of an international task force. *Ann. Rheum. Dis.* **2010**, *69*, 631–637. [CrossRef]
3. Smolen, J.S.; Breedveld, F.C.; Burmester, G.R.; Bykerk, V.P.; Dougados, M.; Emery, P.; Kvien, T.K.; Navarro-Compán, M.V.; Oliver, S.; Schoels, M.; et al. Treating rheumatoid arthritis to target: 2014 update of the recommendations of an international task force. *Ann. Rheum. Dis.* **2016**, *75*, 3–15. [CrossRef]
4. Prevoo, M.L.; van 't Hof, M.A.; Kuper, H.H.; van Leeuwen, M.A.; van de Putte, L.B.; van Riel, P.L. Modified disease activity scores that include twenty-eight-joint counts. Development and validation in a prospective longitudinal study of patients with rheumatoid arthritis. *Arthritis Rheum.* **1995**, *38*, 44–48. [CrossRef]
5. Fransen, J.; Welsing, P.M.; de Keijzer, R.M.; Van Riel, P.L.C.M. Disease activity scores using C-reactive protein: CRP may replace ESR in the assessment of RA disease activity. *Ann. Rheum. Dis.* **2004**, *62*, 151.
6. Aletaha, D.; Smolen, J. The Simplified Disease Activity Index (SDAI) and the Clinical Disease Activity Index (CDAI): A review of their usefulness and validity in rheumatoid arthritis. *Clin. Exp. Rheumatol.* **2005**, *23*, S100–S108.
7. Smolen, J.S.; Landewé, R.B.M.; Bergstra, S.A.; Kerschbaumer, A.; Sepriano, A.; Aletaha, D.; Caporali, R.; Edwards, C.J.; Hyrich, K.L.; E Pope, J.; et al. EULAR recommendations for the management of rheumatoid arthritis with synthetic and biological disease-modifying antirheumatic drugs: 2022 update. *Ann. Rheum. Dis.* **2023**, *82*, 3–18. [CrossRef]
8. Fraenkel, L.; Bathon, J.M.; England, B.R.; St Clair, E.W.; Arayssi, T.; Carandang, K.; Deane, K.D.; Genovese, M.; Huston, K.K.; Kerr, G.; et al. American College of Rheumatology guideline for the treatment of rheumatoid arthritis. *Arthritis Rheumatol.* **2021**, *73*, 924–939. [CrossRef]
9. Singh, J.A.; Furst, D.E.; Bharat, A.; Curtis, J.R.; Kavanaugh, A.F.; Kremer, J.M.; Moreland, L.W.; O'Dell, J.; Winthrop, K.L.; Beukelman, T.; et al. Update of the 2008 American College of Rheumatology recommendations for the use of disease-modifying antirheumatic drugs and biologic agents in the treatment of rheumatoid arthritis. *Arthritis Care Res.* **2012**, *64*, 625–639. [CrossRef]
10. Hyrich, K.L.; Watson, K.D.; Silman, A.J.; Symmons, D.P.; British Society for Rheumatology Biologics Register. Predictors of response to anti-TNF-alpha therapy among patients with rheumatoid arthritis: Results from the British Society for Rheumatology Biologics Register. *Rheumatology* **2006**, *45*, 1558–1565. [CrossRef]
11. Tanaka, Y.; Takeuchi, T.; Inoue, E.; Saito, K.; Sekiguchi, N.; Sato, E.; Nawata, M.; Kameda, H.; Iwata, S.; Amano, K.; et al. Retrospective clinical study on the notable efficacy and related factors of infliximab therapy in a rheumatoid arthritis management group in Japan: One-year clinical outcomes (RECONFIRM-2). *Mod. Rheumatol.* **2008**, *18*, 146–152. [CrossRef]
12. Kvien, T.K.; Uhlig, T.; Ødegård, S.; Heiberg, M.S. Epidemiological aspects of rheumatoid arthritis: The sex ratio. *Ann. N. Y. Acad. Sci.* **2006**, *1069*, 212–222. [CrossRef]
13. Forslind, K.; Hafström, I.; Ahlmén, M.; Svensson, B.; BARFOT Study Group. Sex: A major predictor of remission in early rheumatoid arthritis? *Ann. Rheum. Dis.* **2007**, *66*, 46–52. [CrossRef]
14. Mancarella, L.; Bobbio-Pallavicini, F.; Ceccarelli, F.; Falappone, P.C.; Ferrante, A.; Malesci, D.; Massara, A.; Nacci, F.; Secchi, M.E.; Manganelli, S.; et al. Good clinical response, remission, and predictors of remission in rheumatoid arthritis patients treated with tumor necrosis factor-alpha blockers: The GISEA study. *J. Rheumatol.* **2007**, *34*, 1670–1673.
15. Aletaha, D.; Neogi, T.; Silman, A.J.; Funovits, J.; Felson, D.T.; Bingham, C.O., 3rd; Birnbaum, N.S.; Burmester, G.R.; Bykerk, V.P.; Cohen, M.D.; et al. Rheumatoid arthritis classification criteria: An American College of Rheumatology/European League Against Rheumatism collaborative initiative. *Ann. Rheum. Dis.* **2010**, *69*, 1580–1588. [CrossRef]
16. England, B.R.; Tiong, B.K.; Bergman, M.J.; Curtis, J.R.; Kazi, S.; Mikuls, T.R.; O'Dell, J.R.; Ranganath, V.K.; Limanni, A.; Suter, L.G.; et al. Update of the American College of Rheumatology Recommended Rheumatoid Arthritis Disease Activity Measures. *Arthritis Care Res.* **2019**, *71*, 1540–1555. [CrossRef]
17. Ebina, K.; Hirano, T.; Maeda, Y.; Yamamoto, W.; Hashimoto, M.; Murata, K.; Onishi, A.; Jinno, S.; Hara, R.; Son, Y.; et al. Factors affecting drug retention of Janus kinase inhibitors in patients with rheumatoid arthritis: The ANSWER cohort study. *Sci. Rep.* **2022**, *12*, 134. [CrossRef]
18. Pombo-Suarez, M.; Sanchez-Piedra, C.; Gómez-Reino, J.; Lauper, K.; Mongin, D.; Iannone, F.; Pavelka, K.; Nordström, D.C.; Inanc, N.; Codreanu, C.; et al. After JAK inhibitor failure: To cycle or to switch, that is the question -data from the JAK-pot collaboration of registries. *Ann. Rheum. Dis.* **2023**, *82*, 175–181. [CrossRef]
19. Martinez-Molina, C.; Gich, I.; Diaz-Torné, C.; Park, H.S.; Feliu, A.; Vidal, S.; Corominas, H. Patient-related factors influencing the effectiveness and safety of Janus Kinase inhibitors in rheumatoid arthritis: A real-world study. *Sci. Rep.* **2024**, *14*, 172. [CrossRef]
20. Miller, A.; Green, M.; Robinson, D. Simple rule for calculating normal erythrocyte sedimentation rate. *Br. Med. J. (Clin. Res. Ed.)* **1983**, *286*, 266. [CrossRef]

21. Alende-Castro, V.; Alonso-Sampedro, M.; Vazquez-Temprano, N.; Tuñez, C.; Rey, D.; García-Iglesias, C.; Sopeña, B.; Gude, F.; Gonzalez-Quintela, A. Factors influencing erythrocyte sedimentation rate in adults: New evidence for an old test. *Medicine* **2019**, *98*, e16816. [CrossRef]
22. Sokka, T.; Toloza, S.; Cutolo, M.; Kautiainen, H.; Makinen, H.; Gogus, F.; Skakic, V.; Badsha, H.; Peets, T.; Baranauskaite, A.; et al. QUEST-RA Group. Women, men, and rheumatoid arthritis: Analyses of disease activity, disease characteristics, and treatments in the QUEST-RA study. *Arthritis Res. Ther.* **2009**, *11*, R7. [CrossRef]

Disclaimer/Publisher's Note: The statements, opinions and data contained in all publications are solely those of the individual author(s) and contributor(s) and not of MDPI and/or the editor(s). MDPI and/or the editor(s) disclaim responsibility for any injury to people or property resulting from any ideas, methods, instructions or products referred to in the content.

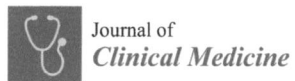 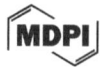

Article

Incidence Rates of Infections in Rheumatoid Arthritis Patients Treated with Janus Kinase or Interleukin-6 Inhibitors: Results of a Retrospective, Multicenter Cohort Study

Shuhei Yoshida [1], Masayuki Miyata [2], Eiji Suzuki [3], Takashi Kanno [3], Yuya Sumichika [1], Kenji Saito [1], Haruki Matsumoto [1], Jumpei Temmoku [1], Yuya Fujita [1], Naoki Matsuoka [1], Tomoyuki Asano [1], Shuzo Sato [1] and Kiyoshi Migita [1,*]

[1] Department of Rheumatology, Fukushima Medical University School of Medicine, 1 Hikarigaoka, Fukushima 960-1295, Japan; shuhei-y@fmu.ac.jp (S.Y.); ysumiti@fmu.ac.jp (Y.S.); s3xbck2p@fmu.ac.jp (K.S.); haruki91@fmu.ac.jp (H.M.); temmoku@fmu.ac.jp (J.T.); fujita31@fmu.ac.jp (Y.F.); naoki-11@fmu.ac.jp (N.M.); asanovic@fmu.ac.jp (T.A.); shuzo@fmu.ac.jp (S.S.)

[2] Department of Rheumatology, Fukushima Red Cross Hospital, Yashima 7-7, Fukushima 960-8136, Japan; fukuintyoumm@fukushima-med-jrc.jp

[3] Department of Rheumatology, Ohta Nishinouchi General Hospital Foundation, 2-5-20 Nishinouchi, Koriyama 963-8558, Japan; azsuzuki@ohta-hp.or.jp (E.S.); t-kanno@ohta-hp.or.jp (T.K.)

* Correspondence: migita@fmu.ac.jp; Tel.: +81-24-547-1171; Fax: +81-24-547-1172

Abstract: Objective: This study aimed to compare the incidence rates (IRs) of infections, including herpes zoster (HZ), in rheumatoid arthritis (RA) patients treated with Janus kinase inhibitors (JAKis) or interleukin-6 inhibitors (IL-6is). **Methods:** We retrospectively analyzed 444 RA patients treated using IL-6is (n = 283) or JAKis (n = 161). After adjusting for clinical characteristic imbalances by propensity score matching (PSM), we compared the IRs of infections including HZ between the JAKi and IL-6i groups. **Results:** Observational period: 1423.93 patient years (PY); median observational period: 2.51 years. After PSM, incidence rate ratios comparing JAKi with IL-6i were 3.45 (95% confidence interval [CI]: 1.48–9.04) for serious infections other than HZ indicating that the JAKi-treated group was more likely to develop serious infection than the IL-6i-treated group. Multivariate Cox regression analyses revealed that the use of prednisolone > 5.0 mg/day, coexisting interstitial lung disease (ILD), and diabetes mellitus (DM) were independent risk factors for serious infections. The crude IR for HZ was significantly higher in the JAKi group, but the difference between groups was not significant (IRR: 2.83, 95% CI: 0.87–10.76) in PSM analysis. Unadjusted and PSM analyses performed in our study showed increased IRs of serious infections in patients with RA treated with JAKis compared with those treated with IL-6is. **Conclusions:** The presence of ILD or DM and the use of prednisolone were found to be independent risk factors for serious infection in RA patients treated using JAKis. Whereas the IRs for HZ after PSM were not significantly different between the JAKi and IL-6i groups.

Keywords: rheumatoid arthritis; Janus kinase inhibitor; interleukin-6 inhibitor; infection; tofacitinib; baricitinib; interstitial lung disease

Citation: Yoshida, S.; Miyata, M.; Suzuki, E.; Kanno, T.; Sumichika, Y.; Saito, K.; Matsumoto, H.; Temmoku, J.; Fujita, Y.; Matsuoka, N.; et al. Incidence Rates of Infections in Rheumatoid Arthritis Patients Treated with Janus Kinase or Interleukin-6 Inhibitors: Results of a Retrospective, Multicenter Cohort Study. *J. Clin. Med.* **2024**, *13*, 3000. https://doi.org/10.3390/jcm13103000

Academic Editors: Santos Castañeda, Sadiq Umar and Blanca Hernández-Cruz

Received: 21 March 2024
Revised: 28 April 2024
Accepted: 15 May 2024
Published: 20 May 2024

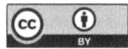

Copyright: © 2024 by the authors. Licensee MDPI, Basel, Switzerland. This article is an open access article distributed under the terms and conditions of the Creative Commons Attribution (CC BY) license (https://creativecommons.org/licenses/by/4.0/).

1. Introduction

Targeting the Janus kinase (JAK) family with small-molecule inhibitors has proven effective in the treatment of various autoimmune diseases [1]. JAK inhibitors (JAKis) with different specificities for each JAK family have been approved for treating rheumatoid arthritis (RA) [2]. In the recent European Alliance of Associations for Rheumatology (EULAR) recommendations for RA management, JAKis are advised in patients who fail to respond to initial treatment with methotrexate (MTX) or other conventional synthetic disease-modifying antirheumatic drugs (csDMARDs) and have poor prognostic factors [3].

However, the safety concerns associated with JAKis, including infections and malignancies, should be carefully addressed. The risk of contracting serious infections or infections that require hospitalization is 1.5 to 2 times higher in patients with RA compared to the general population [4,5]. Similar to biological DMARDs (bDMARDs), JAKis can lead to serious and opportunistic infections including viral infections. Previous studies of JAKi have revealed elderly age, glucocorticoid usage (prednisolone $\geq$ 7.5 mg/day), diabetes mellitus, and high JAKi dosages as risk factors for infection [6]. However, the relative risk of infection in patients receiving JAKis was reported to be comparable to that in patients taking bDMARDs [7]. One retrospective cohort study revealed no significantly increased risk of serious infectious diseases related to the use of tofacitinib, a JAKi, compared with that associated with the use of a tumor necrosis factor inhibitor (TNFi) [8]. The infection profiles of TNFis and JAKis have been found to be similar with regard to serious infections [9,10]. Compared with bDMARDs, JAKis were found to be more frequently associated with the development of HZ [6,11,12]. In patients with RA who received tofacitinib in two phase I, nine phase II, six phase III, and two long-term extension (LTE) studies, the crude incidence rate (IR) of HZ was found to be 4.0 (95% confidence interval [CI]: 3.7, 4.4) per 100 patient years (PY) [13].

Given the widespread use of JAKis in the treatment of RA, the risk of infections, including HZ, in real-world settings should be addressed. Furthermore, it would be of great interest to compare the risks of infection between patients with RA receiving non-TNFi bDMARDs and those receiving JAKis in real-world clinical practice. Therefore, we conducted this multicenter cohort study to determine and compare the IRs of infection in patients with RA treated with an interleukin-6 inhibitor (IL-6i) or a JAKi in real-world settings.

2. Materials and Methods

2.1. Patients and Study Design

We have previously conducted a cohort study involving patients with RA attending our institution from April 2012 to December 2022 to compare the incidence of malignancy and major adverse cardiovascular events [14]. In the present study, we extended the inclusion period by 8 months until August 2023 and collected data on the incidence of serious infections and HZ. The cohort comprised patients treated at the Department of Rheumatology of Fukushima Medical University Hospital, Japanese Red Cross Fukushima Hospital, and Ohta Nishinouchi General Hospital Foundation. The study was approved by the institutional review boards of these institutions (approval Nos. 2021-157, 55, and 2022–8, respectively).

Between April 2012 and August 2023, IL-6i or JAKi therapy was initiated in 473 patients with RA. Among them, 450 started receiving IL-6i or JAKi therapy at our institution, and 444 with sufficient clinical data were enrolled. All patients were diagnosed with RA according to the 2010 American College of Rheumatology/European League Against Rheumatism classification criteria for RA [15]. At treatment initiation, the collected demographic information included age, sex, disease duration, rheumatoid factor, anti-citrullinated protein antibodies, prior use of bDMARDs, presence of comorbidities such as DM or lung disease, and concurrent medications. Patients in the IL-6i group were administered tocilizumab either through intravenous infusion at a dosage of 8 mg/kg every 4 weeks or subcutaneous injection at 162 mg every other week, or sarilumab via subcutaneous injection at 200 mg every 2 weeks. Patients in the JAKi-treated group received the following dosages based on their specific conditions: those with renal impairment were given baricitinib 2 or 4 mg once daily, those with liver impairment received tofacitinib 5 mg twice or once daily, those with renal impairment were administered upadacitinib 15 mg once daily, and filgotinib was given at 100 or 200 mg once daily. The study employed an opt-out approach, and participants who refused to provide informed consent were not included. The full recruitment process is depicted in Figure 1.

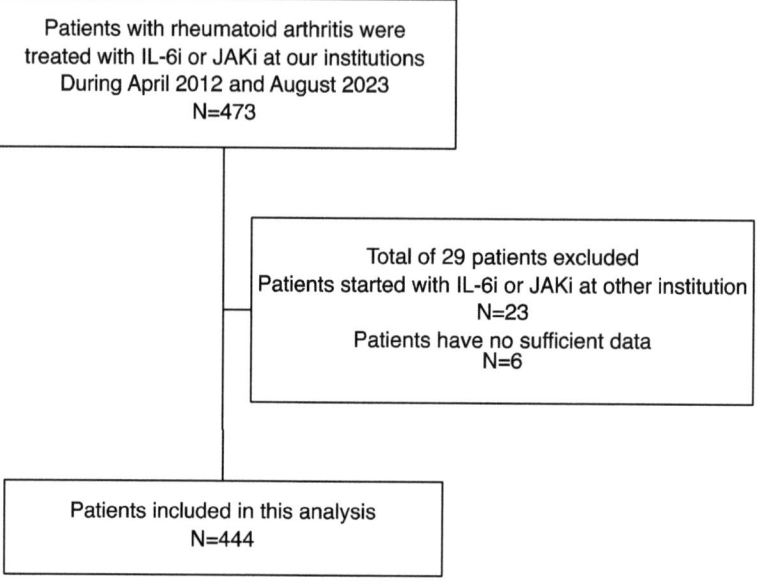

Figure 1. Flow chart showing patient enrollment. Among the 473 patients with RA who received initial treatment with IL-6i or JAKi at our institution between April 2012 and August 2023, 444 patients with sufficient clinical data were enrolled in the study. IL-6i: interleukin-6 inhibitor; JAKi: Janus kinase inhibitor; RA: rheumatoid arthritis.

2.2. Definitions of Exposure and Outcomes

"Exposure" was defined as the period from the initiation of IL-6i or JAKi treatment until treatment discontinuation, patient transfer to another hospital, death, or the end of the study period, whichever occurred first. Serious infections were defined as infections other than HZ that required hospitalization, as determined by treating physicians based on a comprehensive evaluation, including physical, laboratory, and radiological examinations, and the need for hospitalization. HZ was diagnosed by the treating physician based on the observation of skin lesions. The censoring time of the above-described adverse events was defined as the time from the administration of the first dose of JAKi or IL-6i until the end of treatment or the last observation point (31 August 2023).

2.3. Statistical Analysis

Data are presented as median and interquartile range for continuous variables and frequency and percentage for qualitative variables. The Mann–Whitney U test was employed to compare continuous variables, and Fisher's exact test was used to compare categorical variables. Statistical significance was determined by a two-tailed p-value of <0.05.

To calculate the propensity scores, multivariable logistic regression analysis was performed with JAKi use as the dependent variable and the following as independent variables: patient age and sex, disease duration, RF and ACPA positivity, GC and MTX use, and co-occurrence of ILD and DM. Patient backgrounds of the treatment groups were adjusted via propensity score matching. The number of adverse events, PY at risk, and incidence rate ratio (IRR) with 95% CI were determined for each outcome.

The time to serious infection in the treatment groups was calculated using Kaplan–Meier analysis, and log-rank tests were employed to compare the cumulative IRs between the groups. Univariate and multivariate Cox regression analyses were conducted to identify variables related to the occurrence of serious infections. Factors with a *p*-value < 0.05 were included in the multivariate Cox regression analysis. The receiver operating characteristic (ROC) curve was used to determine the cut-off value for the steroid dose that impacted the risk of serious infection.

Statistical analyses were performed using R (version 4.1.2; R Foundation for Statistical Computing, Vienna, Austria, http://www.R-project.org/ [accessed on 23 June 2023]) and IBM SPSS Statistics software (version 29.0.1.0; IBM Co., Armonk, NY, USA).

3. Results

3.1. Patients' Baseline Characteristics

Among the 473 patients with RA in whom IL-6i or JAKi treatment was initiated at our institutions between April 2012 and August 2023, 444 were enrolled. Table 1 presents the background characteristics of patients in the IL-6i- and JAKi-treated groups before and after propensity score matching (PSM). In the IL-6i-treated group, 277 and 6 patients received tocilizumab and sarilumab, respectively. The JAKi-treated group included 95, 43, 15, and 8 patients who received baricitinib, tofacitinib, upadacitinib, and filgotinib, respectively. None of the patients had a history of using JAKi. Before PSM, the IL-6i-treated group showed significantly higher concomitant GC use, GC and MTX doses, and longer observation periods compared to the JAKi-treated group. In contrast, the JAKi-treated group had significantly higher age at tsDMARD introduction and rates of DM coexistence. The observational period for the 444 patients (306 females) examined herein was 1423.93 PY, with a median (interquartile range) duration of 2.51 (1.20–4.22) years. After PSM, 236 patients with RA (165 females) were observed for 650.49 PY, with a median (interquartile range) length of 2.24 (1.22–3.97) years. Following PSM, no significant intergroup differences were observed, except for the history of bDMARD use and observational period.

Table 1. Comparisons of clinical features between IL-6i group and JAKi group.

Characteristics	All Patients			Propensity-Matched Patients			
	IL-6i (*n* = 283)	JAKi (*n* = 161)	*p* Value	IL-6i (*n* = 118)	JAKi (*n* = 118)	*p* Value	SMD
Male, *n* (%)	89 (31.4)	49 (30.4)	0.92	34 (28.8)	37 (31.4)	0.78	0.06
Age at b/ts DMARDs introduction, † years	61 (51–69)	72 (65–81)	<0.001 *	68 (58–76)	69 (60–75)	0.59	0.07
Disease duration, † years	8.7 (3.5–15.4)	7.6 (3.5–15.9)	0.51	9.0 (3.3–15.7)	9.2 (4.2–16.8)	0.39	0.17
Steinbrocker's stage, I/II/III/IV	105/79/37/45 no data, 17	62/41/16/34 no data, 8		35/40/13/23 no data, 7	48/27/10/29 no data, 4		
Steinbrocker's class, I/II/III/IV	30/168/62/8 no data, 15	17/93/45/4 no data, 2		14/70/25/2 no data, 7	7/73/34/2 no data, 2		
RF positivity, *n* (%)	207 (73.1)	109 (67.7)	0.23	85 (72.0)	84 (71.2)	1.00	0.02
ACPA positivity, *n* (%)	212 (74.9)	112 (69.6) no data, 2	0.32	87 (73.7)	89 (75.4)	0.88	0.04
Concomitant GC use, *n* (%)	134 (47.3)	41 (25.5)	<0.001 *	38 (32.2)	37 (31.4)	1.00	0.02
Concomitant GC dose, † mg/day	0.0 (0–5.0)	0.0 (0–0)	<0.001 *	0.0 (0.0–5.0)	0.0 (0.0–6.0)	0.55	0.09
Concomitant MTX use, *n* (%)	148 (52.3)	73 (45.3)	0.17	57 (48.3)	58 (49.2)	1.00	0.02
Concomitant MTX dose, † mg/week	4.0 (0.0–8.0)	0 (0–6)	0.04 *	0.0 (0.0–6.0)	0.0 (0.0–6.0)	0.91	0.03
Coexisting ILD, *n* (%)	37 (13.1)	21 (13.0)	1.0	14 (11.9)	15 (12.7)	1.00	0.03
Coexisting DM, *n* (%)	26 (9.2)	26 (16.1)	0.03 *	17 (14.4)	16 (13.6)	1.00	0.02
Previous use of bDMARDs, *n* (%)	113 (39.9)	76 (47.2)	0.16	44 (37.3)	61 (51.7)	0.04 *	0.29
Observational period, † years	3.0 (1.4–5.2)	1.8 (1.2–3.3)	<0.001 *	2.9 (1.4–4.7)	1.9 (1.2–3.3)	0.01 *	0.45

† Values are the median with interquartile range. * means there is a significant difference at *p* < 0.05. IL-6i: interleukin-6 receptor inhibitors, JAKi: Janus kinase inhibitors, RF: rheumatoid factor, ACPA: anti-citrullinated peptide antibody, GC: glucocorticoid, MTX: methotrexate, ILD: interstitial lung disease, DM: diabetes mellitus, b/ts DMARD: biologic/targeted synthetic disease-modifying anti-rheumatic drug, SMD: standardized mean difference.

3.2. IRs of Serious Infections

The IRs for infectious diseases are listed in Table 2. We identified 27 and 25 cases of serious infections (16.8%; IR: 7.52/100 PY; 8.8%; IR: 2.35/100 PY) among 161 and 283 JAKi- and IL-6i-treated patients, respectively. Serious infections in the IL-6i group included bacterial pneumonia (n = 12), soft tissue infection (n = 6), pyelonephritis (n = 2), diverticulitis (n = 2), sinus mycosis (n = 1), pyothorax (n = 1), and bacterial enteritis (n = 1). In the JAKi group, these included bacterial pneumonia (n = 15), soft tissue infections (n = 5), bacterial enteritis (n = 2), pyelonephritis (n = 2), diverticulitis (n = 1), perforated peritonitis (n = 1), and cholecystitis (n = 1). Pneumonia (n = 27; 51.9% of all infections) was the most frequent serious infection in both groups. Before PSM, the IRR for the JAKi to the IL-6i group was 3.20 (95% CI: 1.85–5.56, p < 0.001), indicating that the former was more likely to develop serious infections. After PSM, the JAKi group was still more likely to develop serious infections (IRR: 3.45, 95% CI: 1.48–9.04, p = 0.004). However, the observational period for the JAKi group was shorter than that for the IL-6i group. Owing to this, we evaluated the time-to-event outcomes (serious infections) using Kaplan–Meier analysis. To this end, serious infections were more frequent in the JAKi group (p = 0.01, log-rank test; Figure 2).

Table 2. Incidence rate of infectious diseases.

	All Patients			Propensity-Matched Patients		
	IL-6i (n = 283)	JAKi (n = 161)	p Value	IL-6i (n = 118)	JAKi (n = 118)	p Value
Serious infectious diseases other than HZ	25 (8.8)	27 (16.8)		7 (5.9)	17 (14.4)	
IR per 100 PY (95%CI)	2.35 (1.42–3.28)	7.52 (4.73–10.31)		1.89 (0.50–3.28)	6.61 (3.57–9.65)	
IRR (95%CI)	1 [reference]	3.20 (1.85–5.56)	<0.001 *	1 [reference]	3.45 (1.48–9.04)	0.004 *
HZ	12 (4.2)	10 (6.2)		4 (3.4)	8 (6.8)	
IR per 100 PY (95%CI)	1.13 (0.48–1.78)	2.91 (1.13–4.69)		1.08 (0.03–2.13)	3.11 (0.99–5.23)	
IRR (95%CI)	1 [reference]	2.49 (1.04–5.83)	0.041 *	1 [reference]	2.83 (0.87–10.96)	0.084

* means there is a significant difference at p < 0.05. IL-6i: interleukin-6 inhibitor; JAKi: Janus kinase inhibitor; HZ: herpes zoster, IR: incidence rate, PY: patient years, IRR: incidence rate ratio, CI: confidence interval.

3.3. Risk Factors for Serious Infections in JAKi-Treated Patients

To establish risk factors associated with serious infections, patient baseline characteristics were analyzed using univariate and multivariate Cox regression analyses (Table 3). Univariate Cox regression analysis revealed a significantly increased risk of serious infections associated with glucocorticoid (GC) use, interstitial lung disease (ILD), and diabetes mellitus (DM). In the multivariate Cox hazard model, prednisolone dose, ILD, and DM emerged as independent risk factors for serious infections in JAKi-treated patients. We analyzed the cut-off value for the GC dose associated with risk of serious infection by obtaining the ROC curve, which revealed a dose of 5.0 mg (Supplementary Figure S1). Therefore, Kaplan–Meier survival curves were plotted for occurrence of the first serious infection stratified by GC use (>5.0 mg/day) or the existence of ILD (Figure 3). The frequency of occurrence of the first serious infection was significantly higher in patients with ILD or those receiving high-dose GCs (>5.0 mg/day).

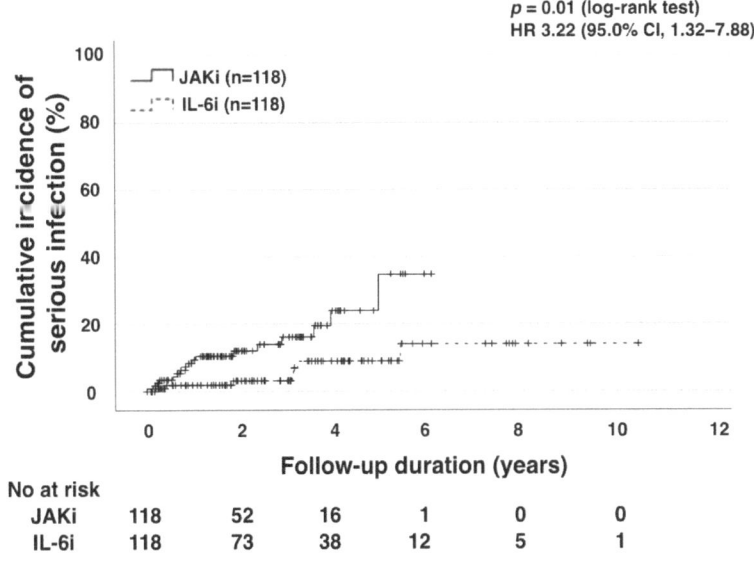

Figure 2. Cumulative incidence curves of serious infection in IL-6i-treated and JAKi-treated patients after propensity score matching. Kaplan–Meier curves show the cumulative incidence of serious infection in patients treated with IL-6is ($n = 118$) and JAKis ($n = 118$). Significant differences were observed between IL-6i-treated and JAKi-treated groups ($p = 0.01$). The starting point (0 years) was the date on which the observations began. HR: hazard ratio; CI: confidence interval; JAKi: Janus kinase inhibitor; IL-6i: interleukin-6 inhibitor; No: number.

Table 3. Independent risk factors of serious infectious diseases in rheumatoid arthritis patients treated with JAKi.

Variavle	Risk Factors for Serious Infectious Diseases			
	Univariate Model		Multivariable Model	
	HR (95%CI)	p-Value	HR (95%CI)	p-Value
Age, >65 years or not	2.00 (0.69–5.81)	0.20		
Disease duration, per 1-year increase	0.98 (0.94–1.03)	0.42		
RF positive or negative	1.50 (0.63–3.56)	0.36		
ACPA positive or negative	1.88 (0.71–4.98)	0.21		
GC dose, per 1 mg increase	1.012 (1.01–1.02)	<0.001 *	1.01 (1.01–1.02)	<0.001 *
MTX dose, per 1 mg increase	0.956 (0.85–1.07)	0.45		
Coexisting ILD, yes/no	4.00 (1.62–9.86)	0.003 *	3.72 (1.48–9.35)	0.01 *
Coexisting DM, yes/no	2.68 (1.20–5.97)	0.02 *	2.53 (1.11–5.75)	0.03 *
No. of previous use of bDMARDs, per drug	1.10 (0.79–1.49)	0.63		
Reduced dose of JAKi, yes/no	0.74 (0.35–1.59)	0.44		

* means there is a significant difference at $p < 0.05$. JAKi: Janus kinase inhibitor, RF: rheumatoid factor, ACPA: anti-citrullinated peptide antibody, GC: glucocorticoid, MTX: methotrexate, ILD: interstitial lung disease, DM: diabetes mellitus, No: number, bDMARDs: biological disease-modifying antirheumatic drugs, HR: hazard ratio, CI: confidence interval.

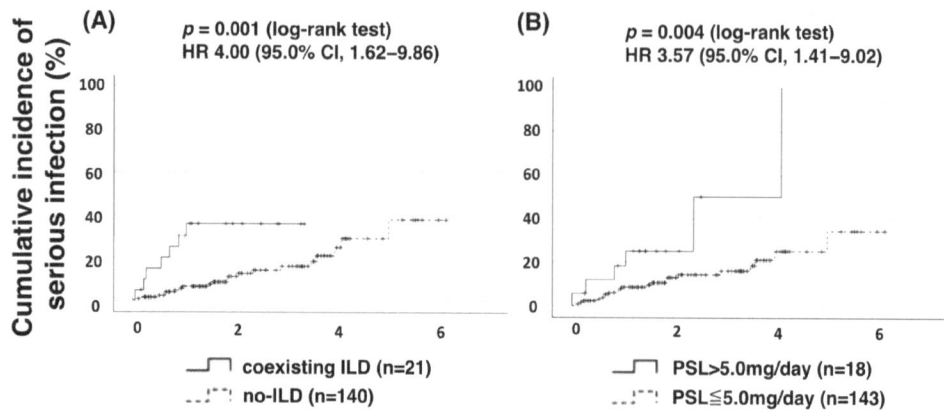

Figure 3. Cumulative incidence curves of serious infections in JAKi-treated patients with or without ILD and with PSL above and below 5.0 mg/day. Kaplan–Meier curves show the cumulative incidence of serious infections in RA patients treated with JAKis, stratified by (**A**) ILD status and (**B**) PSL > 5.0 mg/day and ≤5.0 mg/day. Significant differences were observed between the groups with and without ILD ($p = 0.001$). There was also a significant difference between the two groups in the dosage of PSL (PSL > 5.0 mg and PSL ≤ 5.0 mg) ($p = 0.004$). The starting point (0 years) was the date on which the observations began. HR: hazard ratio; CI: confidence interval; ILD: interstitial lung disease; PSL: prednisolone; JAKi: Janus kinase inhibitor.

3.4. IR for HZ

The IRs for infectious diseases are listed in Table 2. The crude IRs for HZ were higher in the JAKi group (6.2%; IR: 2.91/100 PY) than in the IL-6i group (4.2%; IR: 1.13/100 PY). The crude IRs of HZ were significantly higher in the JAKi group compared to the IL-6i group (IRR = 2.49, 95% CI: 1.04–5.83, $p = 0.041$). After PSM, there was no significant difference in the IRR of HZ between the two groups (IRR = 2.83, 95% CI: 0.87–10.96, $p = 0.084$).

3.5. Comparison of Infectious Diseases between Each JAKi

The baseline demographic and clinical features of patients treated with each JAKi are summarized in Table 4. All "Serious infections other than HZ" and "HZ" in the table are those that occurred during JAKi administration. Among the JAKi group, serious infections occurred only in patients treated with baricitinib and tofacitinib. The baricitinib and tofacitinib groups are presented in Table 5. The crude IRs for serious infections or HZ were higher in the tofacitinib group than in the baricitinib group. However, there was no significant difference in the IRs for serious infection and HZ between these two groups (serious infection IRR = 1.33, 95% CI: 0.59–2.85, $p = 0.48$/HZ IRR = 1.92, 95% CI: 0.43–8.51, $p = 0.38$).

Table 4. Clinical features of RA patients treated with each JAKi.

	Baricitinib (n = 95)	Tofacitinib (n = 43)	Upadacitinib (n = 15)	Filgotinib (n = 8)
Male, n (%)	25 (26.3)	12 (27.9)	8 (53.3)	4 (50.0)
Age at JAKi introduction, † years	74 (68–84)	72 (66–79)	61 (56–68)	64 (61–68)
Disease duration, † years	7.3 (3.1–16.5)	8.7 (4.1–15.6)	6.4 (3.8–8.6)	6.6 (4.2–12.2)
Steinbrocker's stage, I/II/III/IV	36/21/12/20 no data 6	18/13/1/9 no data 2	5/6/2/2	3/1/1/3
Steinbrocker's class, I/II/III/IV	15/53/23/3 no data 1	2/21/18/1 no data 1	0/11/4/0	0/8/0/0
RF positivity, n (%)	65 (68.4)	26 (60.5)	12 (80.0)	6 (75.0)
ACPA positivity, n (%)	68 (71.6) no data 1	26 (60.5) no data 1	12 (80.0)	6 (75.0)
Concomitant GC use, n (%)	18 (18.9)	11 (25.6)	9 (60.0)	3 (37.5)
Concomitant GC dose, † mg/day	0.0 (0.0–0.0)	0.0 (0.0–1.8)	2.0 (0.0–2.5)	0.0 (0.0–5.5)
Concomitant MTX use, n (%)	35 (36.8)	27 (62.8)	6 (40.0)	5 (62.5)
Concomitant MTX dose, † mg/week	0.0 (0.0–6.0)	4.0 (0.0–7.0)	0.0 (0.0–5.0)	5.0 (0.0–6.5)
Coexisting ILD, n (%)	13 (13.7)	6 (14.0)	2 (13.3)	0
Coexisting DM, n (%)	15 (15.8)	9 (20.9)	2 (13.3)	0
Previous use of bDMARDs, n (%)	44 (46.3)	23 (53.5)	8 (53.3)	1 (12.5)
Observation period, † years	1.8 (1.2–3.3)	2.1 (1.0–3.6)	1.9 (1.5–2.1)	1.3 (1.0–1.4)
Serious infectious diseases other than HZ, n (%)	16 (16.8)	11 (25.6)	0	0
HZ	4 (4.2)	4 (9.3)	2 (13.3)	0

† Values are the median with interquartile range. JAKi: Janus kinase inhibitors, RF: rheumatoid factor, ACPA: anti-citrullinated peptide antibody, GC: glucocorticoid, MTX: methotrexate, ILD: interstitial lung disease, DM: diabetes mellitus, bDMARD: biologic disease-modifying anti-rheumatic drug, HZ: herpes zoster.

Table 5. Incidence rates of serious infections, HZ.

	Baricitinib (n = 95)	Tofacitinib (n = 43)	p-Value
Serious infectious diseases other than HZ	16 (16.8%)	11 (25.6%)	
IR per 100 PY (95%CI)	7.54 (3.93–11.15)	9.95 (4.14–15.76)	
IRR (95%CI)	1 [reference]	1.33 (0.59–2.85)	0.48
HZ	4 (4.2%)	4 (9.3%)	
IR per 100 PY (95%CI)	1.89 (0.03–3.75)	3.62 (0.00–7.24)	
IRR (95%CI)	1 [reference]	1.92 (0.43–8.51)	0.38

HZ: herpes zoster, IR: incidence rate, PY: patient years, IRR: incidence rate ratio, CI: confidence interval.

4. Discussion

In this study, we focused on patients with RA treated using targeted DMARDs and compared the incidences of infectious events, including HZ, between patients treated with JAKis and those treated with IL-6is. Despite the different baseline characteristics, our data demonstrated that JAKi-treated patients had a higher risk of serious infections than those treated with IL-6is. Although we could not completely exclude residual or unmeasured confounding factors, we also found increased IRs of serious infectious diseases in JAKi-treated patients with RA compared with those in IL-6i-treated patients with RA in our propensity score-matching comparisons.

The pooled data of baricitinib clinical trials showed that the IR for serious infectious diseases was 2.9/100 PY (95% CI: 2.5–3.4) [16]. In tofacitinib-treated patients with RA in phase I, phase II, phase III, and LTE studies, the IR for serious infections was reported to be 2.7/100 PY (95% CI: 2.5, 3.0), and the most common infection was pneumonia [17]. Elderly age, diabetes mellitus, corticosteroid use (>7.5 mg/day of prednisolone), and tofacitinib dosage (10 mg bid vs. 5 mg bid) were identified as risk factors for serious infections in patients treated with tofacitinib [6]. In contrast to these previous studies, in our study, the IR for serious infection (7.52/100 PY) was higher in patients treated with JAKis. Patients with RA at risk for infections, including elderly patients and those with diabetes or ILD, were enrolled in our real-world study, which could have contributed to the increased IRs for serious infections in JAKi-treated patients compared with those in clinical trial data. In general, GC use is associated with increased susceptibility to infection [18]. However, there are inadequate data on the effects of ILD on infection. We also evaluated the risk factors for serious infections in patients with RA receiving these targeted DMARDs. Our study clearly demonstrates that ILD is an independent risk factor for serious infectious diseases in JAKi-treated RA patients.

Controversy exists as to whether the use of JAKis for patients with RA-ILD can be challenging. Cronin et al. reported that the use of JAKis for the treatment of patients with RA and existing ILD did not increase the rate of hospitalization due to respiratory causes compared with rituximab treatment, suggesting that JAKi is a safe treatment strategy for RA patients with ILD [19]. However, the incidence rates of serious infectious diseases including pneumonia were significantly higher in JAKi-treated patients than in those treated with IL-6i in our study. Furthermore, the presence of ILD has been shown to be an independent risk factor for serious infectious diseases in JAKi-treated patients. Kalyoncu et al. found that in a controlled real-world study on tofacitinib-treated RA patients, infection was the most common cause of drug discontinuation in RA-ILD patients (more so than in non-RA-ILD patients) [20]. They also reported that RA patients with ILD are older than those without ILD. In general, elderly RA patients have a higher rate of comorbid ILDs than younger patients [21]. The possibility that older age and ILD comorbidity are confounding factors cannot be ruled out. In addition to old age, coexisting lung diseases and GC use were associated with the development of pneumocystis pneumonia in JAKi-treated patients [22]. Collectively, these data suggest that clinicians should be concerned about the risk of serious infections, including unusual infections, in patients receiving JAKis. Larger prospective studies are required to determine whether JAKis affect the risk of serious infections in RA patients with or without ILD.

A previous study on younger RA patients (<65 years) initiated on b/tsDMARDs, revealed that patients with frailty were at a significantly higher risk of serious infections than those without frailty [23]. Diabetes and interstitial lung disease are closely associated with patient frailty [24,25]. Therefore, RA patients with DM or ILD, even at a young age, should be cautious with JAKi treatment due to the close association between risk of developing serious infections and JAKi treatment.

Patients with RA have an approximately two- to three-fold increased risk of HZ compared with the general population [26]. In a systematic review and meta-analysis of JAKi-treated patients with RA, Bechman et al. demonstrated that the incidence of HZ was higher than that in the pooled placebo group (3.23/100 PY vs. 1.05/100 PY) [27]. Although the pathogenic mechanism by which JAKis increase the risk of HZ has not yet been completely elucidated, it is hypothesized that the inhibitory effect of JAKis on the intracellular signaling of cytokines acting via the JAK/signal transducer and activator of transcription (STAT) signaling pathway may contribute to the increased risk for HZ through the impairment of cell-mediated immunity [28]. In our study, the estimated IRs of HZ in patients receiving JAKi was 2.91/100 PY, (95% CI: 1.13–4.69) and was higher in the patients treated with JAKis than in those treated with IL-6is. This finding is consistent with those of previous studies, whereas the intergroup difference in our study was not significant. Given the lack of direct comparisons between JAKi-treated patients with RA and IL-6i-treated patients with RA with the same demographic background, we are limited in drawing conclusions regarding the relative risk of HZ linked to JAKis compared with that linked to IL-6is. However, a time-to-event analysis for HZ by using Kaplan–Meier curves showed that HZ developed more frequently in JAKi-treated patients compared with that in

IL-6i-treated patients (Supplementary Figure S2). Therefore, physicians should be aware of the risk of HZ in JAKi-treated patients with RA, particularly those with risk factors.

Our study has several limitations. First, the number of patients ($n = 473$) and the duration of follow-up periods (median; 1.8 years in JAKi and 3.0 years in IL-6i) were not sufficient to detect any adverse events. Second, the choice of treatment and decision to discontinue treatment was made at the discretion of each rheumatologist, with no standardized protocol. Third, adverse events, including infections, were investigated at each patient visit, and the possibility that some cases were treated in the community and events were missed cannot be completely ruled out. Fourth, RA disease activity, HZ history, rate of vaccination, and parameters of a smoking history were not investigated in our study. Although high disease activity in RA has been reported to increase the risk of infection [29], it has been difficult to obtain information on disease activity from medical records. Vaccination for diseases such as HZ, influenza, and pneumococcal vaccines may interact with the IR of infection. Finally, the follow-up period was shorter for the JAKi group than for the IL-6i group.

5. Conclusions

In conclusion, our study demonstrated increased IRs for serious infectious diseases in JAKi-treated patients with RA compared with those in IL-6i-treated patients with RA in unadjusted and propensity score-matching analysis. Furthermore, we found that the presence of ILD or DM and the use of GCs (>5.0 mg/day) might be predictors of serious infections in JAKi-treated patients with RA. However, the IRs for HZ after PSM were not significantly different between the JAKi and IL-6i groups. More safety studies with long-term follow-ups in real-world settings are needed to fully elucidate the safety profile of JAKi for the management of patients with RA in clinical practice.

Supplementary Materials: The following supporting information can be downloaded at: https://www.mdpi.com/article/10.3390/jcm13103000/s1, Supplementary Figure S1. The receiver operating characteristic curve representing the cut-off value of glucocorticoid dose in the prediction of serious infections. AUC: area under the curve. Supplementary Figure S2. Cumulative incidence curves of HZ in IL-6i-treated and JAKi-treated patients after propensity score matching. Kaplan–Meier curves show the cumulative incidence of HZ in patients treated with IL-6is ($n = 118$) and JAKis ($n = 118$). Significant differences were observed between IL-6i-treated and JAKi-treated groups ($p = 0.024$). The starting point (0 years) was the date on which the observations began. HZ: herpes zoster; JAKi: Janus kinase inhibitor; IL-6i: interleukin-6 inhibitor; CI: confidence interval; No: number.

Author Contributions: S.Y. had full access to all of the data in the study and takes responsibility for the integrity of the data and the accuracy of the data analysis. Study design: S.Y. and K.M.; acquisition of data: S.Y., M.M., E.S., T.K., Y.S., K.S., H.M., J.T., Y.F., N.M., T.A., S.S. and K.M.; analysis and interpretation of data: S.Y. and K.M.; manuscript preparation: S.Y., M.M., E.S., T.K. and K.M.; statistical analysis: S.Y. All authors have read and agreed to the published version of the manuscript.

Funding: The study was supported by the Japan Grant-in-Aid for Scientific Research (20K08777).

Institutional Review Board Statement: This study was conducted in accordance with the Declaration of Helsinki and approved by the institutional review boards of Fukushima Medical University (No. 2021-157/22 September 2021), Japanese Red Cross Fukushima Hospital (No. 55/7 February 2022), and Ohta Nishinouchi Hospital (No. 2022–8/31 May 2022).

Informed Consent Statement: Fukushima Medical University Ethics Review Committee, Fukushima Red Cross Hospital Ethics Committee, and Ota General Hospital Bioethics Committee waived the requirement of written informed consent for participation from the participants or the participants' legal guardians/next of kin because an opt-out strategy was chosen for the participants, and those who declined to provide informed consent were excluded.

Data Availability Statement: The raw data supporting the conclusions of this article will be made available by the authors, without undue reservation.

Acknowledgments: We are grateful to Sachiyo Kanno for her technical assistance in this study.

Conflicts of Interest: K.M. has received research grants from Chugai Pharmaceutical Co., Ltd., Taisho Pharmaceutical Holdings Co., Ltd., and Novartis Pharma K.K. The above-mentioned pharmaceutical companies were not involved in the study design, data collection and analysis, manuscript writing, and manuscript submission. The remaining authors declare that they have no conflicts of interests.

Abbreviations

ACPA	Anti-citrullinated protein antibodies
bDMARDs	Biologic disease-modifying antirheumatic drugs
CI	Confidence interval
csDMARDs	Bonventional synthetic disease-modifying antirheumatic drugs
DM	Diabetes mellitus
DMARDs	Disease-modifying antirheumatic drugs
EULAR	European Alliance of Associations for Rheumatology
GC	Glucocorticoid
HR	Hazard ratio
HZ	Herpes zoster
IL	Interleukin
IL-6i	Interleukin-6 inhibitor
ILD	Interstitial lung disease
IR	Incidence rate
IRR	Incidence rate ratio
JAK	Janus kinase
JAKi	Janus kinase inhibitor
MTX	Methotrexate
PSM	Propensity score matching
PY	Patient years
RA	Rheumatoid arthritis
RF	Rheumatoid factor
ROC	Receiver operating characteristic
STAT	Signal transducer and activator of transcription
TNFis	Tumor necrosis factor inhibitors
tsDMARDs	Targeted synthetic disease-modifying antirheumatic drugs

References

1. Nash, P.; Kerschbaumer, A.; Dörner, T.; Dougados, M.; Fleischmann, R.M.; Geissler, K.; McInnes, I.; Pope, J.E.; van der Heijde, D.; Stoffer-Marx, M.; et al. Points to consider for the treatment of immune-mediated inflammatory diseases with Janus kinase inhibitors: A consensus statement. *Ann. Rheum. Dis.* **2021**, *80*, 71–87. [CrossRef] [PubMed]
2. O'Shea, J.J.; Gadina, M. Selective Janus kinase inhibitors come of age. *Nat. Rev. Rheumatol.* **2019**, *15*, 74–75. [CrossRef]
3. Smolen, J.S.; Landewé, R.B.M.; Bijlsma, J.W.J.; Burmester, G.R.; Dougados, M.; Kerschbaumer, A.; McInnes, I.B.; Sepriano, A.; van Vollenhoven, R.F.; de Wit, M.; et al. EULAR recommendations for the management of rheumatoid arthritis with synthetic and biological disease-modifying antirheumatic drugs: 2019 update. *Ann. Rheum. Dis.* **2020**, *79*, 685–699. [CrossRef] [PubMed]
4. Doran, M.F.; Crowson, C.S.; Pond, G.R.; O'Fallon, W.M.; Gabriel, S.E. Frequency of infection in patients with rheumatoid arthritis compared with controls: A population-based study. *Arthritis Rheum.* **2002**, *46*, 2287–2293. [CrossRef]
5. Crowson, C.S.; Hoganson, D.D.; Fitz-Gibbon, P.D.; Matteson, E.L. Development and validation of a risk score for serious infection in patients with rheumatoid arthritis. *Arthritis Rheum.* **2012**, *64*, 2847–2855. [CrossRef]
6. Cohen, S.; Radominski, S.C.; Gomez-Reino, J.J.; Wang, L.; Krishnaswami, S.; Wood, S.P.; Soma, K.; Nduaka, C.I.; Kwok, K.; Valdez, H.; et al. Analysis of infections and all-cause mortality in phase II, phase III, and long-term extension studies of tofacitinib in patients with rheumatoid arthritis. *Arthritis Rheumatol.* **2014**, *66*, 2924–2937. [CrossRef] [PubMed]
7. Strand, V.; Ahadieh, S.; French, J.; Geier, J.; Krishnaswami, S.; Menon, S.; Checchio, T.; Tensfeldt, T.G.; Hoffman, E.; Riese, R.; et al. Systematic review and meta-analysis of serious infections with tofacitinib and biologic disease-modifying antirheumatic drug treatment in rheumatoid arthritis clinical trials. *Arthritis Res. Ther.* **2015**, *17*, 362. [CrossRef] [PubMed]
8. Uchida, T.; Iwamoto, N.; Fukui, S.; Morimoto, S.; Aramaki, T.; Shomura, F.; Aratake, K.; Eguchi, K.; Ueki, Y.; Kawakami, A. Comparison of risks of cancer, infection, and MACEs associated with JAK inhibitor and TNF inhibitor treatment: A multicenter cohort study. *Rheumatology* **2023**, *62*, 3358–3365. [CrossRef]
9. Ytterberg, S.R.; Bhatt, D.L.; Mikuls, T.R.; Koch, G.G.; Fleischmann, R.; Rivas, J.L.; Germino, R.; Menon, S.; Sun, Y.; Wang, C.; et al. Cardiovascular and Cancer Risk with Tofacitinib in Rheumatoid Arthritis. *N. Engl. J. Med.* **2022**, *386*, 316–326. [CrossRef]

10. Kremer, J.M.; Bingham, C.O., 3rd; Cappelli, L.C.; Greenberg, J.D.; Madsen, A.M.; Geier, J.; Rivas, J.L.; Onofrei, A.M.; Barr, C.J.; Pappas, D.A.; et al. Postapproval Comparative Safety Study of Tofacitinib and Biological Disease-Modifying Antirheumatic Drugs: 5-Year Results from a United States-Based Rheumatoid Arthritis Registry. *ACR Open Rheumatol.* **2021**, *3*, 173–184. [CrossRef]
11. Curtis, J.R.; Xie, F.; Yun, H.; Bernatsky, S.; Winthrop, K.L. Real-world comparative risks of herpes virus infections in tofacitinib and biologic-treated patients with rheumatoid arthritis. *Ann. Rheum. Dis.* **2016**, *75*, 1843–1847. [CrossRef]
12. Song, Y.J.; Cho, S.K.; Kim, H.; Kim, H.W.; Nam, E.; Jeon, J.Y.; Yoo, H.J.; Choi, C.B.; Kim, T.H.; Jun, J.B.; et al. Increased risk of herpes zoster with tofacitinib treatment in Korean patients with rheumatoid arthritis: A single-center prospective study. *Sci. Rep.* **2023**, *13*, 7877. [CrossRef] [PubMed]
13. Winthrop, K.L.; Curtis, J.R.; Lindsey, S.; Tanaka, Y.; Yamaoka, K.; Valdez, H.; Hirose, T.; Nduaka, C.I.; Wang, L.; Mendelsohn, A.M.; et al. Herpes Zoster and Tofacitinib: Clinical Outcomes and the Risk of Concomitant Therapy. *Arthritis Rheumatol.* **2017**, *69*, 1960–1968. [CrossRef] [PubMed]
14. Yoshida, S.; Miyata, M.; Suzuki, E.; Kanno, T.; Sumichika, Y.; Saito, K.; Matsumoto, H.; Temmoku, J.; Fujita, Y.; Matsuoka, N.; et al. Safety of JAK and IL-6 inhibitors in patients with rheumatoid arthritis: A multicenter cohort study. *Front. Immunol.* **2023**, *14*, 1267749. [CrossRef]
15. Aletaha, D.; Neogi, T.; Silman, A.J.; Funovits, J.; Felson, D.T.; Bingham, C.O., 3rd; Birnbaum, N.S.; Burmester, G.R.; Bykerk, V.P.; Cohen, M.D.; et al. 2010 Rheumatoid arthritis classification criteria: An American College of Rheumatology/European League Against Rheumatism collaborative initiative. *Arthritis Rheum.* **2010**, *62*, 2569–2581. [CrossRef] [PubMed]
16. Smolen, J.S.; Genovese, M.C.; Takeuchi, T.; Hyslop, D.L.; Macias, W.L.; Rooney, T.; Chen, L.; Dickson, C.L.; Riddle Camp, J.; Cardillo, T.E.; et al. Safety Profile of Baricitinib in Patients with Active Rheumatoid Arthritis with over 2 Years Median Time in Treatment. *J. Rheumatol.* **2019**, *46*, 7–18. [CrossRef] [PubMed]
17. Cohen, S.B.; Tanaka, Y.; Mariette, X.; Curtis, J.R.; Lee, E.B.; Nash, P.; Winthrop, K.L.; Charles-Schoeman, C.; Wang, L.; Chen, C.; et al. Long-term safety of tofacitinib up to 9.5 years: A comprehensive integrated analysis of the rheumatoid arthritis clinical development programme. *RMD Open* **2020**, *6*, e001395. [CrossRef]
18. Aucott, J.N. Glucocorticoids and infection. *Endocrinol. Metab. Clin. N. Am.* **1994**, *23*, 655–670. [CrossRef]
19. Cronin, O.; McKnight, O.; Keir, L.; Ralston, S.H.; Hirani, N.; Harris, H. A retrospective comparison of respiratory events with JAK inhibitors or rituximab for rheumatoid arthritis in patients with pulmonary disease. *Rheumatol. Int.* **2021**, *41*, 921–928. [CrossRef]
20. Kalyoncu, U.; Bilgin, E.; Erden, A.; Satış, H.; Tufan, A.; Tekgöz, E.; Ateş, A.; Coşkun, B.N.; Yağız, B.; Küçükşahin, O.; et al. Efficacy and safety of tofacitinib in rheumatoid arthritis-associated interstitial lung disease: TReasure real-life data. *Clin. Exp. Rheumatol.* **2022**, *40*, 2071–2077.
21. Messina, R.; Guggino, G.; Benfante, A.; Scichilone, N. Interstitial Lung Disease in Elderly Rheumatoid Arthritis Patients. *Drugs Aging* **2020**, *37*, 11–18. [CrossRef]
22. Sonomoto, K.; Tanaka, H.; Nguyen, T.M.; Yoshinari, H.; Nakano, K.; Nakayamada, S.; Tanaka, Y. Prophylaxis against pneumocystis pneumonia in rheumatoid arthritis patients treated with b/tsDMARDs: Insights from 3787 cases in the FIRST registry. *Rheumatology* **2022**, *61*, 1831–1840. [CrossRef]
23. Singh, N.; Gold, L.S.; Lee, J.; Wysham, K.D.; Andrews, J.S.; Makris, U.E.; England, B.R.; George, M.D.; Baker, J.F.; Jarvik, J.; et al. Frailty and Risk of Serious Infections in Patients With Rheumatoid Arthritis Treated With Biologic or Targeted-Synthetic Disease-Modifying Antirheumatic Drugs. *Arthritis Care Res.* **2023**, *76*, 627–635. [CrossRef]
24. Hanlon, P.; Fauré, I.; Corcoran, N.; Butterly, E.; Lewsey, J.; McAllister, D.; Mair, F.S. Frailty measurement, prevalence, incidence, and clinical implications in people with diabetes: A systematic review and study-level meta-analysis. *Lancet Healthy Longev.* **2020**, *1*, e106–e116. [CrossRef] [PubMed]
25. Farooqi, M.A.M.; O'Hoski, S.; Goodwin, S.; Makhdami, N.; Aziz, A.; Cox, G.; Wald, J.; Ryerson, C.J.; Beauchamp, M.K.; Hambly, N.; et al. Prevalence and prognostic impact of physical frailty in interstitial lung disease: A prospective cohort study. *Respirology* **2021**, *26*, 683–689. [CrossRef]
26. Smitten, A.L.; Choi, H.K.; Hochberg, M.C.; Suissa, S.; Simon, T.A.; Testa, M.A.; Chan, K.A. The risk of herpes zoster in patients with rheumatoid arthritis in the United States and the United Kingdom. *Arthritis Rheum.* **2007**, *57*, 1431–1438. [CrossRef] [PubMed]
27. Bechman, K.; Subesinghe, S.; Norton, S.; Atzeni, F.; Galli, M.; Cope, A.P.; Winthrop, K.L.; Galloway, J.B. A systematic review and meta-analysis of infection risk with small molecule JAK inhibitors in rheumatoid arthritis. *Rheumatology* **2019**, *58*, 1755–1766. [CrossRef]
28. O'Shea, J.J.; Schwartz, D.M.; Villarino, A.V.; Gadina, M.; McInnes, I.B.; Laurence, A. The JAK-STAT pathway: Impact on human disease and therapeutic intervention. *Annu. Rev. Med.* **2015**, *66*, 311–328. [CrossRef] [PubMed]
29. Au, K.; Reed, G.; Curtis, J.R.; Kremer, J.M.; Greenberg, J.D.; Strand, V.; Furst, D.E. High disease activity is associated with an increased risk of infection in patients with rheumatoid arthritis. *Ann. Rheum. Dis.* **2011**, *70*, 785–791. [CrossRef]

Disclaimer/Publisher's Note: The statements, opinions and data contained in all publications are solely those of the individual author(s) and contributor(s) and not of MDPI and/or the editor(s). MDPI and/or the editor(s) disclaim responsibility for any injury to people or property resulting from any ideas, methods, instructions or products referred to in the content.

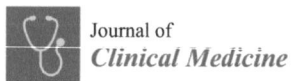

Review

Moving forward in Rheumatoid Arthritis-Associated Interstitial Lung Disease Screening

Javier Narváez

Department of Rheumatology, Hospital Universitario de Bellvitge & Bellvitge Biomedical Research Institute (IDIBELL), Feixa Llarga, s/n. Hospitalet de Llobregat, 08907 Barcelona, Spain; fjnarvaez@bellvitgehospital.cat

Abstract: Patients with rheumatoid arthritis (RA) are at increased risk of developing interstitial lung disease compared to the general population, a complication that is associated with significant morbidity and high mortality. Given its frequency and severity, ILD should always be considered during both the initial assessment and follow-up of RA patients. However, there is currently no consensus on which RA patients should be screened for ILD. In recent years, several scientific societies have developed specific screening proposals. According to the recommendations of the Spanish, American, and Austrian rheumatology societies, it is not necessary to screen all individuals with RA, and it should be tailored to each patient based on clinical risk factors. In contrast, the Portuguese Societies of Rheumatology and Pulmonology advocate for systematic screening of all RA patients. Risk factors for the development of ILD in RA patients are well identified, and several screening tools for RA-ILD based on these risk factors have been developed. However, all of these tools still require further validation. To address this issue, the ANCHOR-RA study, a multinational cross-sectional initiative, has been launched to develop a multivariable model for predicting RA-ILD, which could provide valuable guidance for screening practices in clinical settings. In addition to certain biochemical and genetic predictive markers, lung ultrasound appears to be a useful screening tool. When combined with clinical evaluation and risk factor assessment, it can help identify which patients require a thoracic HRCT evaluation, which remains the gold standard for confirming an ILD diagnosis.

Keywords: rheumatoid arthritis; interstitial lung disease; screening; risk factors; lung ultrasonography

1. Introduction

Interstitial lung disease (ILD) is one of the most prevalent and severe extra-articular manifestations of rheumatoid arthritis (RA), significantly contributing to both morbidity and mortality [1–7]. In patients with RA, the most frequent subtypes of ILD are usual interstitial pneumonia (UIP) and non-specific interstitial pneumonia (NSIP). UIP associated with RA-ILD phenotypically resembles UIP associated with idiopathic pulmonary fibrosis (IPF), both of which carry a high risk of progressive pulmonary fibrosis (PPF) and increased short-term mortality. Additionally, some RA patients with NSIP-type ILD may also experience progressive fibrosis [7].

The clinical course of RA-ILD is highly variable (8–10). In some patients, the disease progresses to PPF, characterized by a rapid decline in lung function, rapid progression to chronic respiratory failure, and increased risk of premature mortality. Although RA-ILD can significantly impact patient prognosis, there is ongoing debate about when, whom, and how to screen for this complication. This review examines the current landscape of RA-ILD screening practices, highlights recent advancements, and explores future directions in this area.

2. Why Is Screening Necessary? Understanding the Extent of the Problem

ILD can develop at any point during the course of RA. In more than half of the cases, ILD occurs after the diagnosis of RA, typically within the first 5 to 10 years [1–10]. In these cases, late diagnosis is not uncommon, as lung involvement is often asymptomatic or presents with only mild symptoms in its early stages. Indeed, when all individuals with RA were screened for ILD using thoracic high-resolution computed tomography (HRCT), a significant percentage of subclinical disease was detected (ranging from 11.9% to 55.7%), confirming that this complication is frequently underdiagnosed [11,12]. Less frequently, ILD may manifest at the onset of RA or even precede the joint manifestations by several months or years. Data from our early RA cohort indicate that these situations occur in 32.5% and 17.5% of cases, respectively [13]. In the latter circumstance, RA-ILD is often misdiagnosed as an idiopathic form, despite the differences in prognosis and treatment [1–3,6,14].

Although there have been significant improvements in prognosis over the past 25 years [15], ILD remains the second leading cause of death in RA patients, following cardiovascular complications. Approximately 55% of RA-ILD patients experience disease progression [16,17], with an estimated 40% meeting the criteria for PPF within 5 years of onset [18,19]. Patients with RA-ILD have an adjusted mortality risk that is 3- to 10-fold higher than that of RA patients without this complication, regardless of follow-up duration or the presence of comorbidities [4,6,20]. The average survival time following an RA-ILD diagnosis ranges from 2.6 to 8.1 years [5].

3. Screening for RA-ILD: Recommendations by Scientific Societies

Rheumatologists play a crucial role in screening patients with RA for ILD. Early detection and assessment of RA-ILD are essential for initiating treatment promptly, as patients may already have significantly impaired lung function at the time of RA-ILD diagnosis. A pivotal study with 167 patients revealed that, at the time of diagnosis, 14% of RA-ILD patients had a forced vital capacity (FVC) below 50% of the predicted value, and 29% had a hemoglobin-corrected diffusing capacity for carbon monoxide (DLCO) below 40% of the predicted value [16]. Another recent study showed that delayed diagnosis of RA-ILD was linked to higher mortality rates [21]. However, there is still no consensus on which RA patients should be screened for ILD.

In the absence of evidence supporting the effectiveness of universal screening, a reasonable strategy is to implement selective screening based on clinical risk factors.

This approach was exemplified by the AR-EPIDSER Project, a collaborative effort between the Spanish Society of Rheumatology (SER) and the Spanish Society of Pulmonology and Thoracic Surgery (SEPAR). The project developed a multidisciplinary proposal for screening criteria aimed at the early identification of patients with RA-ILD [22].

Based on published evidence and using consensus-based techniques (Delphi method), screening for ILD was proposed in three scenarios: (1) patients with a history of respiratory symptoms (cough and/or dyspnea) lasting more than 3 months; (2) patients with dry "velcro-like" crackles on respiratory auscultation, even if asymptomatic; and (3) in patients without respiratory symptoms and with normal respiratory auscultation, screening will be based on the score obtained according to their number of risk factors for developing this complication [22]. Details of the proposal and the frequency of screening are shown in Tables 1 and 2.

Table 1. The AR-EPIDSER Project: proposed screening criteria for interstitial lung disease in patients with rheumatoid arthritis [22].

ILD Screening Will Be Conducted in These Three Clinical Scenarios	
(1) Patients with respiratory symptoms (such as cough and/or dyspnea) lasting for more than 3 months. (2) Patients with dry, "velcro-like" crackles on respiratory auscultation, even if they are asymptomatic. (3) For patients without respiratory symptoms and with normal respiratory auscultation, screening will be based on the score calculated from the number of risk factors present for developing this complication. Any patient with a score of ≥ 5 points will be considered eligible for screening.	
List of variables and the suggested score for each variable used in the overall calculation	*Score*
Older age ($\geq$60 years)	2
Male sex	1
Tobacco exposure (active or ex-smoker)	
$\leq$20 pack-years	2
>20 pack-years	3
RA duration of more than 5 years	1
Persistent moderate to high disease activity: an average DAS28-ESR > 3.2 from the time of diagnosis in early RA (defined as symptom duration $\leq$ 12 months) or a DAS28-ESR > 3.2 for at least 6 months in established RA	1
Serology (only the criterion with the highest weighting is counted towards the total score):	
RF positive > 3 times the ULN	1
ACPA-positive $\leq$ 3 times above the ULN	2
ACPA-positive > 3 times the ULN	3
Family history of ILD	1
Screening approach For patients with cough and/or dyspnea >3 months, start with CXR and PFTs (spirometry, %pDLCO). Based on results, consider thoracic HRCT * For patients with dry 'velcro-like' crackles on auscultation, perform HRCT directly. In asymptomatic patients with normal auscultation, if the risk score is 5–6, start with CXR and PFTs (spirometry and %pDLCO); consider thoracic HRCT based on results *. If score $\geq$7, perform HRCT directly	

Abbreviations: ACPA: anti-cyclic citrullinated peptide antibodies; CXR: chest X ray; DAS: Disease Activity Score; HRCT: high-resolution computed tomography; ILD: diffuse interstitial lung disease; %pDLCO: predicted diffusing capacity for carbon monoxide corrected for hemoglobin; PFTs: pulmonary function tests; RA: rheumatoid arthritis; RF: rheumatoid factor; ULN: upper normal limit. * If PFTs are unavailable or there is a long waiting list, consider thoracic HRCT directly to expedite diagnosis. Direct HRCT doesn't exclude PFTs for ILD severity assessment.

Table 2. Frequency of screening for interstitial lung disease in patients with rheumatoid arthritis according to the recommendations of the AR-EPIDSER Project [22].

Frequency of Screening
During the follow-up of RA patients, auscultation should be performed at least annually, along with specific questioning about respiratory symptoms and an assessment of risk factors for ILD, based on the scoring system outlined above. If 'Velcro-like' crackles or respiratory symptoms (cough and/or dyspnea >3 months) are detected during follow-up, repeat screening tests as recommended, regardless of prior negative results For asymptomatic patients with normal respiratory auscultation and a total score of $\geq$5, repeat screening tests (including spirometry and %pDLCO) after one year, even if the initial results are negative.

Abbreviations: ILD: diffuse interstitial lung disease; %pDLCO: predicted diffusing capacity for carbon monoxide corrected for hemoglobin.

This initiative is based on the consensus of a national panel of experts, and its effectiveness in identifying these patients in clinical practice will need to be confirmed through future validation studies. To address this, a multicenter study sponsored by the SER is currently underway to evaluate its clinical utility. While awaiting the results, which may take some time to become available, we conducted an external validation study of the AR-EPIDSER criteria in our cohort of early RA patients diagnosed between 2003 and

2023 [23]. In all cases, systematic screening for ILD was performed at diagnosis using a targeted medical history, respiratory auscultation, chest X-ray (CXR), and pulmonary function tests (PFTs), including %pFVC and %pDLCO. In cases of respiratory symptoms, velcro-like dry crackles, or abnormalities on CXR or PFTs, a thoracic HRCT was performed. Of the 146 patients included, 28 (19.1%) were finally diagnosed with ILD by HRCT. Ninety patients (61.6%) met the AR-EPIDSER screening criteria for ILD at the time of RA diagnosis. Among these patients, 28.8% had either clinical or subclinical ILD. Of the 56 patients who did not meet the screening criteria at the onset of RA, only 1.3% developed ILD during follow-up. The sensitivity of the criteria in our cohort was 92.8%, and the specificity was 45.7% (data pending publication). In 12 patients, ILD preceded the onset of joint symptoms. Excluding these cases, where screening would not have been necessary, the sensitivity was 87.5%, while specificity remained at 45.7%. If the threshold is lowered to a score of ≥ 4 (instead of the cut-off of ≥ 5 established in the original document), sensitivity increases to 90.91%, but specificity decreases to 23.8%.

Based on these results, the AR-EPIDSER criteria for ILD screening demonstrate a sensitivity greater than 90% in patients with early RA, supporting their use in daily clinical practice. Given that the primary goal of screening is the early detection of this complication, it is essential to employ a highly sensitive test in the initial phase to identify as many cases as possible. This approach is consistent with the recommendations outlined in the policy framework for population screening by the Public Health Committee of the Spanish Ministry of Health [24].

After the publication of the AR-EPIDSER criteria, various scientific societies drafted specific recommendations for ILD screening in patients with RA. Consistent with the SER/SEPAR proposal, neither the American College of Rheumatology (ACR) nor the Austrian Society of Rheumatology recommends universal screening for ILD in RA patients. The recently published 2023 ACR/American College of Chest Physicians (CHEST) Guideline for the Screening and Monitoring of ILD in People with Systemic Autoimmune Rheumatic Diseases emphasizes that screening should be tailored to individual RA patients at high risk for ILD [25]. Risk factors that may warrant screening include high titers of rheumatoid factor (RF) or anti-cyclic citrullinated peptide antibodies (ACPA), cigarette smoking, older age at RA onset, and high disease activity. Screening should be conducted using PFTs and thoracic HRCT. If the initial screening is negative, it may be repeated annually. If ILD is confirmed, it is recommended to repeat PFTs every 3 to 12 months during the first year and adjust the frequency thereafter based on the patient's clinical progression.

In the recommendations of the Austrian Society of Rheumatology, developed through a Delphi consensus, no agreement was reached on the specific combination of risk factors that would justify screening in asymptomatic patients [26]. The panel concluded that there is currently insufficient evidence to support any specific scoring or weighting of these risk factors. Consequently, they left the decision to the physician's discretion, emphasizing that the assessment of risk factors and the decision to initiate continuous RA-ILD screening should be made on a case-by-case basis.

In contrast, the recommendations of the Portuguese Societies of Rheumatology and Pulmonology [27] advocate for systematic screening of all RA patients using PFTs and CXR. If abnormalities are detected, a thoracic HRCT should be conducted. The frequency of reevaluation depends on the presence or absence of risk factors. For high-risk patients, it is recommended to perform PFTs annually and HRCT every two years. In low-risk patients, PFTs should only be repeated if symptoms develop.

4. Tools for Estimating the Risk of ILD in RA Patients

The main recognized risk factors for the development of ILD in RA include male sex, older age, late disease onset, duration of RA, tobacco exposure, moderate or high sustained RA activity, seropositivity for RF and/or ACPA, and polymorphisms in the MUC5B gene [4,7,15,22,28]. In addition to the Delphi panel AR-EPIDSER proposal, several

RA-ILD screening tools based on these risk factors have been developed. However, all of these tools require further validation.

Paulin et al. [29] proposed a risk score model based on five variables: male sex (1 point), smoking status (2 points), the presence of extra-articular manifestations (1 point), Clinical Disease Activity Index (CDAI > 28: 1 point), and erythrocyte sedimentation rate (ESR > 80 mm/h: 4 points). A total score of 2 points yields a sensitivity of 90.3% and a specificity of 63.64% for identifying RA-ILD. When the score increases to 4 points, sensitivity decreases to 51.9% while specificity rises to 90.9%.

A simpler risk estimation model, the Four Factor Risk Score, was proposed by Koduri et al. [30]. This model is based on 4 risk factors: smoking (current or past), advanced age, RF, and ACPA. By incorporating these factors, a risk score system was developed using multivariate logistic regression models, which classifies patients as low- or high-risk on a scale of 0 to 9 points. A threshold of 5 points provides a sensitivity of 86%, a specificity of 85%, and an area under the curve (AUC) of 0.76 (Table 3).

Table 3. Four Factor Risk Score model [30].

	Score		
	0	1	2
Age at onset of RA	<40	40–70	>70
Tobacco exposure	Never	Ex-smoker or current smoker	
RF titer	Negative	Weak positive	Positive
ACPA titer	Negative	Weak positive	Positive

Abbreviations: ACPA, anti–citrullinated peptide antibody; RA: rheumatoid arthritis; RF: rheumatoid factor.

Another model, which incorporates factors such as sex, tobacco exposure, RF, C-reactive protein, and plasma matrix metalloproteinase (MMP)-3, showed a C-index of 0.826 for accuracy in detecting RA-ILD compared to evaluations conducted by a multidisciplinary team [31].

The VECTOR algorithm, designed to detect velcro-like crackles in lung sounds recorded by an electronic stethoscope, demonstrated 93% sensitivity and 77% specificity for identifying ILD on HRCT in RA patients [32]. However, the availability of such equipment is limited.

A predictive score based on sex, age at RA onset, the RA Disease Activity Score in 28 joints using ESR (DAS28-ESR), and the MUC5B rs35705950 risk allele showed 75% sensitivity and 85% specificity for identifying RA-ILD when compared to HRCT [33] but this tool may be challenging to implement in clinical practice.

Finally, the VARA-ILD Combined Risk Score model was developed using data from a North American cohort of veterans with RA. This model integrates five single nucleotide polymorphisms (MUC5B, DSP, LRRC34, OBFC1, and FAM13A) along with male sex, age, smoking status, disease activity assessed by DAS-CRP, and RF positivity, achieving an AUC of 0.67 [34].

The ANCHOR-RA study is a multinational, cross-sectional study designed to create a multivariable model for predicting RA-ILD, which could be applied to guide screening for RA-ILD in clinical practice [35]. The study will enroll 1200 participants from USA, UK, Germany, France, Italy, and Spain, all of whom will present with at least two risk factors for ILD, such as male gender, smoking history, older age at RA diagnosis, or high disease activity. This study will assess the prevalence of RA-ILD and investigate the effectiveness of lung ultrasound as a screening tool, comparing its accuracy to HRCT for detecting ILD.

5. Biochemical and Genetic Markers

In the search for biochemical markers to predict the development of ILD in RA, neither Krebs von den Lungen 6 (KL-6) nor anticarbamylated protein antibodies have demonstrated predictive value superior to that of ACPA or RF [36–38].

Preliminary data suggest that angiogenic T cells could serve as a useful biomarker for this purpose [39]. Additionally, findings from a recent multicentre, prospective RA cohort study have revealed that elevated concentrations of MMPs, particularly MMP-7 and MMP-9, are associated with both the presence of RA-ILD and an increased risk of developing incident ILD [40]. This association was especially strong for MMP-7, with participants in the highest quartile of MMP-7 concentrations having nearly fourfold increased odds of prevalent ILD and a twofold increased risk of incident ILD, typically developing within an average of four years following cohort enrolment. Notably, higher plasma MMP-7 concentrations were predominantly observed in cases of prevalent RA-ILD with a UIP pattern, while MMP-9 showed a modest correlation with impaired %pFVC. In recent years, accumulating clinical evidence has supported the role of MMPs in the pathogenesis of RA-ILD, independent of articular disease activity [40,41].

Regarding genetic biomarkers, the gain-of-function MUC5B rs35705950 promoter variant has been identified as a significant risk factor for both IPF and RA-ILD with a UIP phenotype [42]. Additionally, mutations in telomere-related genes such as DSP, LRRC34, OBFC1, and FAM13A, which are associated with accelerated telomere shortening, have also been implicated [34]. As previously mentioned, these genetic factors are beginning to be incorporated into predictive risk models [33,34].

6. Usefulness of Lung Ultrasound

The role of lung ultrasound in screening for ILD in various systemic autoimmune rheumatic diseases, including RA, has been increasingly investigated in recent years. This technique is based on interpreting findings related to changes in the lung's physical properties, which are detected as artifacts rather than anatomical structures. Studies assessing the usefulness of lung ultrasound for ILD screening have primarily focused on evaluating B-lines and the pleural line. More recently, research has begun to explore diaphragm function [43,44].

The B lines are reverberation artifacts associated with septal thickening. They appear as well-defined hyperechoic vertical lines that begin at the pleural line and extend to the bottom of the screen without fading. B lines, also referred to as "comet-tails," are artefacts that occur when the air content in the pulmonary parenchyma partially decreases and/or the interstitial space expands in volume. They move synchronically with lung sliding. B lines are not exclusive to ILD, as they can also be observed in other conditions such as pulmonary oedema, and they do not allow for differentiation between the inflammatory or fibrotic phases of ILD [43,44]. The presence of multiple B-lines is a key ultrasound indicator of lung interstitial syndrome. In 2012, efforts to standardize this finding resulted in a consensus definition, establishing the diagnostic criterion as the detection of three or more B-lines in at least two areas on each side of the chest [45]. Pleural line abnormalities include irregularities, thickening, microscopic consolidation, fragmentation, and subpleural nodules. The cut-off for considering a pleural line as thickened is generally set at 2.4 mm, although some authors suggest 2.8 mm [43,44]. For diaphragm evaluation, it is necessary to assess diaphragmatic dysfunction, inspiratory thickness, expiratory thickness, and the thickening fraction.

The strongest evidence supporting the use of lung ultrasound has been published in systemic sclerosis (SSc), where the assessment of appearance, criterion, and construct validity is more advanced, both in the early and advanced stages of the disease. In this context, a strong correlation has been observed between B lines and thoracic HRCT or PFTs (including %pFVC and %pDLCO) [43,44]. In terms of pleural line evaluation, some researchers suggest it has a higher negative predictive value for ILD than B lines and better differentiation from healthy controls [44].

To date, seven published studies [46–52] have evaluated the usefulness of pulmonary ultrasound in screening for ILD in RA (see Table 4). In cases where ILD is suspected, mainly because of respiratory symptoms and/or dry crackles on auscultation, the sensitivity of pulmonary ultrasound compared with thoracic HRCT ranges from 62.2% to 98.3%.

Specificity ranges from 14.7% to 97.6%, positive predictive value from 42.2% to 88.4%, and negative predictive value from 69.5% to 87.5%. When the technique is used to detect asymptomatic or subclinical DILD, sensitivity ranges from 90.6% to 97.1%, specificity from 73% to 97.3%, positive predictive value from 59.2% to 94.3%, and negative predictive value from 94.7% to 98.6%.

Thus, lung ultrasound has proven to be a valuable tool for systematic screening of ILD in patients with RA, demonstrating very high sensitivity and negative predictive value. It serves as a useful complement to clinical information in identifying patients who are candidates for thoracic HRCT, which remains the gold standard for confirming the diagnosis of ILD. Moreover, Otaola et al. [46] found the diagnostic sensitivity of pulmonary ultrasound to be higher than that of PFT and of dry crackles on auscultation.

Table 4. Studies on the usefulness of lung ultrasound in detecting interstitial lung disease in patients with rheumatoid arthritis.

	Number of Patients	Population	Number of Intercostal Spaces Evaluated	Diagnostic Criteria for ILD	Results (Compared with Chest HRCT)
Cogliati C et al. [46]	39 RA	Suspected ILD	72 and 8	72 IS >17 B-lines 8 IS >10 B-lines	*8 IS >10 B-lines* Sensitivity 69% Specificity 88% *72 IS >17 B-lines* Sensitivity 92% Specificity 56%
Moazedi-Fuerst FC et al. [47]	64 RA and 40 healthy controls	No respiratory symptoms, normal PFTs findings	18	B-lines in ≥2 chest areas Pleural thickening >2.8 mm and at least 1 subpleural nodule	Sensitivity 97.1% Specificity 97.3% PPV: 94.3% NPV: 98.6%
Otaola M et al. [48]	106	No respiratory symptoms (ILD detected by thoracic HRCT in 32)	14	≥5 B-lines	Sensitivity: 90.6% Specificity: 73% PPV: 59.2% NPV: 94.7% AUC: 0.82 *PFTs* Sensitivity %pFVC: 28.1% Specificity %pDLCO: 63.3% *Crackles on auscultation* Sensitivity: 68.8%
Santos Moreno P et al. [49]	192	Respiratory symptoms and/or crackles on auscultation	72	>11 B-lines	Sensitivity: 98.3% Specificity: 14.7% PPV: 64.2% NPV: 84.6% AUC: 0.63

Table 4. Cont.

	Number of Patients	Population	Number of Intercostal Spaces Evaluated	Diagnostic Criteria for ILD	Results (Compared with Chest HRCT)
Mena Vázquez N et al. [50]	71	35 with ILD and 36 without ILD	72 y 8	72 IS > 5 B-lines 8 IS > 5 B-lines	A 8-space reduced score showed a similar total predictive capacity than 72-space score. *8 IS >5 B lines* Sensitivity: 62.2% Specificity: 91.3% PPV: 88.4 NPV: 69.5%
Di Carlo M et al. [51]	72	Suspected ILD	14	>9 B-lines	Sensitivity: 70% Specificity: 97.6% AUC: 0.83 Positive likelihood ratio of 29.4
Sofíudóttir BK et al. [52]	77	Respiratory symptoms	14	≥10 B-lines or pleural line abnormalities (thickening and fragmentation)	Sensitivity: 82.6% Specificity: 51.9% PPV: 42.2% NPV: 87.5%

Abbreviations: AUC: area under the curve; HRCT: high-resolution computed tomography; ILD: interstitial lung disease; IS: intercostal space; NPV: negative predictive value; %pDLCO: predicted diffusing capacity for carbon monoxide corrected for hemoglobin; %pFVC: predicted forced vital capacity; PFTs: pulmonary function tests; PPV: positive predictive value.

Major limitations of the technique include the considerable heterogeneity in the published evidence, particularly regarding B line echographic counts and indexes, the cut-off points set to define the disease, and the types of equipment used (from high-range ultrasound devices to pocket-size devices), probes (cardiac, linear, or convex), and the examiner's experience. Since the first index based on 72 intercostal spaces, counts have gradually decreased to 8 intercostal spaces in the search for easier performance while maintaining precision. However, there is still no consensus on the learning curve, procedural steps, or validated index needed to ensure its effective and reliable use in clinical practice.

Funding: This research received no external funding.

Conflicts of Interest: The author declares no conflict of interest.

References

1. Farquhar, H.; Vassallo, R.; Edwards, A.L.; Matteson, E.L. Pulmonary complications of rheumatoid arthritis. *Semin. Respir. Crit. Care Med.* **2019**, *40*, 194–207. [CrossRef] [PubMed]
2. Yunt, Z.X.; Solomon, J.J. Lung disease in rheumatoid arthritis. *Rheum. Dis. Clin. N. Am.* **2015**, *41*, 225–236. [CrossRef] [PubMed]
3. Spagnolo, P.; Lee, J.S.; Sverzellati, N.; Rossi, G.; Cottin, V. The lung in rheumatoid arthritis: Focus on interstitial lung disease. *Arthritis Rheumatol.* **2018**, *70*, 1544–1554. [CrossRef]
4. Bongartz, T.; Nannini, C.; Medina-Velasquez, Y.F.; Achenbach, S.J.; Crowson, C.S.; Ryu, J.H.; Vassallo, R.; Gabriel, S.E.; Matteson, E.L. Incidence and mortality of interstitial lung disease in rheumatoid arthritis: A population-based study. *Arthritis Rheum.* **2010**, *62*, 1583–1591. [CrossRef]
5. Assayag, D.; Lubin, M.; Lee, J.S.; King, T.E.; Collard, H.R.; Ryerson, C.J. Predictors of mortality in rheumatoid arthritis-related interstitial lung disease. *Respirology* **2014**, *19*, 493–500. [CrossRef]
6. Hyldgaard, C.; Hilberg, O.; Pedersen, A.B.; Ulrichsen, S.P.; Løkke, A.; Bendstrup, E.; Ellingsen, T. A population-based cohort study of rheumatoid arthritis-associated interstitial lung disease: Comorbidity and mortality. *Ann. Rheum. Dis.* **2017**, *76*, 1700–1706. [CrossRef]

7. Koduri, G.; Solomon, J.J. Identification, monitoring, and management of rheumatoid arthritis-associated interstitial lung disease. *Arthritis Rheumatol.* **2023**, *75*, 2067–2077. [CrossRef]
8. Shidara, K.; Hoshi, D.; Inoue, E.; Yamada, T.; Nakajima, A.; Taniguchi, A.; Hara, M.; Momohara, S.; Kamatani, N.; Yamanaka, H. Incidence of risk factors for interstitial pneumonia in patients with rheumatoid arthritis in a large Japanese observational cohort, I.O.R.R.A. *Mod. Rheumatol.* **2010**, *20*, 280–286. [CrossRef]
9. Koduri, G.; Norton, S.; Young, A.; Cox, N.; Davies, P.; Devlin, J.; Dixey, J.; Gough, A.; Prouse, P.; Winfield, J.; et al. ERAS (Early Rheumatoid Arthritis Study). Interstitial lung disease has a poor prognosis in rheumatoid arthritis: Results from an inception cohort. *Rheumatology* **2010**, *49*, 1483–1489. [CrossRef]
10. Duarte, A.C.; Porter, J.C.; Leandro, M.J. The lung in a cohort of rheumatoid arthritis patients—An overview of different types of involvement and treatment. *Rheumatology* **2019**, *58*, 2031–2038. [CrossRef]
11. Bilgici, A.; Ulusoy, H.; Kuru, O.; Celenk, C.; Unsal, M.; Danaci, M. Pulmonary involvement in rheumatoid arthritis. *Rheumatol. Int.* **2005**, *25*, 429–435. [CrossRef] [PubMed]
12. Mori, S.; Cho, I.; Koga, Y.; Sugimoto, M. Comparison of pulmonary abnormalities on high-resolution computed tomography in patients with early versus longstanding rheumatoid arthritis. *J. Rheumatol.* **2008**, *35*, 1513–1521. [PubMed]
13. Aguilar, M.; Narváez, J.; Robles Pérez, A.; Luburich, P.; Vicens, V.; Bermudo, G.; Bolivar, S.; Maymó, P.; Palacios, J.; Roig, M.; et al. Primary lung involvement in early-onset rheumatoid arthritis [Abstract 312]. *Reumatol. Clínica* **2024**, *20* (Suppl. 2), S409.
14. Gizinski, A.M.; Mascolo, M.; Loucks, J.L.; Kervitsky, A.; Meehan, R.T.; Brown, K.K.; Holers, V.M.; Deane, K.D. Rheumatoid arthritis (RA)-specific autoantibodies in patients with interstitial lung disease absence of clinically apparent articular RA. *Clin. Rheumatol.* **2009**, *28*, 611–613. [CrossRef]
15. Kelly, C.A.; Nisar, M.; Arthanari, S.; Carty, S.; Woodhead, F.A.; Price-Forbes, A.; Middleton, D.; Dempsey, O.; Miller, D.; Basu, N.; et al. Rheumatoid arthritis related interstitial lung disease—Improving outcomes over 25 years: A large multicentre UK study. *Rheumatology* **2021**, *60*, 1882–1890. [CrossRef]
16. Zamora-Legoff, J.A.; Krause, M.L.; Crowson, C.S.; Ryu, J.H.; Matteson, E.L. Progressive decline of lung function in rheumatoid arthritis-associated interstitial lung disease. *Arthritis Rheumatol.* **2017**, *69*, 542–549. [CrossRef]
17. Hyldgaard, C.; Ellingsen, T.; Hilberg, O.; Bendstrup, E. Rheumatoid arthritis-associated interstitial lung disease: Clinical characteristics and predictors of mortality. *Respiration* **2019**, *98*, 455–460. [CrossRef]
18. Spagnolo, P.; Distler, O.; Ryerson, C.J.; Tzouvelekis, A.; Lee, J.S.; Bonella, F.; Bouros, D.; Hoffmann-Vold, A.M.; Crestani, B.; Matteson, E.L. Mechanisms of progressive fibrosis in connective tissue disease (CTD)-associated interstitial lung diseases (ILDs). *Ann. Rheum. Dis.* **2021**, *80*, 143–150. [CrossRef]
19. Olson, A.; Hartmann, N.; Patnaik, P.; Wallace, L.; Schlenker-Herceg, R.; Nasser, M.; Richeldi, L.; Hoffmann-Vold, A.M.; Cottin, V. Estimation of the prevalence of progressive fibrosing interstitial lung diseases: Systematic literature review and data from a physician survey. *Adv. Ther.* **2021**, *38*, 854–867. [CrossRef]
20. Kim, D.; Cho, S.K.; Choi, C.B.; Choe, J.Y.; Chung, W.T.; Hong, S.J.; Jun, J.B.; Jung, Y.O.; Kim, T.H.; Kim, T.J.; et al. Impact of interstitial lung disease on mortality of patients with rheumatoid arthritis. *Rheumatol. Int.* **2017**, *37*, 1735–1745. [CrossRef]
21. Cano-Jiménez, E.; Vázquez Rodríguez, T.; Martín-Robles, I.; Castillo Villegas, D.; Juan García, J.; Bollo de Miguel, E.; Robles-Pérez, A.; Ferrer Galván, M.; Mouronte Roibas, C.; Herrera Lara, S.; et al. Diagnostic delay of associated interstitial lung disease increases mortality in rheumatoid arthritis. *Sci. Rep.* **2021**, *11*, 9184. [CrossRef] [PubMed]
22. Narváez, J.; Aburto, M.; Seoane-Mato, D.; Bonilla, G.; Acosta, O.; Candelas, G.; Cano-Jiménez, E.; Castellví, I.; González-Ruiz, J.M.; Corominas, H.; et al. Screening criteria for interstitial lung disease associated to rheumatoid arthritis: Expert proposal based on Delphi methodology. *Reumatol. Clin.* **2023**, *19*, 74–81. [CrossRef] [PubMed]
23. Aguilar, M.; Narváez, J.; Roig, M.; Maymó, P.; Palacios, J.; Nolla, J.M. Validation Study in Early-Onset Rheumatoid Arthritis of the SER/SEPAR Criteria for Screening Interstitial Lung Disease [Abstract 328]. *Reumatol. Clínica* **2024**, *20* (Suppl. 2), S422–S423.
24. Documento Marco Sobre Cribado Poblacional de la Comisión de Salud Pública del Ministerio de Sanidad. Available online: https://www.sanidad.gob.es/areas/promocionPrevencion/cribado/documentosTecnicos/docs/Cribado_poblacional.pdf (accessed on 16 August 2024).
25. Johnson, S.R.; Bernstein, E.J.; Bolster, M.B.; Chung, J.H.; Danoff, S.K.; George, M.D.; Khanna, D.; Guyatt, G.; Mirza, R.D.; Aggarwal, R.; et al. 2023 American College of Rheumatology (ACR)/American College of Chest Physicians (CHEST) Guideline for the Screening and Monitoring of Interstitial Lung Disease in People with Systemic Autoimmune Rheumatic Diseases. *Arthritis Care Res.* **2024**, *76*, 1070–1082. [CrossRef]
26. Hackner, K.; Hütter, L.; Flick, H.; Grohs, M.; Kastrati, K.; Kiener, H.; Lang, D.; Mosheimer-Feistritzer, B.; Prosch, H.; Rath, E.; et al. Screening for rheumatoid arthritis-associated interstitial lung disease-a Delphi-based consensus statement. *Z. Rheumatol.* **2024**, *83*, 160–168. [CrossRef]
27. Morais, A.; Duarte, A.C.; Fernandes, M.O.; Borba, A.; Ruano, C.; Marques, I.D.; Calha, J.; Branco, J.C.; Pereira, J.M.; Salvador, M.J.; et al. Early detection of interstitial lung disease in rheumatic diseases: A joint statement from the Portuguese Pulmonology Society, the Portuguese Rheumatology Society, and the Portuguese Radiology and Nuclear Medicine Society. *Pulmonology*, 2023; *online ahead of print*. [CrossRef]
28. Rodríguez Portal, J.A.; Brito García, N.; Díaz Del Campo Fontecha, P.; Valenzuela, C.; Ortiz, A.M.; Nieto, M.A.; Mena-Vázquez, N.; Cano-Jiménez, E.; Castellví, I.; Aburto, M.; et al. SER-SEPAR recommendations for the management of rheumatoid arthritis-related interstitial lung disease. Part 1, Epidemiology, risk factors and prognosis. *Reumatol. Clin.* **2022**, *18*, 443–452. [CrossRef]

29. Paulin, F.; Doyle, T.J.; Mercado, J.F.; Fassola, L.; Fernández, M.; Caro, F.; Alberti, M.L.; Espíndola, M.E.C.; Buschiazzo, E. Development of a risk indicator score for the identification of interstitial lung disease in patients with rheumatoid arthritis. *Reumatol. Clin.* **2021**, *17*, 207–211. [CrossRef]
30. Koduri, G.M.; Podlasek, A.; Pattapola, S.; Zhang, J.; Laila, D.; Nandagudi, A.; Dubey, S.; Kelly, C. Four-factor risk score for the prediction of interstitial lung disease in rheumatoid arthritis. *Rheumatol. Int.* **2023**, *43*, 1515–1523. [CrossRef]
31. Xue, J.; Hu, W.; Wu, S.; Wang, J.; Chi, S.; Liu, X. Development of a risk nomogram model for identifying interstitial lung disease in patients with rheumatoid arthritis. *Front. Immunol.* **2022**, *13*, 823669. [CrossRef]
32. Manfredi, A.; Cassone, G.; Cerri, S.; Venerito, V.; Fedele, A.L.; Trevisani, M.; Furini, F.; Addimanda, O.; Pancaldi, F.; Della Casa, G.; et al. Diagnostic accuracy of a velcro sound detector (VECTOR) for interstitial lung disease in rheumatoid arthritis patients: The InSPIRAtE validation study (INterStitial pneumonia in rheumatoid ArThritis with an electronic device). *BMC Pulm. Med.* **2019**, *19*, 111. [CrossRef]
33. Juge, P.A.; Granger, B.; Debray, M.P.; Ebstein, E.; Louis-Sidney, F.; Kedra, J.; Doyle, T.J.; Borie, R.; Constantin, A.; Combe, B.; et al. A risk score to detect subclinical rheumatoid arthritis-associated interstitial lung disease. *Arthritis Rheumatol.* **2022**, *74*, 1755–1765. [CrossRef] [PubMed]
34. Wheeler, A.M.; Baker, J.F.; Riley, T.; Yang, Y.; Roul, P.; Wysham, K.D.; Cannon, G.W.; Kunkel, G.; Kerr, G.; Ascherman, D.P.; et al. Development and internal validation of a clinical and genetic risk score for rheumatoid arthritis-associated interstitial lung disease. *Rheumatology* **2024**, keae001. [CrossRef] [PubMed]
35. Sparks, J.A.; Dieudé, P.; Hoffmann-Vold, A.M.; Burmester, G.R.; Walsh, S.L.; Kreuter, M.; Stock, C.; Sambevski, S.; Alves, M.; Emery, P. Design of ANCHOR-RA: A multi-national cross-sectional study on screening for interstitial lung disease in patients with rheumatoid arthritis. *BMC Rheumatol.* **2024**, *8*, 19. [CrossRef] [PubMed]
36. Oka, S.; Higuchi, T.; Furukawa, H.; Shimada, K.; Okamoto, A.; Hashimoto, A.; Komiya, A.; Saisho, K.; Yoshikawa, N.; Katayama, M.; et al. Serum rheumatoid factor IgA, anti-citrullinated peptide antibodies with secretory components, and anti-carbamylated protein antibodies associate with interstitial lung disease in rheumatoid arthritis. *BMC Musculoskelet. Disord.* **2022**, *23*, 46. [CrossRef] [PubMed]
37. Dong, R.; Sun, Y.; Xu, W.; Xiang, W.; Li, M.; Yang, Q.; Zhu, L.; Ma, Z. Distribution and clinical significance of anti-carbamylation protein antibodies in rheumatological diseases among the Chinese Han population. *Front. Immunol.* **2023**, *14*, 1197458. [CrossRef]
38. Fotoh, D.S.; Helal, A.; Rizk, M.S.; Esaily, H.A. Serum Krebs von den Lungen-6 and lung ultrasound B lines as potential diagnostic and prognostic factors for rheumatoid arthritis-associated interstitial lung disease. *Clin. Rheumatol.* **2021**, *40*, 2689–2697. [CrossRef]
39. Pulito-Cueto, V.; Remuzgo-Martínez, S.; Genre, F.; Atienza-Mateo, B.; Mora-Cuesta, V.M.; Iturbe-Fernández, D.; Lera-Gómez, L.; Rodriguez-Carrio, J.; Prieto-Peña, D.; Portilla, V.; et al. Angiogenic T cells: Potential biomarkers for the early diagnosis of interstitial lung disease in autoimmune diseases? *Biomedicines* **2022**, *10*, 851. [CrossRef]
40. Luedders, B.A.; Wheeler, A.M.; Ascherman, D.P.; Baker, J.F.; Duryee, M.J.; Yang, Y.; Roul, P.; Wysham, K.D.; Monach, P.; Reimold, A.; et al. Plasma Matrix Metalloproteinase Concentrations and Risk of Interstitial Lung Disease in a Prospective Rheumatoid Arthritis Cohort. *Arthritis Rheumatol.* **2024**, *76*, 1013–1022. [CrossRef]
41. Van Kalsbeek, D.; Brooks, R.; Shaver, D.; Ebel, A.; Hershberger, D.; Schmidt, C.; Poole, J.A.; Ascherman, D.P.; Thiele, G.M.; Mikuls, T.R.; et al. Peripheral Blood Biomarkers for Rheumatoid Arthritis-Associated Interstitial Lung Disease: A Systematic Review. *ACR Open Rheumatol.* **2023**, *5*, 201–226. [CrossRef]
42. Juge, P.A.; Solomon, J.J.; van Moorsel, C.H.M.; Garofoli, R.; Lee, J.S.; Louis-Sidney, F.; Rojas-Serrano, J.; González-Pérez, M.I.; Mejia, M.; Buendia-Roldán, I.; et al. MUC5B promoter variant rs35705950 and rheumatoid arthritis associated interstitial lung disease survival and progression. *Semin. Arthritis Rheum.* **2021**, *51*, 996–1004. [CrossRef]
43. Velázquez Guevara, B.A.; Abud Mendoza, C.; Avilés Ramírez, L.R.J.; Santillán Guerrero, E. Utilidad del ultrasonido para el diagnóstico de enfermedad pulmonar intersticial en enfermedades difusas del tejido conectivo. *Reumatol. Clin.* **2023**, *19*, 455–462. [CrossRef] [PubMed]
44. Vicente-Rabaneda, E.F.; Bong, D.A.; Busquets-Pérez, N.; Möller, I. Ultrasound evaluation of interstitial lung disease in rheumatoid arthritis and autoimmune diseases. *Eur. J. Rheumatol.* 2022; *online ahead of print*. [CrossRef]
45. Volpicelli, G.; Elbarbary, M.; Blaivas, M.; Lichtenstein, D.A.; Mathis, G.; Kirkpatrick, A.W.; Melniker, L.; Gargani, L.; Noble, V.E.; Via, G.; et al. International evidence-based recommendations for point-of-care lung ultrasound. *Intensive Care Med.* **2012**, *38*, 577–591. [CrossRef]
46. Cogliati, C.; Antivalle, M.; Torzillo, D.; Birocchi, S.; Norsa, A.; Bianco, R.; Costantino, G.; Costantino, G.; Ditto, M.C.; Battellino, M.; et al. Standard and pocket-size lung ultrasound devices can detect interstitial lung disease in rheumatoid arthritis patients. *Rheumatology* **2014**, *53*, 1497–1503. [CrossRef]
47. Moazedi-Fuerst, F.C.; Kielhauser, S.M.; Scheidl, S.; Tripolt, N.J.; Lutfi, A.; Yazdani-Biuki, B.; Dejaco, C.; Graninger, W.B. Ultrasound screening for interstitial lung disease in rheumatoid arthritis. *Clin. Exp. Rheumatol.* **2014**, *32*, 199–203. [PubMed]
48. Otaola, M.; Paulin, F.; Rosemffet, M.; Balcazar, J.; Perandones, M.; Orauscio, E.; Cazenave, T.; Rossi, S.; Marciano, S.; Schneeberger, E.; et al. Lung ultrasound is a promising screening tool to rule out interstitial lung disease in patients with rheumatoid arthritis. *Respirology*, 2024; *online ahead of print*. [CrossRef]
49. Santos-Moreno, P.; Linares-Contreras, M.F.; Rodríguez-Vargas, G.S.; Rodríguez-Linares, P.; Mata-Hurtado, A.; Ibatá, L.; Martínez, S.; Rojas-Villarraga, A.; Diaz, M.; Vicente-Rabaneda, E.F.; et al. Usefulness of lung ultrasound as a method for early diagnosis of interstitial lung disease in patients with rheumatoid arthritis. *Open Access Rheumatol.* **2024**, *16*, 9–20. [CrossRef] [PubMed]

50. Mena-Vázquez, N.; Jimenez-Núñez, F.G.; Godoy-Navarrete, F.J.; Manrique-Arija, S.; Aguilar-Hurtado, M.C.; Romero-Barco, C.M.; Ureña-Garnica, I.; Espildora, F.; Padin-Martín, M.I.; Fernández-Nebro, A. Utility of pulmonary ultrasound to identify interstitial lung disease in patients with rheumatoid arthritis. *Clin. Rheumatol.* **2021**, *40*, 2377–2385. [CrossRef]
51. Di Carlo, M.; Tardella, M.; Filippucci, E.; Carotti, M.; Salaffi, F. Lung ultrasound in patients with rheumatoid arthritis: Definition of significant interstitial lung disease. *Clin. Exp. Rheumatol.* **2022**, *40*, 495–500. [CrossRef]
52. Sofíudóttir, B.K.; Harders, S.; Laursen, C.B.; Lage-Hansen, P.R.; Nielsen, S.M.; Just, S.A.; Christensen, R.; Davidsen, J.R.; Ellingsen, T. Detection of interstitial lung disease in rheumatoid arthritis by thoracic ultrasound. A diagnostic test accuracy study. *Arthritis Care Res.* **2024**; *online ahead of print.* [CrossRef]

Disclaimer/Publisher's Note: The statements, opinions and data contained in all publications are solely those of the individual author(s) and contributor(s) and not of MDPI and/or the editor(s). MDPI and/or the editor(s) disclaim responsibility for any injury to people or property resulting from any ideas, methods, instructions or products referred to in the content.

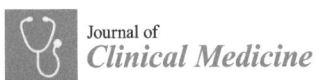

Article

Neutropenia and Felty Syndrome in the Twenty-First Century: Redefining Ancient Concepts in Rheumatoid Arthritis Patients

Jorge Luis Rodas Flores [1], Blanca Hernández-Cruz [1,*], Víctor Sánchez-Margalet [2], Ana Fernández-Reboul Fernández [1], Esther Fernandez Panadero [1], Gracia Moral García [1] and José Javier Pérez Venegas [1]

1. Rheumatology Department, Virgen Macarena University Hospital, Health Service of Andalucian, 41009 Seville, Spain; jorgel.rodas.sspa@juntadeandalucia.es (J.L.R.F.); ana.fernandez.sspa@juntadeandalucia.es (A.F.-R.F.); esther.fernandez.panadero.sspa@juntadeandalucia.es (E.F.P.); gracia.moral.sspa@juntadeandalucia.es (G.M.G.); jjavier.perez.sspa@juntadeandalucia.es (J.J.P.V.)
2. Department of Medical Biochemistry and Molecular Biology and Immunology, School of Medicine, Virgen Macarena University Hospital, 41009 Seville, Spain; margalet@us.es
* Correspondence: blancae.hernandez.sspa@juntadeandalucia.es

Abstract: Objectives: To describe the frequency of neutropenia and Felty syndrome in patients with rheumatoid arthritis (RA) attended in routine clinical practice. **Methods:** We selected by randomization a sample of 270 RA patients attended from January 2014 to November 2022. Demographic, clinical, and neutropenia-related variables were collected from the electronic medical records. Neutropenia was defined as having an absolute neutrophil count (ANC) of less than $1500/mm^3$ once, and acute if it persisted for <3 months. Felty syndrome was defined as RA-related neutropenia, rheumatoid factor (RF) and/or anti citrullinated protein antibody (ACPA) positivity. **Results:** We found 50 patients who had at least one neutropenia episode, with an incidence of 18.5% (14.0–25.6%). Most were women, with age (mean, p25–p75) at the time of neutropenia of 61.5 (57.4–69.3) years, 85% RF+ and 76% ACPA+. The demographic and RA characteristics of patients with and without neutropenia were very similar, except for sex: most patients with neutropenia were women. The 50 patients had 99 episodes of neutropenia; 59% were acute. The lower ANC was 1240 (1000–1395) mm^3, and most of the episodes were mild (74%). In 32% of cases, there was other cytopenia. The RA activity measured by DAS28 in patients with neutropenia was low, at 2.18 (1.75–2.97). A total of 82 of 99 neutropenia episodes were related to DMARDs, 60% to Anti-IL6 drugs in monotherapy, 13% to RA activity, 3% to infectious diseases and 1% to hematologic malignancy. There were five (1.8%) cases with Felty syndrome, but only one woman with the classic combination of RA, positivity of autoantibodies (RF and ACPA), neutropenia and splenomegaly. **Conclusions:** In the 21st century, neutropenia in RA patients is most commonly related to biologics, mostly IL6 inhibitors and methotrexate. Episodes are mild, acute, with low RA activity, and associated with severe infections in few cases. Felty syndrome is rare.

Keywords: rheumatoid arthritis; neutropenia; DMARDs; Felty syndrome

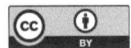

1. Introduction

Neutropenia in patients with rheumatoid arthritis (RA) occurs in 0.5 to 37% of cases depending on several variables, mainly involving treatment with disease-modifying anti-rheumatic drugs (DMARDs) [1–4]. In patients with early untreated RA, the frequency of neutropenia is as low as 0.65–1.4% [3,4]. For RA patients treated with synthetic conventional DMARDs (scDMARDs), this rate is about 8% (2–12%) [1]. In those treated with biologics (bDMARDs), it is 14–19%, with higher values for IL6-inhibitors (IL6i) like tocilizumab (1–10%) and anti-CD20 drugs like rituximab (3–27%) and lower ones for tumoral necrosis factor inhibitors (TNFi) (2–3%) [1,2]. In those treated with Janus Kinase inhibitors (JAKi), the rate is about 5% [1,2]. A recent study estimated the frequency of neutropenia in early

AR, finding a value of 7.5% [1]. Neutropenia increases with the combination of scDMARDs and bDMARDs, and significantly increases comorbidity and complicates the management of the disease with DMARDs within the treat-to-target strategy [3,4]. The most common complication of neutropenia, whatever the cause, is infection, which can be serious [1–3]. The risk of severe infection is greater if neutropenia is severe, if it appears quickly and with a longer duration, if it is associated with chronic foci of infections, previous infections, anemia or other cytopenia and if it occurs in the presence of certain comorbidities (chronic kidney disease, lung pathology, heart failure or chronic infections). And the risk is mainly for bacterial infections [1–3].

The etiology of neutropenia in RA patients is complex. Neutropenia can be congenital, a very rare condition that occurs with the same frequency as in individuals without RA, or acquired, which is the most common. The causes of acquired neutropenia are i. peripheral destruction by an autoimmune reaction or toxics (drugs as DMARDs or others); ii. sequestration, either splenic (hypersplenism), in reticuloendothelial tissue or excess of vascular marginalization of neutrophils; and iii. inadequate neutrophil production in hematopoietic organs due to vitamin deficiency (i.e., folic acid deficiency in patients treated with methotrexate), tumor invasion or toxicity (drugs as DMARDS or others) [1–4].

A special form of RA was described in 1924 as a combination of RA, leucopenia and splenomegaly by Augustus Felty [5]. Currently, Felty syndrome is defined as the presence of neutropenia (absolute neutrophil counts of less than $1500 \times mm^3$), splenomegaly and typical antibodies (RF and/or ACPA) in RA patients. Although it has been described in association with other autoimmune conditions as systemic lupus erythematosus; in these cases, the term autoimmune neutropenia is preferred. Its prevalence is low and decreasing: 1% in 1985 to 0.5% in the 21st century [6]. Other common signs are extra-articular RA manifestations, fever, anemia, mucosal and skin ulcers, respiratory tract infections, thrombocytopenia and lymphadenopathy. These patients have poor prognostics [5,6].

The treatment of neutropenia depends on its etiology. If related to toxics, withdrawal of the drug or toxic substance or material is recommended. In some cases, the addition of folic acid supplementation is pursued. Optimizing the treatment of RA is useful, as in Felty syndrome. Neoplasia should be looked for and treated, for example, by the screening and treatment of large granular lymphocyte leukemia. In addition, the correct prevention of infections with vaccination or antibiotic prophylaxis must be pursued in specific cases, as well as the early treatment of associated infections [1–3].

The objectives of our study were to determine the frequency of neutropenia and Felty syndrome, and to determine its clinical characteristics.

2. Materials and Methods

An observational, retrospective and analytical study was designed. From a database of 858 patients with adult RA diagnosed according to ACR/EULAR criteria [7] treated in usual clinical practice in the Rheumatology Department of the Virgen Macarena University Hospital (a tertiary level hospital belonging to the Public Health System of Andalusia, in Seville, Spain) from January 2014 to November 2022, we selected a sample. The sample size was calculated based on an estimated prevalence of neutropenia of 10%, and the patients were selected by randomization with a computer program. Patients without an accurate RA diagnosis, those under 18 years of age, those with overlapping syndromes and those with other immune mediated diseases were excluded. Demographic, clinical, laboratory and neutropenia-specific data were collected from electronic medical records, with emphasis on the identification of neutropenia. Neutropenia information was cross-checked with electronic laboratory records. Data on treatment were reviewed in the electronic prescription, and its relationship with neutropenia was defined by the treating rheumatologist.

Definitions: Neutropenia was when the absolute neutrophil count (ANC) was $\leq 1500/mm^3$ in a determination. Mild neutropenia (grade II) was diagnosed in patients with an ANC of 1500 to $1000/mm^3$; moderate (grade III) of 1000 to $500/mm^3$; and severe (grade IV) < $500/mm^3$. Neutropenia was considered acute if it persisted <3 months and chronic if it persisted

≥3 months. Anemia was defined as having a hemoglobin level <13 g/dL (men) and <12 g/dL (women). Lymphopenia was defined as having an absolute lymphocyte count of <1000/mm^3. Thrombocytopenia was defined as having an absolute platelet count of <140,000/mm^3 (men) and <130,000/mm^3 (women) [8,9]. Infection associated with the neutropenia process was that present within 3 months of the detected neutropenia episode. Felty syndrome was diagnosed if patients had rheumatoid factor positivity (RF+) and/or anti-citrullinated protein antibody positivity (ACPA+) and/or neutropenia attributed to RA activity; and classic Felty syndrome was if splenomegaly plus typical signs and symptoms were present.

Statistical analysis was performed by descriptive statistics with calculation of median and percentiles 25 and 75, percentages, and 95% confidence intervals. Nonparametric tests were used to calculate p values (Xi^2 and Mann–Whitney U tests), assuming non-normal distribution of variables and unequal sample sizes. A logistic regression was performed to determinate the variables related to neutropenia. In them, the dependent variable was neutropenia, and the independent variables were those with clinical relevance and those that, in the univariate analysis, showed a p value ≤ 0.2. Analyses were performed using Stata version 13.1 (StataCorp LP, College Station, TX, USA). The study was approved by the regional Ethics and Clinical Research Committee of the Andalusian Health Service.

3. Results

Out of a base of 858 patients with RA who attended usual clinical practice, 270 (30%) were randomly selected. The sample included 213 (79%) women. The median age (percentile 25–percentile 75) at the time of the study was 61.5 (53.0–69.3) years. They had an RA of 10.5 (6.6–18.2) years; 84% had RF+, 78% ACPA+ and 72% both FR+ and ACPA+.

Of the 270 patients included, 50 (18.5% CI95% 14.0–25.6%) had at least one episode of neutropenia. The demographic and RA characteristics of both groups, with and without neutropenia, were very similar, except for sex, since most patients with neutropenia were women. Patients with neutropenia had other cytopenias, mainly thrombocytopenia. They used bDMARDs most frequently, without statistical differences, as shown in Table 1.

Table 1. Clinical characteristics of patients with neutropenia.

Variable	Neutropenia		Without Neutropenia		p Value
	n	%	n	%	
	50	19	220	81	
Female sex	45	90	168	76	0.03
RF+	43	86	184	84	0.6
ACPA+	36	73	175	80	0.3
ACPA+ and RF+	32	65	163	74	0.06
Other cytopenia	21	48	57	27	0.006
Anemia	19	38	47	21	0.01
Thrombocytopenia	11	22	12	5	0.0001
Lymphopenia	2	5	3	1	0.1
Splenomegaly	1	2	0	0	
Felty syndrome	1	2	0	0	
Deaths	2	4	2	1	0.1
DMARD	48	96	205	94	0.5
scDMARD	27	54	140	64	0.1
One	26	52	136	62	0.4
Two	1	2	4	2	0.1

Table 1. Cont.

Variable	Neutropenia		Without Neutropenia		p Value
	n	%	n	%	
MTX	19	68	102	73	0.1
bDMARD	35	71	128	58	0.08
Monotherapy	1	2	20	7	0.09
Combo with scDMARD	16	32	73	33	0.09
sdDMARD	1	2	20	9	0.09
Combo with scDMARD	0	0	6	3	0.2
	Median	p25–p75	Median	p25–p75	
Age at diagnosis, years	45.7	38.2–53.7	48.5	39.1–57.9	0.1
Age (at time of neutropenia or cut off), years	61.6	49.8–69.2	61.4	53.0–69.5	0.2
Disease duration, (at time of neutropenia or cut off) years	11.6	6.4–21.3	10.4	6.6–17.7	0.5
RF title, U/mL	274	96.2–591.2	236	119.2–367.7	0.2
ACPA title, U/mL	299	87–343.5	340	113.7–359	0.2

RF: rheumatoid factor, ACPA: anti-citrullinated protein antibody positivity, DMARD: disease-modifying anti-rheumatic drugs, scDMARD: synthetic conventional disease-modifying anti rheumatic drugs, MTX: methotrexate, Combo: in combination with, sdDMARD: synthetic directed disease-modifying anti-rheumatic drugs. Data are presented as median and percentiles 25 and 75 (p25 and p75).

3.1. Multivariate Analysis

In the best logistic regression model, the variables that were associated with neutropenia were treatment with IL6i, the presence of other cytopenias, and female sex. Neither activity according DAS28, age or the duration of the RA showed association. The data are shown in Table 2.

Table 2. Logistic regression model.

Variable	Odds Ratio	95% Confidence Interval	n = 256 p = 0.0001 LR Chi^2 42.5 p Value
IL6 inhibitors	10.73	3.56–32.2	0.0001
Other cytopenia *	3.83	1.93–7.60	0.0001
Gender, female	5.10	1.36–19.18	0.01
TNF inhibitors	2.50	1.0–6.29	0.05
Rituximab	4.18	0.32–62.8	0.2
DAS28	1.35	0.95–1.90	0.08
Age	0.99	0.95–1.02	0.6
Disease duration	1.01	0.97–1.05	0.5

* includes anemia, thrombocytopenia or lymphopenia. LR Likelihood ratio. DAS28 Disease activity score with 28 joint count.

3.2. Neutropenia Episodes Features

A total of 50 patients had 99 episodes of neutropenia (Table 3); 59% episodes were acute and 41% chronic. The lower ANC was 1240 (1000–1395) mm^3, and most of the episodes were mild (74%). In 32%, there was other cytopenia: anemia in 19%, thrombocytopenia in 14% and lymphopenia in 9%.

Table 3. Main characteristics of neutropenia episodes.

Variable	n	%
Patients	50	18.5
Number of episodes of neutropenia		
1	26	53
2	7	14
3	9	18
4	5	10
5	1	2
7	1	2
Total	99	100
Duration of neutropenia		
Acute	58	59
Chronic	41	41
Severity of neutropenia		
Mild	73	74
Moderate	20	20
Severe	6	6
Cause of neutropenia		
Drugs	78	78
RA activity	13	13
Systemic viral infections	3	3
Hematologic cancer	1	1

Neutropenic episodes occurred in older patients with long-standing illnesses. Interestingly, the RA activity measured by DAS28 at each neutropenia episode was low, at 2.18 (1.75–2.97). The most common adverse event related to neutropenia was infection in 12 (12%) cases. Most infections were mild, auto-limited and resolved with symptomatic or oral antibiotic therapy; 6% of those were of the upper respiratory tract and 4% of the lower urinary tract. There were two (2%) severe infections: one case of herpes simplex keratitis and another of pneumonia by *K. pneumoniae*, which we describe below.

Regarding etiology, neutropenia drugs (78%) and RA activity (13%) were the most common causes. Biologics were related to 79 episodes of neutropenia: IL6i in 54, with tocilizumab either in monotherapy (40%) or in combination with scDMARDs (19%) as the bDMARD. The second one was TNFi, in 24 episodes, etanercept either in monotherapy (11%) or combination (6%), followed by adalimumab and infliximab. The third was rituximab, with only one case. scDMARDs were, as a group, the second most common cause of neutropenia either in monotherapy or combination with biologics in 44 episodes. Methotrexate in monotherapy caused 20% of episodes, and methotrexate with bDMARDs caused 41% of episodes. The JAKi were related to neutropenia episodes only in 3% of cases. In addition, the treatment of oncologic conditions was related to two episodes (Table 4). In total, 86% of neutropenia episodes were resolved: 59% spontaneously, 31% with reduction in the dose of DMARD, 11% with stopping DMARD, and 4% changing DMARD.

Table 4. Drugs related to neutropenia episodes.

Type	Monotherapy	Combo with Synthetic Conventional DMARDs	Combo with Biologic DMARDs	Total
Synthetic Conventional DMARDs Either in Monotherapy or in Combination with Biologic DMARDs				
Total				
	n (%)	n (%)	n (%)	n (%)
Methotrexate	9 (20)	1 (2)	18 (41)	28 (64)
Leflunomide	3 (7)	1 (2)	6 (14)	10 (23)
Hydroxychloroquine	0	1 (2)	5 (11)	6 (14)
Total	12 (27)	3 (7)	29 (66)	44 (100)
Biologic DMARDs related to neutropenia				
Tocilizumab	32 (40)		15 (19)	47 (59)
Etanercept	9 (11)		5 (6)	14 (18)
Adalimumab	3 (4)		4 (5)	7 (9)
Sarilumab	5 (6)		2 (2)	7 (9)
Infliximab	0		3 (4)	3 (4)
Rituximab	1 (1)		0	1 (1)
Total	49 (62)		29 (37)	79 (100)
Targeted synthetic DMARDs related to neutropenia				
Baricitinib	2 (66)		0	2 (66)
Upadicitinib	1 (33)		0	1 (33)
Total	3 (-)		0	3 (100)
Other treatments				
Rucaparib	1 (50)		0	1 (50
Carboplatin/paclitaxel	1 (50)		0	1 (50)
Total	2 (100)		0	2 (100)

DMARDs: disease-modifying anti rheumatic drugs.

3.2.1. Description of Cases with Severe Infections

- Case 1. The patient is a 79-year-old woman with RA FR+, ACPA+, erosive and sicca symptoms with a duration of 23 years. She had received multiple scDMARDs and, since 2010, tocilizumab monotherapy, maintaining remission with DAS < 2.4. Her co-morbidities include arterial hypertension and stable stage 3a chronic kidney disease. In October 2022, when she was receiving tocilizumab at a reduced dose (162 mg/2 weeks) during an episode of mild acute leucopenia and neutropenia for two months (total leukocytes $3990 \times$ mm^3, total neutrophils $1310 \times$ mm^3, total lymphocytes $1380 \times$ mm^3, platelets $190,000 \times$ mm^3, serum creatinine 1.02 mg/dL, glomerular filtration rate 53 mL/min, erythrocyte sedimentation rate (ESR) 7 mm/hour, C-Reactive protein (CRP) 0.3 mg/L), she was admitted to the emergency room with a red left eye, photophobia plus epiphora. The ophthalmologists established the diagnosis of herpetic keratitis, and she was treated on an outpatient basis with topical ganciclovir with resolution after 7 days, without recurrence. Tocilizumab was discontinued during the infection and restarted in reduced doses, according to the label [10]. She currently remains in remission with tocilizumab (162 mg/2 weeks/SC) and has not had infections, keratitis or neutropenia.

- Case 2. The patient is a 79-year-old woman with RA, FR+ ACPA+, erosive plus fibromyalgia and bronchial asthma of 25 years. After multiple scDMARDs, she started her first biologic, tocilizumab, in 2009, and maintained remission with reduced dose (4 mg/kg/IV each 28 days). The reduction in dose was due to good clinical response but moderate neutropenia. She was admitted due to fever, chills, cough with hemoptoic sputum plus left pleural pain during 5 days. A pulmonary condensation image in the left base and a positive blood culture for *Klebsiella pneumoniae* were confirmed. At the time of pneumonia, RA was in remission (DAS28VSG 2.1) without leukopenia or neutropenia (total leucocytes $6900\times$ mm^3, and total neutrophils $6430\times$ mm^3) but severe lymphopenia ($130\times$ mm^3) and mild thrombocytopenia (total platelets $129,000\times$ mm^3), ESR 2 mm/hour, CRP 46.1 mg/L. After 10 days of IV antibiotic therapy, the condition resolved. Tocilizumab was restarted one month later and was discontinued after 10 months due to chronic moderate neutropenia, according to the label [10]. She was switched to etanercept, which is maintained to date at 50 mg/week SC. She is in remission, without infections and without neutropenia.

3.2.2. Classic Felty Syndrome

Five of fifty (1.8%) patients with neutropenia had characteristics of Felty Syndrome, i.e., neutropenia plus RF+ and/or ACPA+, but just one of the three classic features (RA, FR+ and ACPA+, neutropenia and splenomegaly), for a prevalence of 0.3% of the total of patients.

- Case 3. Felty Syndrome. The patient is a 46-year-old woman with RA according to EULAR/ACR criteria [7], with poor prognostic characteristics (high levels of activity, RF+, ACPA+, erosions and poor physical function) as evaluated in 2011, with poor compliance. From 2011 to 2015, she received irregular treatment with methotrexate, leflunomide, and low doses of oral prednisone and refused bDMARDs. In 2019, she returned to the clinic with six swollen joints, eight tender joints, 6 cm of visual analogue scale of pain (0 = no pain to 10 = maximum pain), and 6 cm of VAS of RA activity (0 = no activity to 10 = maximum activity), with DAS28PCR 5.07, HAQ 1.5 and poor perception of health. We found hand deformity with ulnar burst and swan neck fingers (Figure 1).

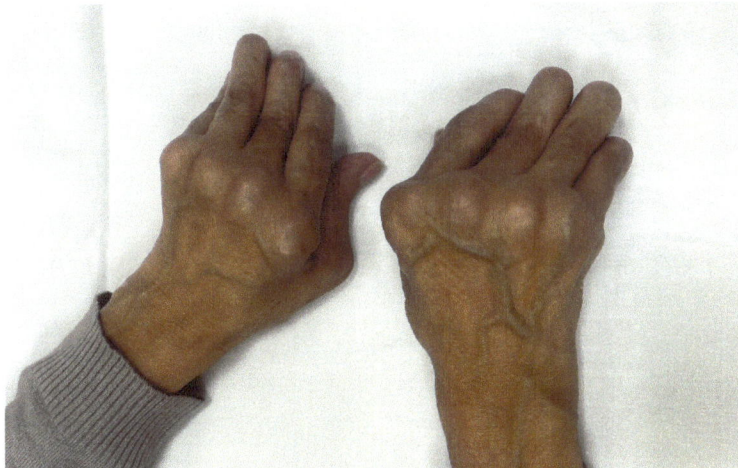

Figure 1. Hands of patient with Felty syndrome. She has characteristics swan neck deformity, metacarpophalangeal subluxation and ulnar blunt.

Her laboratory data were as follows: hemoglobin 10.7 g/dL, total leukocytes 3850× mm^3, total neutrophils 1000× mm^3, serum IgA 693 mg/dL, serum IgG 2706 mg/dL, serum IgM 868 mg/dL, FR 522 UI/dL, ACPA > 340 U/mL, ESR 35 mm/hora, CRP 15 mg/dL. Her X-rays showed ulnar subluxation of bilateral first finger interphalangeal, with erosions in carpals, metacarpophalangeal and proximal interphalangeal (Figure 2) as well as erosions in metatarsal heads.

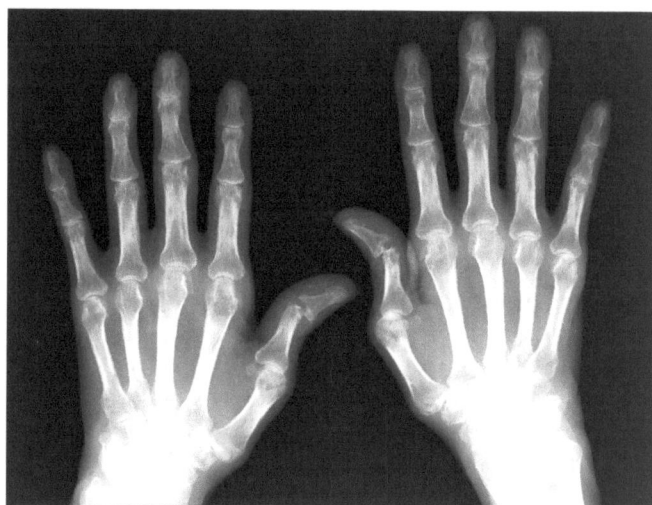

Figure 2. Anteroposterior hand X-ray with subluxation of the metacarpophalangeal and interphalangeal joints of first fingers, and erosions in metacarpal heads and proximal interphalangeal heads.

Treatment was attempted with adalimumab and etanercept, which she did not tolerate and preferred low doses of prednisone (1.25 to 5 mg/day). She evolved poorly with persistent RA activity (DAS28-PCR index between 4.5 to 6.0) and pancytopenia (mild to moderate anemia, neutropenia, lymphopenia, and thrombocytopenia), without clinical manifestations. Abdominal ultrasound was performed for suspected Felty syndrome, confirming 14 cm splenomegaly (Figure 3).

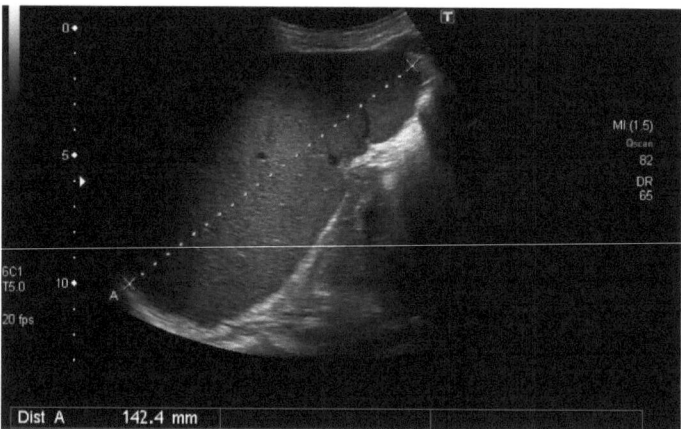

Figure 3. Splenomegaly with spleen of 14 cm.

The patient did not agree to complete the hematological study (bone marrow aspiration and large granular cell leukemia study). After multiple attempts to reach a consensus on diagnostic test and treatment without success, she was admitted due to fever, nosebleeds and anemic syndrome related to severe thrombopenia plus pancytopenia. Upon admission, she had fever without infection. After multiple blood urine cultures and specific serology, her laboratory tests showed Hb 7.9 g/dL, hematocrit 26.4%, total leucocytes 3770× mm^3, total neutrophils 1400× mm^3, platelets 28,000× mm^3, serum IgA 1004 mg/dL, serum IgE 107 UI/mL, serum IgG 6038 mg/dL, serum IgM 611 mg/dL, ESR 125 mm/hora, CRP 22.4 mg/L, serum amyloid 3.34 mg/L, procalcitonin 0.32 ng/mL, RF 5623 U/L and ACPA > 340 U/mL. Multiple myeloma (absence of serum monoclonal protein, heavy chain expression by immunofixation, urinary monoclonal protein) and large granular lymphocyte leukemia (absence of CD8+ cell proliferation by flux cytometry) were ruled out (Figure 4).

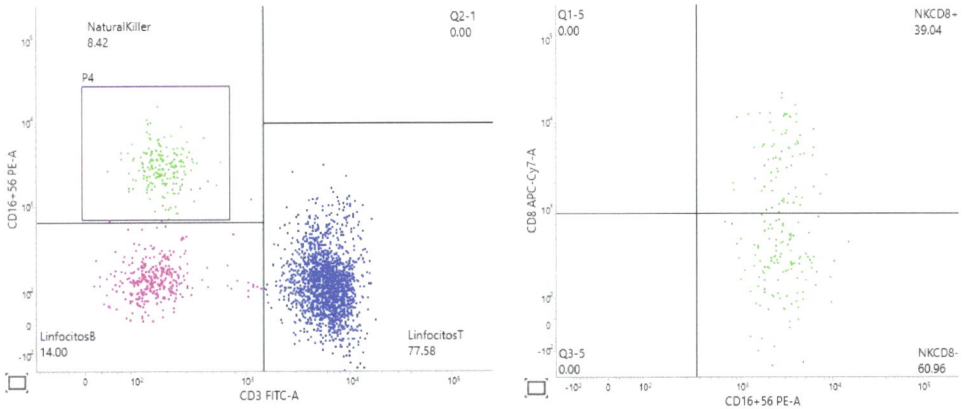

Figure 4. Flow cytometry dot plots that show absence of clonal expansion of NK cells expressing or not CD8+.

She accepted treatment with biannual rituximab. Until the last review, she had received two cycles of 1000 mg IV (day 0 and day 15), with the last one in March 2024, without complications. There was evidence of improvement in inflammatory activity DAS28PCR, 1.8, anemia and thrombocytopenia, but so far, not for the remaining laboratory parameters. She had Hb 14.5 g/dL, total leukocytes 2000× mm^3, total neutrophils 1060× mm^3, platelets 53,000× mm^3, ESR 121 mm/h, CRP 1.3 mg/L, RF 4935 UI/mL and ACPA > 340 U/mL. She had had mild upper respiratory tract infections managed on an outpatient basis and agreed to continue the treatment but not with aggressive diagnostic tests.

4. Discussion

In the 21st century, neutropenia in RA patients is a common finding, with values between 0.5% to 37% (1–3). In our sample of RA patients, it was 18.5% (14.0–25.6%), in agreement with these values. With the introduction of the T2T strategy since 2010 [11], the characteristics and consequences of neutropenia in RA patients have changed. Recent studies report that in early RA without DMARD treatment, neutropenia occurs uncommonly (in less than 1.5% of cases), and congenital neutropenia should be ruled out [1–4]. In established RA, the prevalence is much higher, and the main cause of neutropenia is treatment with DMARDs, mainly bDMARDs with prevalences of 14.3% to 19%, followed by RA activity. Our retrospective series included patients with a mean of 61 years, long-lasting disease and a high proportion of RF and ACPA positivity, and the frequency and causes of neutropenia were like those in other studies [1–3]. Between the biologics, those most common related with neutropenia were IL6i drugs, mainly tocilizumab followed by rituximab, and lastly, by TNFi drugs. scDMARDs were the second most common cause of neutropenia after bDMARDs, mainly methotrexate. And JAKi were the third group related to neutropenia [1–3]. These findings were very similar to ours, with 79% of episodes of neutropenia for bDMARDs mainly involving IL6i (59% tocilizumab and 9% sarilumab), followed by TNFi drugs in 24% (18% etanercept, 9% adalimumab and 4% infliximab), and JAKi in 3%. Maybe rituximab was the last due to the low prevalence of use of rituximab in our cohort. In our series and in the recent literature, no cases were related to NSAIDs, maybe because the prevalence of use of NSAIDs has reduced, according to recommendations for RA treatment [12]. The use of oral or parenteral corticosteroids has not been correlated with neutropenia either in our or in other studies [1].

In multivariate analysis, neutropenia was correlated to drugs, especially bDMARDs, particularly IL6i, and with sex and the presence of other cytopenia [1–3,10,13]. As with the prevalence of neutropenia, the causes of it are different between DMARDs classes, and even within the same class [1–3]. In the case of tocilizumab, moderate (grade III) neutropenia occurred in 7% of RA patients [13]. Although the mechanism of neutropenia associated with tocilizumab is unknown, up-to-date blocking of IL-6 in has an effect on neutrophil recruitment from bone marrow and in the regulation of its selection and expression, but the proposed mechanisms have no effects on the neutrophils function [13,14]. These data are like sarilumab, the other IL6i used in RA patients [15]. For the case of TNFi, the causes of neutropenia are different and varied: decreased upregulation of pro inflammatory cytokines (IL-1, IL-6, IL8 and granulocyte-macrophage colony-stimulating factor), all of them involved in the differentiation and maturation of neutrophils and hematopoietic cells. Also in increases in the peripherical consumption of neutrophils, and imbalances between apoptosis and their survival, mainly accelerated neutrophil apoptosis. Even these effects are different between monoclonal antibodies or soluble receptors against TNF [16,17]. In the case of rituximab, the exact frequency of neutropenia is difficult to estimate due to the highly variable posology in RA patients [1–3]. The onset of neutropenia in rituximab patients is late, after 4 weeks of the last dose, without another identifiable cause, and its frequency is about 1.3% to 6.5% [18,19]. Several mechanisms are postulated, highlighting the interference with the output of neutrophils from the bone marrow during B cell recovering, imbalance between granulopoiesis vs. lymphopoiesis, and arrest in the maturation of promyelocyte stage [18,19].

For csDMARDs the prevalence of neutropenia is about 8%, similar between methotrexate, leflunomide or sulfasalazine. Here, the mechanisms are different [1–3]. Methotrexate was discovered in the mid-20th century and introduced for the treatment of RA between 1951 and the 1970s; after more than 60 years of use, it is the anchor drug treating RA [20]. With the actual dose regimen of a low dose of methotrexate recommended (between 10 and 25 mg/week plus folic acid supplementation of 5 to 15 mg/week), the frequency of neutropenia is about 6.5% [21]. Data confirmed in other cohorts methotrexate-exposed populations [22]. The cause of methotrexate-related neutropenia is not elucidated but may be related to the competitive inhibition of the enzyme dihydrofolate reductase and depleted hepatic folate stores, without effect in the adenosine pathway [20–22]. Whatever the mechanisms of neutropenia associated with DMARDs, in ours and in most of the published works, neutropenia was mild, acute, of a single episode, and was resolved with DMARD dose reductions. As in other series, risk factors of neutropenia were female sex, pre-existing neutropenia, and presence of other cytopenia [1–3,10,13–22]. A specific protocol of cytopenia related to methotrexate [20], IL6i [10,23] and other DMARDs has been developed and should be implemented in clinical practice according to the label. It is simple and includes baseline medical history with emphasis in infection, neutropenia and other medication history; complete blood counts should be taken at 2 to 3 months depending on the clinical condition and type of DMARDs. In addition, vaccination, specific prophylaxis protocols, reduction in the use of steroids, and the management of comorbidities and concomitant drugs related to neutropenia and infection risk (diabetes, lung disease, chronic kidney disease, etc.) should be undertaken. If infection is suspected, early treatment should be initiated to reduce morbidity and mortality [24,25]. In a case of severe neutropenia, either febrile or not, the patient should be hospitalized, and a multidisciplinary team should start the specific protocol [26,27].

Autoimmune causes of neutropenia and Felty syndrome after the introduction of the T2T strategy of RA treatment as cause of neutropenia are rare, as in our series [1–4,6]. However, in our series, the patients with neutropenia were older and had long-lasting disease. Felty syndrome prevalence was 0,3% of the total. Case 3 showed, in addition, poor therapeutic adherence. The diagnosis of RA activity as cause of neutropenia in Felty syndrome is determined by exclusion, after discarding drug toxicity (DMARDs and non-steroid anti-inflammatory drugs (NSAIDs), and painkillers as the most common), followed by infections. Again, baseline medical history with emphasis on RA activity index, physical examination, folic, B12 or cupper deficiencies should be tested. Acute-phase reactants are usually elevated, except in patients treated with IL6i, where they may be decreased [23]. In some cases, if it is possible, antibodies against granulocytes of pan-RF-γIIIB type can be useful [2]. Once toxicity drugs or other toxic materials, infection or neoplasia have been ruled out, RA treatment should be intensified following the T2T strategy [11,12,20,24,25].

Nowadays, the frequency of Felty syndrome is very low at about 0.5% [6]. In these patients, it is relevant to confirm RA treatment adherence. RA activity searches should be completed with image studies to confirm splenomegaly. Of particular interest is ruling out large granular lymphocyte leukemia and multiple myeloma, as well as some uncommon chronic parasitic and fungal infections. In the multidisciplinary team, the inclusion of a hematologist and infectious disease expert is mandatory [2–6]. Some cases of Felty syndrome have been informed by effective treatment with rituximab, tocilizumab, etanercept or abatacept, even intravenous gamma globulins, without consensus about the best one [28–33]. In any case, the intensification of the T2T strategy in consensus with the patient should be implemented.

The study limitations are of course the retrospective design and the absence of a control group. But the results, according to recent previous studies and the scarcity of works with clear prevalence estimations and clinical course of the patients, reinforce the data.

5. Conclusions

In the 21st century, neutropenia associated with RA is common and especially related to T2T strategy and DMARDs. Most of the episodes were mild, of short duration and not related to infections. The frequency of classical Felty syndrome is half that of the last century, with effective therapeutic alternatives.

Author Contributions: Conceptualization, J.L.R.F., B.H.-C. and J.J.P.V.; Data curation, V.S.-M., A.F.-R.F., E.F.P. and G.M.G.; Formal analysis, B.H.-C. and V.S.-M.; Methodology, J.L.R.F., B.H.-C., A.F.-R.F., E.F.P. and G.M.G.; Resources, J.J.P.V.; Software, J.L.R.F.; Supervision, J.J.P.V.; Writing—original draft, J.L.R.F. and B.H.-C.; Writing—review and editing, J.L.R.F., B.H.-C., V.S.-M., A.F.-R.F., E.F.P., G.M.G. and J.J.P.V. All authors have read and agreed to the published version of the manuscript.

Funding: This research received no external funding.

Institutional Review Board Statement: The protocol was presented and approved by the Comité Coordinador de Ética de la Investigación Biomédica en Andalucía, date 29 July 2022 and CODE NUMBER Neutropenia AR-2022-1442-N-22. This was conducted according to Good Clinical Practice https://www.aemps.gob.es/industria/inspeccionBPC/docs/guia-BPC_octubre-2008.pdf (accesed on 17 November 2024) and The International Council for Harmonization of technical requirements for pharmaceuticals for human use https://database.ich.org/sites/default/files/E6_R2_Addendum.pdf (accesed on 17 November 2024).

Informed Consent Statement: Written informed consent has been obtained from the patients to publish this paper.

Data Availability Statement: Data have been stored in our research archives according to local legislation.

Conflicts of Interest: The authors declare no conflicts of interest.

References

1. Fragoulis, G.E.; Paterson, C.; Gilmour, A.; Derakhshan, M.H.; McInnes, I.B.; Porter, D.; Siebert, S. Neutropaenia in early rheumatoid arthritis: Frequency, predicting factors, natural history and outcome. *RMD Open.* **2018**, *4*, e000739. [CrossRef] [PubMed]
2. Lazaro, E.; Morel, J. Management of neutropenia in patients with rheumatoid arthritis. *Jt. Bone Spine* **2015**, *82*, 235–239. [CrossRef]
3. Nikiphorou, E.; de Lusignan, S.; Mallen, C.; Khavandi, K.; Roberts, J.; Buckley, C.D.; Galloway, J.; Raza, K. Haematological abnormalities in new-onset rheumatoid arthritis and risk of common infections: A population-based study. *Rheumatology* **2020**, *59*, 997–1005. [CrossRef] [PubMed]
4. Le Boëdec, M.; Marhadour, T.; Devauchelle-Pensec, V.; Jousse-Joulin, S.; Binard, A.; Fautrel, B.; Flipo, R.M.; Le Loët, X.; Ménard, J.F.; Saraux, A. Baseline laboratory test abnormalities are common in early arthritis but rarely contraindicate methotrexate: Study of three cohorts (ESPOIR, VErA, and Brittany). *Semin. Arthritis Rheum.* **2013**, *42*, 474–481. [CrossRef] [PubMed]
5. Sienknecht, C.W.; Urowitz, M.B.; Pruzanski, W.; Stein, H.B. Felty's syndrome. Clinical and serological analysis of 34 cases. *Ann. Rheum. Dis.* **1977**, *36*, 500–507. [CrossRef] [PubMed]
6. Wegscheider, C.; Ferincz, V.; Schöls, K.; Maieron, A. Felty's syndrome. *Front. Med.* **2023**, *17*, 1238405. [CrossRef]
7. Aletaha, D.; Neogi, T.; Silman, A.J.; Funovits, J.; Felson, D.T.; Bingham, C.O., 3rd; Birnbaum, N.S.; Burmester, G.R.; Bykerk, V.P.; Cohen, M.D.; et al. 2010 Rheumatoid arthritis classification criteria: An American College of Rheumatology/European League Against Rheumatism collaborative initiative. *Arthritis Rheum.* **2010**, *62*, 2569–2581. [CrossRef]
8. Available online: https://admin.new.meddra.org/sites/default/files/guidance/file/intguide_25_1_Spanish.pdf (accessed on 17 November 2024).
9. Available online: https://www.sspa.juntadeandalucia.es/servicioandaluzdesalud/sites/default/files/sincfiles/wsas-media-pdf_publicacion/2020/Enfermedades_Sangre.pdf (accessed on 17 November 2024).
10. Available online: https://cima.aemps.es/cima/dochtml/ft/108492007/FT_108492007.html (accessed on 12 October 2024).
11. Smolen, J.S.; Aletaha, D.; Bijlsma, J.W.; Breedveld, F.C.; Boumpas, D.; Burmester, G.; Combe, B.; Cutolo, M.; de Wit, M.; Dougados, M.; et al. T2T Expert Committee. Treating rheumatoid arthritis to target: Recommendations of an international task force. *Ann. Rheum. Dis.* **2010**, *69*, 631–637. [CrossRef]
12. Smolen, J.S.; Landewé, R.B.M.; Bergstra, S.A.; Kerschbaumer, A.; Sepriano, A.; Aletaha, D.; Caporali, R.; Edwards, C.J.; Hyrich, K.L.; Pope, J.E.; et al. EULAR recommendations for the management of rheumatoid arthritis with synthetic and biological disease-modifying antirheumatic drugs: 2022 update. *Ann. Rheum. Dis.* **2023**, *82*, 3–18. [CrossRef] [PubMed]
13. Kim, Y.E.; Ahn, S.M.; Oh, J.S.; Kim, Y.G.; Lee, C.K.; Yoo, B.; Hong, S. Clinical significance of tocilizumab-related neutropenia in patients with rheumatoid arthritis. *Jt. Bone Spine* **2023**, *90*, 105510. [CrossRef]
14. Moots, R.J.; Sebba, A.; Rigby, W.; Ostor, A.; Porter-Brown, B.; Donaldson, F.; Dimonaco, S.; Rubbert-Roth, A.; van Vollenhoven, R.; Genovese, M.C. Effect of tocilizumab on neutrophils in adult patients with rheumatoid arthritis: Pooled analysis of data from phase 3 and 4 clinical trials. *Rheumatology* **2017**, *56*, 541–549. [CrossRef]
15. Emery, P.; Rondon, J.; Parrino, J.; Lin, Y.; Pena-Rossi, C.; van Hoogstraten, H.; Graham, N.M.H.; Liu, N.; Paccaly, A.; Wu, R.; et al. Safety and tolerability of subcutaneous sarilumab and intravenous tocilizumab in patients with rheumatoid arthritis. *Rheumatology* **2019**, *58*, 849–858. [CrossRef]
16. Rajakulendran, S.; Gadsby, K.; Allen, D.; O'Reilly, S.; Deighton, C. Neutropenia while receiving anti-tumour necrosis factor treatment for rheumatoid arthritis. *Ann. Rheum. Dis.* **2006**, *65*, 1678–1679. [CrossRef] [PubMed]
17. Hastings, R.; Ding, T.; Butt, S.; Gadsby, K.; Zhang, W.; Moots, R.J.; Deighton, C. Neutropenia in patients receiving anti-tumor necrosis factor therapy. *Arthritis Care Res.* **2010**, *62*, 764–769. [CrossRef]
18. Monaco, W.E.; Jones, J.D.; Rigby, W.F. Rituximab associated late-onset neutropenia-a rheumatology case series and review of the literature. *Clin. Rheumatol.* **2016**, *35*, 2457–2462. [CrossRef] [PubMed]
19. Salmon, J.H.; Cacoub, P.; Combe, B.; Sibilia, J.; Pallot-Prades, B.; Fain, O.; Cantagrel, A.; Dougados, M.; Andres, E.; Meyer, O.; et al. Late-onset neutropenia after treatment with rituximab for rheumatoid arthritis and other autoimmune diseases: Data from the AutoImmunity and Rituximab registry. *RMD Open* **2015**, *30*, e000034. [CrossRef] [PubMed]
20. García González, C.M.; Baker, J. Treatment of early rheumatoid arthritis: Methotrexate and beyond. *Curr. Opin. Pharmacol.* **2022**, *64*, 102227. [CrossRef]
21. Malley, T.; Corfield, G.; Fung, P.; Heneghan, D.; Kitchen, J. Transaminitis and neutropenia are rare in patients on methotrexate: Evidence from a large cohort of inflammatory arthritis patients. *Rheumatology* **2019**, *58*, 2061–2062. [CrossRef]
22. Solomon, D.H.; Glynn, R.J.; Karlson, E.W.; Lu, F.; Corrigan, C.; Colls, J.; Xu, C.; MacFadyen, J.; Barbhaiya, M.; Berliner, N.; et al. Adverse Effects of Low-Dose Methotrexate: A Randomized Trial. *Ann. Intern. Med.* **2020**, *172*, 369–380. [CrossRef]
23. Aletaha, D.; Kerschbaumer, A.; Kastrati, K.; Dejaco, C.; Dougados, M.; McInnes, I.B.; Sattar, N.; Stamm, T.A.; Takeuchi, T.; Trauner, M.; et al. Consensus statement on blocking interleukin-6 receptor and interleukin-6 in inflammatory conditions: An update. *Ann. Rheum. Dis.* **2023**, *82*, 773–787. [CrossRef]
24. Fraenkel, L.; Bathon, J.M.; England, B.R.; St Clair, E.W.; Arayssi, T.; Carandang, K.; Deane, K.D.; Genovese, M.; Huston, K.K.; Kerr, G.; et al. 2021 American College of Rheumatology Guideline for the Treatment of Rheumatoid Arthritis. *Arthritis Care Res* **2021**, *73*, 924–939. [CrossRef] [PubMed]

25. Holroyd, C.R.; Seth, R.; Bukhari, M.; Malaviya, A.; Holmes, C.; Curtis, E.; Chan, C.; Yusuf, M.A.; Litwic, A.; Smolen, S.; et al. The British Society for Rheumatology biologic DMARD safety guidelines in inflammatory arthritis. *Rheumatology* **2019**, *58*, e3–e42. [CrossRef]
26. Nucci, M. How I Treat Febrile Neutropenia. *Mediterr. J. Hematol. Infect. Dis.* **2021**, *13*, e2021025. [CrossRef]
27. Keck, J.M.; Wingler, M.J.B.; Cretella, D.A.; Vijayvargiya, P.; Wagner, J.L.; Barber, K.E.; Jhaveri, T.A.; Stover, K.R. Approach to fever in patients with neutropenia: A review of diagnosis and management. *Ther. Adv. Infect. Dis.* **2022**, *9*, 20499361221138346. [CrossRef]
28. Chandra, P.A.; Margulis, Y.; Schiff, C. Rituximab is useful in the treatment of Felty's syndrome. *Am. J. Ther.* **2008**, *15*, 321–322. [CrossRef]
29. Wang, C.R.; Chiu, Y.C.; Chen, Y.C. Successful treatment of refractory neutropenia in Felty's syndrome with rituximab. *Scand. J. Rheumatol.* **2018**, *47*, 340–341. [CrossRef]
30. Li, R.; Wan, Q.; Chen, P.; Mao, S.; Wang, Q.; Li, X.; Yang, Y.; Dong, L. Tocilizumab treatment in Felty's syndrome. *Rheumatol. Int.* **2020**, *40*, 1143–1149. [CrossRef] [PubMed]
31. Ghavami, A.; Genevay, S.; Fulpius, T.; Gabay, C. Etanercept in treatment of Felty's syndrome. *Ann. Rheum. Dis.* **2005**, *64*, 1090–1091. [CrossRef] [PubMed]
32. Chin, R.V.; Serin, S.; Khan, A.; Smith, K.; Kumar, S. The Use of Abatacept for the Treatment of Felty Syndrome in Rheumatoid Arthritis. *Cureus* **2023**, *15*, e46086. [CrossRef] [PubMed]
33. Jeong, M.; Kolovos, P.; Taper, J.; Yun, J. The role of intravenous immunoglobulin in treatment of refractory Felty syndrome c. *Intern. Med. J.* **2021**, *51*, 303–304. [CrossRef] [PubMed]

Disclaimer/Publisher's Note: The statements, opinions and data contained in all publications are solely those of the individual author(s) and contributor(s) and not of MDPI and/or the editor(s). MDPI and/or the editor(s) disclaim responsibility for any injury to people or property resulting from any ideas, methods, instructions or products referred to in the content.

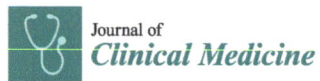

Article

Radiographic Progression in Patients with Rheumatoid Arthritis in Clinical Remission or Low Disease Activity: Results from a Swiss National Registry (SCQM)

Lena L. N. Brandt [1,2], Hendrik Schulze-Koops [2], Thomas Hügle [3], Michael J. Nissen [4], Johannes von Kempis [5] and Ruediger B. Mueller [1,2,*]

1. Rheumazentrum Ostschweiz, 9000 St. Gallen, Switzerland; lena.brandt@fen-net.de
2. Division of Rheumatology and Clinical Immunology, Department of Internal Medicine IV, Ludwig-Maximilians-University Munich, 80539 Munich, Germany; hendrik.schulze-koops@med.uni-muenchen.de
3. Division of Rheumatology, University Hospital Lausanne (CHUV), University Lausanne, 1015 Lausanne, Switzerland; thomas.hugle@chuv.ch
4. Rheumatology, Geneva University Hospital, 1205 Geneva, Switzerland; michaelnissen@gmail.com
5. Clinic for Rheumatology, Kantonsspital St. Gallen, 9007 St. Gallen, Switzerland; johannes.vonkempis@kssg.ch
* Correspondence: ruediger.mueller@hin.ch

Abstract: Background/Objectives: The therapeutic aim for rheumatoid arthritis (RA) is to control disease activity and prevent radiographic progression. Various clinical scores are used to assess disease activity in RA patients. The DAS 28 score can define states of low disease activity (LDA) and remission. Despite achieving LDA or remission, radiographic progression may, nevertheless, occur. However, the rates and frequency of this occurrence have not been analyzed in detail. (1) To characterize radiographic progression in patients with persistent DAS 28-defined LDA or remission. (2) Analyze the potential benefits of modifying therapeutic strategies in response to observed radiographic progression in patients with persistent LDA or remission. **Methods:** An analysis was conducted on RA patients enrolled in the SCQM (Swiss Clinical Quality Management) cohort. Persistent LDA or remission was defined as DAS 28 $\leq$ 3.2 or <2.6, respectively, recorded at two consecutive follow-up time points. Inclusion criteria involved patients with a minimum of two sets of radiographs taken during these LDA and/or remission periods. Radiographic progression was measured using the Ratingen score, a numerical scale ranging from 0 to 190, which quantifies joint erosions. Repair was defined as a decrease in the Ratingen score > 5 points/year, while progression was characterized by an increase of >1, >2, or >5 points change in the Ratingen score within a one-year timeframe. **Results:** Among 10′141 RA patients, there were 1′447 episodes of remission and 2′614 episodes of LDA, with two sets of X-rays available for assessment during these episodes. The rates of radiographic progression (>5 points change in the Ratingen score per year) were 11.2% for LDA and 8.8% for remission. Therapeutic adaptations were made in 7.0% of patients in remission and 12.9% of patients in LDA following radiographic progression. After radiographic progression despite LDA, loss of LDA was observed in 19% of patients with treatment intensification versus in 8.5% under continued treatment during follow-up within 36 months. **Conclusions:** We report a considerable rate of radiographic progression occurring in RA patients with LDA or clinical remission. Notwithstanding minor radiographic progression, maintaining therapeutic continuity seemed more favorable than altering the therapeutic regimen.

Keywords: rheumatoid arthritis; disease activity; radiographic progression; remission

1. Introduction

Rheumatoid Arthritis (RA) is a chronic inflammatory disease leading to joint damage [1]. Treatment decisions for RA patients, as recommended by the European League Against Rheumatism (EULAR), should consider disease activity, progression of structural damage, comorbidities, and safety concerns [2]. Conventional radiographs of the hands and feet are crucial for assessing radiographic damage progression, both in clinical trials and routine practice [3,4]. Over the past two decades, an encouraging effect on radiographic progression has been reported for various conventional, biological, and targeted synthetic DMARDs (disease-modifying anti-rheumatic drugs). The majority of clinical studies have shown inhibition or at least a deceleration in radiographic progression for all therapeutic compounds [5–8].

Disease activity can be measured by various scores, such as the Disability Assessment Score 28 (DAS 28) [9], Clinical/Simplified Disease Activity Index (C/SDAI) [10], and others not listed here. Radiographic progression is measured as a continuous variable, e.g., by the Sharp van der Heijde [11] or the Ratingen score [12], among many others. For pragmatic reasons, it can only be dichotomized into progression or non-progression. Clinical disease activity scores, continuous variables, can categorize patients as high, moderate, or low disease activity (LDA) or remission.

As defined by the EULAR recommendations, "inhibition of damage progression by radiography is still a pivotal outcome for the classification of a drug as a DMARD" [2,9,13]. However, little is known about the management approach when radiographic progression occurs despite clinically assessed LDA or remission. Several studies have shown that patients can experience radiographic disease progression despite achieving good clinical outcomes, such as low DAS 28 scores [14–18]. The question remains open whether radiographic progression is a good reason for a therapeutic change and whether treatment adaptions lead to a beneficial outcome considering the patient's disease activity.

Hypothesis: this study analyzed whether changing therapy in patients with radiographic progression despite LDA or remission is beneficial.

2. Materials and Methods

2.1. Study Population

The analysis included all rheumatoid arthritis (RA) patients from the SCQM RA cohort who achieved a disease activity score (DAS 28)-defined low disease activity (LDA) ($\leq$3.2) or remission (<2.6) designation at two consecutive follow-up visits, with a minimum interval of 90 days. Intervals of LDA or remission were defined between the first and the last documented time point in LDA or remission without any visits in between indicating loss of LDA or remission. Within intervals of LDA or remission, we searched for the first radiographic interval ($\geq$2 sets of radiographs of hands and feet) to derive radiographic progression during LDA.

Radiographs were scored using the Ratingen score [12]. The Ratingen score is an erosion score ranging from 0 to 190, allowing the classification of joint destruction from 0 to 5 per joint. Each grade represents 20% of joint surface destruction. It is assessed in a total of 38 joints. The changes in Ratingen scores were standardized to describe yearly progression: Ratingen scores time difference between the radiographs in days $\times$365.25 days/year.

The patients/episodes were grouped according to their radiographical progression.

Repair: reduction of Ratingen score >5 points/year, no change: $\pm$1, $\pm$2, $\pm$5 Ratingen points/year, progression: 5–10, 10–20, 20–40, >40 Ratingen points/year for patients in LDA or remission.

Demographic and clinical data including age, sex, time to diagnosis, rheumatoid factor positivity, anti-cyclic citrullinated peptide antibody (ACPA) positivity, body mass index, DAS 28, erythrocyte sedimentation rate (ESR), C-reactive protein (CRP), Health Assessment Questionnaire-Disability Index (HAQ-DI), and smoking status were analyzed for each patient group separately.

Clinical progression in relation to therapeutic continuity or adaptation was also assessed.

Patients in LDA or remission with radiographical progression were followed and observed for increases (number and time to increase) in DAS 28 $\geq$ 2.6 $\geq$ 3.2, grouped depending on their subsequent treatment scheme (adaptation vs. continuity approach).

The administered medicinal agents resulting in therapeutic change after radiographic progression in LDA or remission were analyzed independently for patients in LDA, remission, and radiographic progression. If a therapeutic change was introduced 20 days prior to 100 days after a radiographic progression, this patient was grouped as an intervention due to radiographic progression.

2.2. Statistical Analysis

The descriptive analyses of patient disease characteristics were compared using standard descriptive statistics. Continuous variables were compared using a Student's t-test and categorical variables with a Chi^2 (χ^2) test. All statistical analyses were 2-sided at the 0.05 significance level. The analyses have been performed using GraphPad Prism 5 software and R.

Radiographic progression was analyzed as a continuous outcome (i.e., the yearly rate of damage progression).

Multivariate analysis was conducted, adjusting for potential confounders and including various clinical, radiological, and patient-centered functional scores. The confounders considered were age, sex, disease duration, rheumatoid factor and ACPA positivity, DAS 28 level, disease duration, and number of previously used DMARDs.

The baseline disease characteristics were compared using standard descriptive statistics. Ratingen scores, DAS 28, and HAQ-DI scores were analyzed with the Wilcoxon signed-rank tests.

3. Results

3.1. Group Definition

Out of 10'141 RA patients in the SCQM cohort (1998–2020), 5'525 patients were selected, with 6'962 episodes in LDA. Within these 6'962 episodes in LDA, 11'803 sets of hand and foot X-rays of hands and feet were taken, and 2'614 periods of LDA were available with ≥2 sets of radiographs to analyze radiographic progression during LDA.

Similarly, 4'051 episodes of remission in 4'051 RA patients were found. Within these episodes of remission, 9'020 sets of hands and feet X-rays were taken, and 1'447 periods in remission with ≥2 radiographs were available for analysis.

3.2. Definition of Radiographical Progression vs. Non-Progression

Radiographic non-progression was significantly more frequent among patients in remission compared to LDA. The radiographic progression was analyzed as a calculated yearly increase in Ratingen scores of >1, 2, or 5 points/year.

In detail, 374 (25.8%), 146 (10.1%), and 128 (8.8%) patients progressed radiographically in remission, as compared to 1075 (38.0%), 739 (26.1%), and 317 (11.2%) in LDA with > 1 (χ^2: 78.5139, $p < 0.00001$), 2 (χ^2: 50.3102, $p < 0.00001$), or 5 points in the Ratingen score/year (χ^2: 5.768, $p = 0.016$), respectively (Table 1, Figure 1).

Table 1. Change in Ratingen scores in patients in LDA or remission.

	LDA (n = 2826)	Remission (n = 1447)
Repair *	4.8%	1.6%
No change ±1 Ratingen points/year	41.2% *	58.7% *
No change ±2 Ratingen points/year	61.0% *	81.8% *
No change ±5 Ratingen points/year	84.0% *	96.5% *
Progress 5–10 Ratingen points/year	7.0% *	1.9% *
Progress 10–20 Ratingen points/year	3.0% *	0.8% *
Progress >40 Ratingen points/year	0.14%	0%

* Statistically significant differences $p < 0.05$.

In parallel, 208 (4.8%) patients in LDA and 23 (1.6%) patients in remission developed repair, as defined by a decrease in Ratingen scores > 5 points (Chi-square 286.7425, $p < 0.00001$, Table 1, Figure 1).

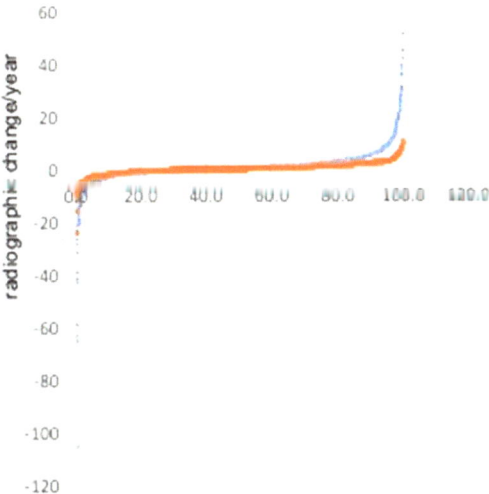

Figure 1. Radiographic-determined change/year within periods of LDA (blue) and remission (red) were analyzed separately for both patient groups. The groups were normalized to reflect progression observed between 2 sets of radiographs: 1447 patients in remission and 2614 patients in LDA.

3.3. Demographic Data

Based on these definitions of radiographic progression in LDA or remission, demographic data were analyzed per group and for the respective subgroups: patient groups were similar for age, sex, BMI, disease duration, DAS 28, HAQ-DI, ACPA, and rheumatoid factor independently, whether their changes in Ratingen scores/year were judged as repair, status quo, or progression independently or whether the patients were in continued remission or LDA. Interestingly, patients developing repair of joint erosions were younger (59.0 years vs. 68.7 years, all patients in remission in the analysis) and less frequent rheumatoid factor positive (60.9 vs. 71.5%, all patients in remission in the analysis, Tables 1 and 2).

Table 2. Demographic data.

Change in Ratingen Score (Points/Year) (Years)	LDA					Remission				
	Repair > −5	No Change, ±1	No Change, ±2	No Change, ±5	Progress >5	Repair >−5	No Change, ±1	No Change, ±2	No Change, ±5	Progress >5
Age (years, av)	50.0	53.8	56.9	56.9	59.0	59.0	69.1	69.0	68.9	67.7
Sex (% female)	69.8	69.6	72.4	72.4	65.2	65.2	70.4	70.1	70.5	78.6
Time to diagnosis (years)	7.4	7.0	6.4	6.4	13.1	13.1	14.2	14.1	14.2	18.1
Rheumatoid factor pos. (%)	70.8	76.7	70.3	71.6	60.9	60.9	69.3	70.5	71.3	92.9
ACPA pos. (%)	57.9	66.3	43.4	40.8	73.7	73.7	70.3	70.8	71.3	84.2
BMI (kg/m², av)	24.7	25.2	25.1	25.1	28.5	28.5	25.6	26.0	26.1	19.0
DAS 28	1.8	1.9	2.3	2.3	2.1	2.1	1.8	1.8	1.8	1.8
ESR (mm/h, av)	8.5	8.7	8.9	8.9	14.7	14.7	11.1	11.4	11.4	10.2
CRP (mg/L, av)	4.6	3.9	4.0	4.3	4.7	4.7	3.7	3.5	3.4	1.0
HAQ-DI	0.4	0.4	0.8	0.8	0.8	0.8	0.4	0.4	0.4	1.2
Smoking current (%)	12.3	12.6	20.8	23.3	22.2	22.2	16.6	15.4	14.7	14.3
Smoking ever (%)	26.9	25.9	29.2	28.8	22.2	22.2	43.6	42.3	41.7	14.3

For patients with double intervals with radiographic change and LDA, the first data entry was used for the analysis to avoid duplicates.

3.4. Therapeutic Changes After Radiographic Progression

A total of 57 patients (7.0%) in remission and 105 patients (12.9%) in LDA underwent therapeutic changes within 90 days following the detection of radiographic progression (χ^2: 4.203, $p < 0.0002$) (Table 3).

Table 3. Change in therapy after radiographic progression.

	LDA		Remission	
	Change Therapy ($n = 105$)	Stay on Therapy ($n = 706$)	Change Therapy ($n = 57$)	Stay on Therapy ($n = 729$)
Age (years)	57.0	56.9	69.1	68.1
Sex (% female)	72.2%	72.4%	77.2%	73.5%
Time to diagnosis (years)	10.2	6.4	15.6	14.3
Rheumatoid factor pos.	74.6%	70.3%	77.2%	77.0%
ACPA pos.	38.5%	43.4%	71.9%	54.6%
BMI (kg/m^2)	25.5	25.1	28.6	25.9
DAS 28	2.3	2.3	1.9	1.8
HAQ-DI	1.0	0.8	0.5	0.5
Smoking current	20.5%	20.8%	19.3%	26.3%
Smoking ever	23.0%	29.2%	19.3%	26.3%
No change +1 Ratingen points	-	-	30 (57.1%)	383 (52.5%)
No change +2 Ratingen points	30 (28.0%)	274 (30.1%)	14 (25.0%)	213 (29.2%)
No change +5 Ratingen points	39 (36.4%)	320 (39.8%)	10 (15.6%)	112 (15.4%)
Progress >5 Ratingen points	38 (35.1%)	210 (25.2%)	3 (4%)	24 (3.3%)

When we analyzed how much progression was required to result in therapeutic change, we found that 57.1% of patients in remission underwent a therapeutic change compared to none in LDA with a radiographic progression with a maximum of 1 Ratingen point/year (Table 3).

Conversely, 71.5% of patients in LDA with radiographic progression > 2 points in the Ratingen score/year underwent a therapeutic change compared to 19.6% of patients in remission (Table 3).

No differences in demographic data were found comparing patients staying in therapy as compared to changing therapy subsequent to radiographic progression in LDA and/or remission (Table 3).

The therapeutic strategies used after radiographic progression were oral glucocorticosteroids in 17.1% and 3.5%, conventional synthetic DMARDs in 46.7% and 35.1%, non-TNF biologic agents in 21.9% and 38.6%, TNF antagonists in 26.7% and 21.1%, and targeted synthetic DMARDs in 4.8% and 1.7% for patients progressing in LDA and remission, respectively (Tables 3 and 4).

Table 4. Therapeutic agents used after radiographic progression in LDA or remission.

	Therapeutic Agent	LDA ($n = 105$) Number	Remission ($n = 57$) Number
csDMARXDs/other drugs	Prednisone	18 *	2 *
	Chloroquine	10 *	- *
	Cyclophosphamide	1	-
	Sulfasalazine	11 *	1 *
	Leflunomide	14	8
	Methotrexate	13	11
Biologics	Abatacept	8	2
	Ixekizumab	1	-
	Rituximab	8	10
	Tocilizumab	6	10
TNF antagonists	Adalimumab	9	4
	Etanercept	7	3
	Golimumab	2	1
	Infliximab	10	2
	Certolizumab	-	2
tsDMARDs	Baricitinib	2	1
	Tofacitinib	3	-

* Statistically significant differences $p < 0.05$.

3.5. Clinical Follow-Up After Therapeutic Changes After Radiographic Progression Despite Remission

The frequency of patients who lost the status of a disease in remission was analyzed, revealing increases in DAS 28 > 2.6 in 15.8% and 4.1% (χ^2: 5.8565, $p = 0.016$), and increases in DAS 28 > 3.2 in 5.3% and 1.9% (χ^2: 0.5863, $p = 0.44$) during the next year of follow-up for patients with radiographic progression despite remission and changes in the therapeutic protocol, compared to patients who stayed on the same therapeutic protocol (Figure 2). The increase in DAS 28 > 2.6 occurred on average after 234.5 and 302.5 days ($p = 0.06$) for patients changing therapy or staying on the same therapeutic protocol, respectively. Likewise, the increase in DAS 28 > 3.2 occurred after 285.5 and 289.4 days ($p = 0.95$), respectively.

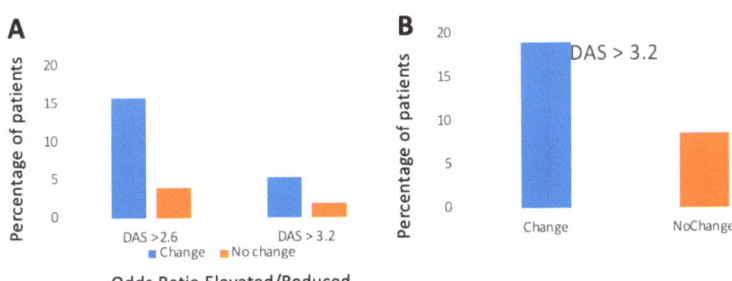

Figure 2. Frequency of radiographic progression: DAS 28 > 2.6 (left) and > 3.2 (right). (**A**) Remission, (**B**) LDA, Orange: No therapeutic regime change, Blue: Therapeutic regime change.

3.6. Clinical Development After Changing or Staying on Therapy Because of Radiographic Progression Despite LDA

The frequency of patients dropping out of LDA was analyzed, revealing rates of 19% and 8.5% (χ^2: 11.0272, $p = 0.0009$) for increases in DAS 28 > 3.2 during the next year of follow-up for patients with radiographic progression despite LDA and changes in the therapeutic protocol, compared to patients who stayed on the same therapeutic protocol. The increase in DAS 28 > 3.2 occurred on average after 208.1 and 294.7 days ($p = 0.06$) for patients changing therapy or staying on the same therapeutic protocol, respectively.

4. Discussion

In summary, we have demonstrated that radiographic progression despite LDA/remission is common. It occurred more frequently in patients in LDA (38.0%) compared to those in remission (25.8%, Figure 1). Therapeutic changes following radiographic progression were infrequent. These changes were more common in patients with LDA (12.9%) than in those with remission (7.0%). When analyzing clinical disease activity after a therapeutic change due to radiographic progression despite LDA or remission, it more frequently worsened compared to patients who remained on the same therapeutic regimen.

The question of whether achieving remission or the lower rate of radiographic progression in patients with remission discouraged rheumatologists from changing therapy remains unanswered and cannot be addressed in this analysis. Surprisingly, smaller changes in Ratingen scores ($\leq$1 point/year) were associated with a therapeutic change in patients in DAS 28-defined remission compared to patients in LDA. On the other hand, higher rates of radiographic progression (>2 points of Ratingen score) were more frequently associated with subsequent therapeutic changes.

Since the percentages of patients with radiographic progression did not differ based on the annual rate of progression when comparing patients with and without subsequent therapeutic changes, we reject the hypothesis that therapeutic change may be influenced by the degree of radiographic progression (Table 3). This rejection of the hypothesis is independent of the achieved clinical status of LDA or remission.

Therefore, whether the detection of smaller radiographic changes in patients in remission may lead to the urge to react to these minor changes remains open. However, our data indicate that patients may benefit if their treatment regime remains unaltered.

Secondly, there is no standardized strategy for how to react to radiographic progression despite LDA/remission (Table 4). Whether a specific strategy may help to prevent clinical progression after therapeutic change remains an open question.

We believe that the problem addressed is challenging to analyze in clinical trials or long-term follow-ups. Therefore, we hope that data from other registries may address the same question, giving us insight into the situation in other countries.

Thirdly, the data show less radiographical progression in remission compared to low disease activity. Thus, aiming for remission is beneficial in inhibiting radiographic progression as compared to LDA.

Interestingly, repair occurred more frequently in LDA than in remission (Figure 1). We hypothesize that minimal inflammation may be beneficial for stimulating the restructuring/repairing of damaged tissue. This hypothesis, suggesting that inflammation may promote repair, is also supported by other studies [19].

Weaknesses

The analysis is based on a registry, and missing data, as with any registry, is a concern. It is conceivable that patients with complex acute issues are less likely to be documented in registries, as the focus is on stabilizing symptoms and not updating databases. It is also feasible that time constraints of medical professionals may also play an important role.

Secondly, we had a central scoring of radiographs, but they were not consecutively scored for all patients.

Like other scoring systems, the Ratingen score only focuses on radiographic destruction and not joint space narrowing. However, radiographic erosions are more accessible to detect than joint space narrowing. It is our believe that incorporating additional information from the Sharp van der Heijde score may not provide substantial benefit for clinical decision making.

A major issue of this paper is the definition of LDA and sustained remission. Other criteria like S/CDAI or Boolean-defined remission were not analyzed in this paper. Furthermore DAS 28 remission defined <2.6 has been discussed as not being a sufficient basis for defining remission [20–22].

Next, the definition of sustained remission as a minimum of three months for the data collection does not suit the requested standard of six months. On the other hand, no patients with sustained LDA/remission shorter than 6 months were included in the analysis.

5. Conclusions

In conclusion, we have demonstrated that radiographic progression despite LDA/remission is frequent. However, reacting to radiographic progression may not be necessary for the patients in LDA/remission.

Author Contributions: Conceptualization, L.L.N.B., T.H., M.J.N., H.S.-K., J.v.K. and R.B.M.; Methodology, L.L.N.B., R.B.M. and J.v.K.; Validation, R.B.M.; Formal analysis, L.L.N.B. and R.B.M.; Writing—original draft, L.L.N.B. and R.B.M.; Writing—review and editing, L.L.N.B., R.B.M., H.S.-K. and J.v.K. All authors have read and agreed to the published version of the manuscript.

Funding: This research received no external funding.

Institutional Review Board Statement: This study was conducted in accordance with the Declaration of Helsinki and approved by the Institutional Review Board (or Ethics Committee, EKNZ, Project ID 2020-01173, approval date: 29 May 2020) of northwest and central Switzerland.

Informed Consent Statement: Informed consent was obtained from all subjects involved in the study.

Data Availability Statement: Study-related data can be made available from the SCQM Foundation according to the SCQM Rules of Research after the publication of all study-related research objectives. Researchers interested in further analyzing the data resulting from this study can contact the SCQM Foundation (scqm@hin.ch). Data can only be used for scientific research. SCQM is an ongoing, long-term registry with no end date for data collection and data provision. The original contributions presented in this study are included in the article; further inquiries can be directed to the corresponding authors.

Acknowledgments: A list of participating practices and hospitals contributing to the SCQM registries can be found on the SCQM website (https://www.scqm.ch/en/about-scqm/active-institutions/). The SCQM Foundation is supported by AbbVie, Biogen, Janssen-Cilag, Eli Lilly, MSD, Novartis, Pfizer, Sandoz, and UCB, as listed on the SCQM website (https://www.scqm.ch/en/partners/). SCQM supporting partners had no role in the study design, the analysis and interpretation of the data, the writing of the manuscript, or the decision to submit the manuscript for publication.

Conflicts of Interest: The authors declare no conflicts of interest.

References

1. Wolfe, F.; Sharp, J.T. Radiographic outcome of recent-onset rheumatoid arthritis: A 19-year study of radiographic progression. *Arthritis Rheum.* **1998**, *41*, 1571–1582. [CrossRef] [PubMed]
2. Smolen, J.S.; Landewé, R.B.M.; Bijlsma, J.W.J.; Burmester, G.R.; Dougados, M.; Chatzidionysiou, M.K.; Nam, J.; Ramiro, S.; Voshaar, M.; van Vollenhoven, R.; et al. EULAR recommendations for the management of rheumatoid arthritis with synthetic and biological disease-modifying anti-rheumatic drugs: 2016 update. *Ann. Rheum. Dis.* **2017**, *76*, 960–977. [CrossRef] [PubMed]
3. Bruynesteyn, K.; Landewé, R.; van der Linden, S.; van der Heijde, D. Radiography as the primary outcome in rheumatoid arthritis: Acceptable sample sizes for trials with 3 months follow up. *Ann. Rheum. Dis.* **2004**, *63*, 1413–1418. [CrossRef] [PubMed]
4. Cohen, S.B.; Dore, R.K.; Lane, N.E.; Ory, P.A.; Peterfy, C.G.; Sharp, J.T.; van der Heijde, D.; Zhou, L.; Tsuji, W.; Newmark, R.; et al. Denosumab treatment effects on structural damage, bone mineral density, and bone turnover in rheumatoid arthritis: A twelve-month, multicenter, randomized, double-blind, placebo-controlled, phase II clinical trial. *Arthritis Rheum.* **2008**, *58*, 1299–1309. [CrossRef] [PubMed]
5. Genant, H.K.; Peterfy, C.G.; Westhovens, R.; Becker, J.-C.; Aranda, R.; Vratsanos, G.; Teng, J.; Kremer, J.M. Abatacept inhibits progression of structural damage in rheumatoid arthritis: Results from the long-term extension of the AIM trial. *Ann. Rheum. Dis.* **2008**, *67*, 1084–1089. [CrossRef]
6. Breedveld, F.C.; Weisman, M.H.; Kavanaugh, A.F.; Cohen, S.B.; Pavelka, K.; van Vollenhoven, R.; Sharp, J.; Perez, J.L.; Spencer-Green, G.T. The PREMIER study: A multicenter, randomized, double-blind clinical trial of combination therapy with adalimumab plus methotrexate versus methotrexate alone or adalimumab alone in patients with early, aggressive rheumatoid arthritis who had not had previous methotrexate treatment. *Arthritis Rheum.* **2006**, *54*, 26–37.
7. Nishimoto, N.; Hashimoto, J.; Miyasaka, N.; Yamamoto, K.; Kawai, S.; Takeuchi, T.; Murata, N.; van der Heijde, D.; Kishimoto, T. Study of active controlled monotherapy used for rheumatoid arthritis, an IL-6 inhibitor (SAMURAI): Evidence of clinical and radiographic benefit from an x-ray reader-blinded randomized controlled trial of tocilizumab. *Ann. Rheum. Dis.* **2007**, *66*, 1162–1167. [CrossRef]
8. Cohen, S.B.; Emery, P.; Greenwald, M.W.; Dougados, M.; Furie, R.A.; Genovese, M.C.; Keystone, E.C.; Loveless, J.E.; Burmester, G.-R.; Cravets, M.W.; et al. Rituximab for rheumatoid arthritis refractory to anti-tumor necrosis factor therapy: Results of a multicenter, randomized, double-blind, placebo-controlled, phase III trial evaluating primary efficacy and safety at twenty-four weeks. *Arthritis Rheum.* **2006**, *54*, 2793–2806. [CrossRef]
9. Prevoo, M.L.; van't Hof, M.A.; Kuper, H.H.; van Leeuwen, M.A.; van de Putte, L.B.; van Riel, P.L. Modified disease activity scores that include twenty-eight-joint counts. Development and validation in a prospective longitudinal study of patients with rheumatoid arthritis. *Arthritis Rheum.* **1995**, *38*, 44–48. [CrossRef]
10. Aletaha, D.; Smolen, J. The Simplified Disease Activity Index (SDAI) and the Clinical Disease Activity Index (CDAI): A review of their usefulness and validity in rheumatoid arthritis. *Clin. Exp. Rheumatol.* **2005**, *23* (Suppl. S39), 100–108.
11. Van der Heijde, D. How to read radiographs according to the Sharp/van der Heijde method. *J. Rheumatol.* **1999**, *26*, 743–745.
12. Rau, R.; Wassenberg, S.; Herborn, G.; Stucki, G.; Gebler, A. A new method of scoring radiographic change in rheumatoid arthritis. *J. Rheumatol.* **1998**, *25*, 2094–2107. [PubMed]
13. Smolen, J.S.; Breedveld, F.C.; Schiff, M.H.; Kalden, J.R.; Emery, P.; Eberl, G.; van Riel, P.L.; Tugwell, P. A simplified disease activity index for rheumatoid arthritis for use in clinical practice. *Rheumatology* **2003**, *42*, 244–257. [CrossRef] [PubMed]
14. Sewerin, P.; Vordenbaeumen, S.; Hoyer, A.; Brinks, R.; Buchbender, C.; Miese, F.; Schleich, C.; Klein, S.; Schneider, M.; Ostendorf, B. Silent progression in patients with rheumatoid arthritis: Is DAS28 remission an insufficient goal in RA? Results from the German Remission-plus cohort. *BMC Musculoskelet. Disord.* **2017**, *18*, 163. [CrossRef] [PubMed]
15. Fonseca, J.E.; Canhão, H.; Tavares, N.J.; Cruz, M.; Branco, J.; Queiroz, M.V. Persistent low-grade synovitis without erosive progression in magnetic resonance imaging of rheumatoid arthritis patients treated with infliximab over 1 year. *Clin. Rheumatol.* **2009**, *28*, 1213–1216. [CrossRef] [PubMed]

16. Soukup, T.; Nekvindova, J.; Dosedel, M.; Brtkova, J.; Toms, J.; Bastecka, D.; Bradna, P.; Vlcek, J.; Pavek, P. Methotrexate impact on radiographic progression in biologic-treated rheumatoid arthritis under clinical remission: A case report on monozygotic Caucasian twins. *Int. J. Immunopathol. Pharmacol.* **2016**, *29*, 790–795. [CrossRef]
17. Rezaei, H.; Saevarsdottir, S.; Forslind, K.; Albertsson, K.; Wallin, H.; Bratt, J.; Ernestam, S.; Geborek, P.; Pettersson, I.F.; van Vollenhoven, R.F. In early rheumatoid arthritis, patients with a good initial response to methotrexate have excellent 2-year clinical outcomes, but radiological progression is not fully prevented: Data from the methotrexate responders population in the SWEFOT trial. *Ann. Rheum. Dis.* **2012**, *71*, 186–191. [CrossRef]
18. Machold, K.P.; Stamm, T.A.; Nell, V.P.K.; Pflugbeil, S.; Aletaha, D.; Steiner, G.; Uffmann, M.; Smolen, J.S. Very recent onset rheumatoid arthritis: Clinical and serological patient characteristics associated with radiographic progression over the first years of disease. *Rheumatology* **2007**, *46*, 342–349. [CrossRef]
19. Takeuchi, T.; Yoshida, H.; Tanaka, S. Role of interleukin-6 in bone destruction and bone repair in rheumatoid arthritis. *Autoimmun. Rev.* **2021**, *9*, 102884. [CrossRef]
20. Felson, D.T.; Smolen, J.S.; Wells, G.; Zhang, B.; van Tuyl, L.H.D.; Funovits, J.; Aletaha, D.; Allaart, C.F.; Bathon, J.; Bombardieri, S.; et al. American College of Rheumatology/European League against Rheumatism provisional definition of remission in rheumatoid arthritis for clinical trials. *Ann. Rheum. Dis.* **2011**, *70*, 404–413. [CrossRef]
21. Smolen, J.S.; Aletaha, D. Scores for all seasons: SDAI and CDAI. *Clin. Exp. Rheumatol.* **2014**, *32* (Suppl. S85), S75–S79.
22. Hèctor, C.; Millan, A.M.; Diaz-Torne, C. Rheumatoid Arthritis: Defining Clinical and Ultrasound Deep Remission. *Mediterr. J. Rheumatol.* **2020**, *31*, 384–388. [CrossRef] [PubMed]

Disclaimer/Publisher's Note: The statements, opinions and data contained in all publications are solely those of the individual author(s) and contributor(s) and not of MDPI and/or the editor(s). MDPI and/or the editor(s) disclaim responsibility for any injury to people or property resulting from any ideas, methods, instructions or products referred to in the content.

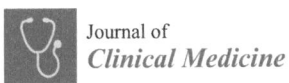

Article

Ultrasound-Guided Injections of HYADD4 for Knee Osteoarthritis Improves Pain and Functional Outcomes at 3, 6, and 12 Months without Changes in Measured Synovial Fluid, Serum Collagen Biomarkers, or Most Synovial Fluid Biomarker Proteins at 3 Months

Richard T. Meehan [1,*], Mary T. Gill [1], Eric D. Hoffman [1], Claire M. Coeshott [1], Manuel D. Galvan [1], Molly L. Wolf [1], Isabelle A. Amigues [1], Liudmila M. Kastsianok [1], Elizabeth A. Regan [1], James L. Crooks [1,2], Gregory J. Czuczman [1,3] and Vijaya Knight [4]

[1] Departments of Medicine, Clinical Labs, Radiology and Divisions of Rheumatology, Immunology/Complement Labs, and Biostatistics and Bioinformatics, National Jewish Health, Denver, CO 80206, USA; gillm@njhealth.org (M.T.G.); ehoffman@arthroventions.org (E.D.H.); coeshottc@njhealth.org (C.M.C.); galvanm@njhealth.org (M.D.G.); molly.wolf@vailhealth.org (M.L.W.); dramigues@unabridgedmd.com (I.A.A.); regane@njhealth.org (E.A.R.); crooksj@njhealth.org (J.L.C.); gregory.czuczman@riao.com (G.J.C.)

[2] Department of Epidemiology, Colorado School of Public Health, CU Anschutz School of Medicine, University of Colorado, Aurora, CO 80045, USA

[3] Radiology Imaging Associates, Englewood, CO 80112, USA

[4] Department of Pediatrics, Section of Allergy and Immunology, CU Anschutz School of Medicine, University of Colorado, Aurora, CO 80045, USA; vijaya.knight@childrenscolorado.org

* Correspondence: meehanr@njhealth.org

Abstract: Background: Prior studies have demonstrated improved efficacy when intra-articular (IA) therapeutics are injected using ultrasound (US) guidance. The aim of this study was to determine if clinical improvement in pain and function after IA hyaluronic acid injections using US is associated with changes in SF volumes and biomarker proteins at 3 months. Methods: 49 subjects with symptomatic knee OA, BMI < 40, and KL radiographic grade II or III participated. Subjects with adequate aspirated synovial fluid (SF) volumes received two US-guided IA-HA injections of HYADD4 (24 mg/3 mL) 7 days apart. Clinical evaluations at 3, 6, and 12 months included WOMAC, VAS, PCS scores, 6 MWD, and US-measured SF depth. SF and blood were collected at 3 months and analyzed for four serum OA biomarkers and fifteen SF proteins. Results: Statistical differences were observed at 3, 6, and 12 months compared to baseline values, with improvements at 12 months for WOMAC scores (50%), VAS (54%), and PCS scores (24%). MMP10 levels were lower at 3 months without changes in SF volumes, serum levels of C2C, COMP, HA, CPII, or SF levels of IL-1 ra, IL-4, 6, 7, 8, 15, 18, ILGFBP-1, 3, and MMP 1, 2, 3, 8, 9. Baseline clinical features or SF biomarker protein levels did not predict responsiveness at 3 months. Conclusions: Clinical improvements were observed at 12 months using US needle guidance for IA HA, whereas only one SF protein biomarker protein was different at 3 months. Larger studies are needed to identify which SF biomarkers will predict which individual OA patients will receive the greatest benefit from IA therapeutics.

Keywords: osteoarthritis; ultrasound; synovial fluid; biomarkers; cytokines

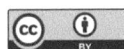

1. Introduction

Knee osteoarthritis (OA) is an increasingly common leading cause of disability and is costly to manage, especially if patients progress and require surgical intervention [1,2]. Unfortunately, there are no effective FDA-approved disease-modifying therapeutic agents that can halt or reverse cartilage loss in knee OA. However, two recently published large cardiovascular treatment trials demonstrated that inhibition of IL-1 beta by canakinumab and low-dose colchicine reduced the incidence of hip and knee arthroplasty compared to the placebo groups [3,4]. Therefore, intra-articular (IA) hyaluronic acid (HA) injections are common treatment options for knee OA patients to provide symptomatic pain relief or for those who are not surgical candidates or choose to defer total joint arthroplasty [5].

Recent studies emphasize the knee as an organ containing important supporting structures, including the subchondral bone, ligaments, joint capsule, meniscus, synovium, and the surrounding musculature, in addition to cartilage [6]. There is also growing evidence that knee OA is associated with chronic inflammation and phenotypes rather than a non-inflammatory degenerative joint disease process. Synovial biopsies revealed synovitis in 50% of patients with early OA, and synovial fluid (SF) analysis revealed cytokines and other inflammatory mediators that distinguish early from advanced knee OA [7,8]. The presence of substantial synovial effusion and synovitis on MRI also correlates with subsequent loss of knee cartilage among OA patients [9]. It has also been reported that OA SF contains a pro-inflammatory cytokine profile [10–14]. We also observed that many OA patients with sufficiently severe knee pain requesting an IA glucocorticoid or HA injection have a pro-inflammatory SF cytokine profile similar to that of many rheumatoid arthritis (RA) patients [15]. SF is also a rich source of potentially valuable biomarkers that may be used to classify different OA endotypes and, hopefully, in the future, may help guide therapy by predicting drug responsiveness for individual patients [16].

There are multiple proposed mechanisms whereby IA HA injections might provide clinical benefit in OA [17–19]. These include anti-inflammatory properties based upon in vitro studies, improved SF viscoelastic, rheologic, and frictional properties of HA, and possible chondroprotection since HA also interacts directly with articular cartilage [20].

The viscosupplement used in this study, HYADD4 (Hymovis® Fidia, Abano Terme, Padova, Italy), is a modified derivative of HA with a molecular weight of 500–730 kDa obtained by a controlled chemical–physical synthesis process with 2% of the carboxyl radicals on the glucuronic acid present in the polysaccharide chain conjugated with an aliphatic amine (hexadexyclamine) [21]. The chemical modification of HA by the addition of hexadecylamine increases the rheological properties of HYADD4, conferring higher viscoelasticity in solution compared to other HA derivatives of the same molecular weight. To confirm delivery of this HA product into the synovial fluid compartment, we utilized ultrasound (US) guidance with direct needle visualization during all injections and aspirations. Other studies have confirmed that US delivery of glucocorticoids into the knee joint space is more effective and less painful than non-image-based injections [22,23].

We chose to use direct needle visualization with US guidance as well as an external pneumatic compression device to enhance the success of aspiration even in patients with very small SF effusions since no OA patients were excluded from this study based upon the size of knee effusions on US [24]. To our knowledge, this is the first study to determine if an IA HA injection alters SF volumes as a surrogate for intra-articular inflammation and if baseline clinical features or SF protein levels predict clinical responsiveness at 3 months when HA is delivered with US guidance.

2. Materials and Methods

2.1. Subjects

This single-center, open-label, prospective, investigator-initiated knee OA biomarker study (HS 3179, ClinicalTrials.gov accessed on 5 July 2023 NCT 04093232) was conducted with all subjects providing informed consent after Institutional Review Board approval. We recruited subjects from National Jewish Health (NJH) clinics, clinical trial notification web sites, and local radio advertisements. Exclusion criteria included age < 21 or >80 years, BMI > 40, pregnancy, knee surgery within one year, IA injectable therapeutics within 3 months, a history of systemic inflammatory or crystal arthritis, prior allergic reactions to chloroprep, lidocaine, or HA products, or any use of oral or systemic immunomodulatory therapeutics. Subjects were also required to ambulate for 6 min without the use of walking assistive devices, and the diagnosis of knee osteoarthritis was confirmed by a NJH study rheumatologist. Weight-bearing tibiofemoral joint radiographs were obtained within 1 year of their first study visit. These images were reviewed by a fellowship-trained musculoskeletal (MSK) radiologist for study inclusion based upon the presence of Kellgren-Lawrence (KL) grade II or III osteoarthritis [25]. Forty-nine eligible subjects had one knee aspirated between 2019 and 2021, and if an adequate SF volume of ≥0.5 mL was aspirated, they received the first of two intra-articular (IA) injections of an HA HYADD 4 (Hymovis® 24 mg/3 mL, Fidia Farmaceutici S.p.A., Abano Terme, Padova, Italy) and provided simultaneous peripheral blood samples.

The study protocol included five visits over 12 months. Baseline visit 1 included clinical assessments, knee aspiration, and an IA HA injection if the SF aspirated volume was ≥0.5 mL. Visit 2 was scheduled 7 days later for a second US-guided IA HA injection and a peripheral blood draw. Three additional visits at 3, 6, and 12 months were for clinical assessments and US-measured SF depth.

2.2. Aspiration and Injection Technique

An external pneumatic compression device (KneeTap™ Arthroventions LLC, Denver, CO, USA) was inflated to 100 mmHg as previously described [24]. Ultrasound images were acquired using a GE LOGIQ e ultrasound (Fairfield, CT, USA) with a 12L-RS linear array probe, as displayed in Figure 1A,B.

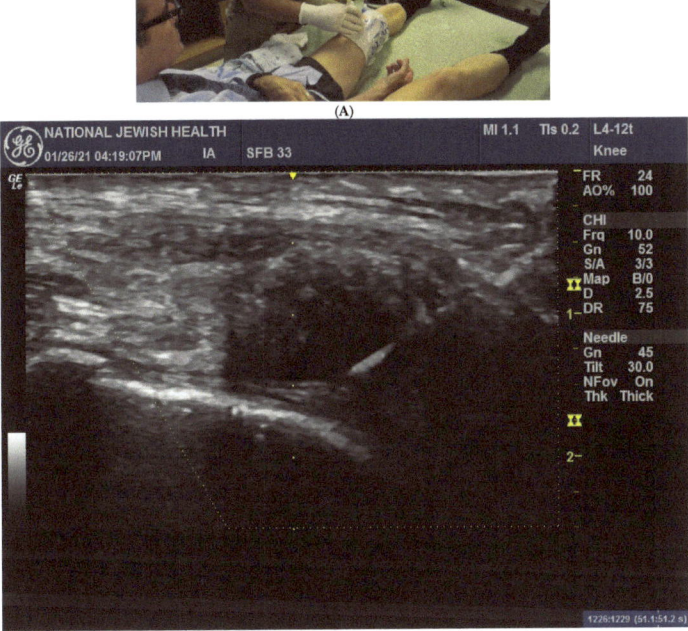

Figure 1. (**A**) An inflated pneumatic compression device with an image displayed on an ultrasound screen prior to successful knee aspiration of synovial fluid. Image courtesy of Dr. R. Meehan and Dr. R. Scheuring. (**B**) US image of a study subject during needle insertion, displaying a bright 20-gauge needle entering from the upper right-hand corner of the image with the tip placed within the intra-synovial space (dark anechoic region) during inflation and prior to injecting IA HA product.

A direct-in-line needle visualization technique was used for all procedures. The probe was covered with gel; a sterile sleeve (CIV-FlexTM Transducer Cover, CIVCO Kalona, IA, USA) and sterile gel were next applied. The injection site was cleansed with ChloroPrep One-Step (2% w/v chlorhexidine gluconate and 70% v/v isopropyl alcohol, Care Fusion, El Paso, TX, USA), and then a sterile drape was placed. All procedures were performed by an American College of Rheumatology (ACR) certified MSK US-trained rheumatologist who used sterile gloves, head coverings, and surgical face masks to reduce the risk of needle entry site contamination and per NJH COVID precaution guidelines. The superior-lateral site was selected most often with the knee in slight flexion during supine positioning. The needle entry site was selected based on the US location of the largest anechoic region in SF. The skin, joint capsule, and anechoic region were then infiltrated with 1–2 mLs of preservative-free 2% lidocaine HCL (40 mg/2 mL) without epinephrine (Hospira Inc., Lake Forest, IL, USA) using a 27-gauge needle with US visualization. Next, also with direct needle visualization, an 18-gauge needle on a syringe was advanced into the anesthetized region to avoid needle tip placement into the joint capsule, synovium, or plica during aspiration and injection. The steer needle image enhancement software program on the GE US instrument was utilized, which allowed visualization of the 27-gauge needle during local infiltration of lidocaine as well as the aspirating and injecting needle during product instillation. If an adequate amount of SF volume was obtained during visit 1, then with the 18-gauge needle remaining in place, HYADD4 (24 mg/3 mL) was injected under direct US visualization. For study visit 2, scheduled for 7 days later, a 20-gauge needle was placed on the IA HA syringe for direct US-visualized injection after local infiltration of lidocaine without an aspiration.

2.3. Sample Preparation and Analysis of SF and Serum Proteins

SF was aspirated into a 5 or 20 mL syringe (Medline Industries Inc., Mundelein, IL, USA) and rapidly transferred into 6 mL plastic tubes containing sodium heparin (BD, Becton Drive, Franklin Lakes, NJ, USA). SF white blood cells (WBCs) were counted on a Beckman Coulter ACT 2 diff hematology analyzer (Beckman Coulter, Loveland, CO, USA). Peripheral blood was then collected into 6 mL plastic vacutainer tubes (BD) without anticoagulant for serum samples. SF and peripheral blood samples were centrifuged at 2000 rpm for 10 min within 45 min of collection and then aliquoted into 200 µL or 50 µL vials for storage at −80 °C until analyzed. All SF analytes were measured by multiplex fluorescent bead (Luminex) immune assays using three separate R&D Systems Inc. kits (Minneapolis, MN, USA). The following analytes were quantitated in pg/mL: IL-1ra (Interleukin 1 receptor antagonist), IL-4 (Interleukin 4), IL-6 (Interleukin 6), IL-7 (Interleukin 7), IL-8 (Interleukin 8), IL-15 (Interleukin 15), IL-18 (Interleukin 18), IGFBP-1 (Insulin-Like Growth Factor Binding Protein 1), IGFBP-3 (Insulin-Like Growth Factor Binding Protein 3), and MMPs (Matrix Metalloproteinases) 1, 2, 3, 8, 9, and 10. The bead multiplex assay was performed as previously described [15]. Cytokine concentrations were calculated with reference to the standard curve for each analyte.

Serum cartilage biomarkers were analyzed in the Duke University Molecular Physiology Institute laboratory (Durham, NC, USA), under the direction of Virginia Kraus, MD, PhD. These included Collagen Type II cleavage product (C2C), Hyaluronic acid (HA), procollagen II C-propeptide (CP II), and cartilage oligomeric matrix protein (COMP). These were quantitated in ng/mL as previously described using various enzyme-linked immunosorbent assays (ELISA) as either competitive inhibition or sandwich protein binding [26]. In general, C2C, HA, and COMP levels reflect cartilage degeneration, whereas CPII levels correlate with type II collagen synthesis. All samples were analyzed in duplicate and paired at baseline, and samples from visit 3 at 3 months were run simultaneously.

2.4. Clinical Efficacy Variables

Four clinical variables were measured at baseline, 3, 6, and 12 months: Western Ontario and McMaster Universities Index (WOMAC) total scores, Visual Analog Pain Score (VAS

0–10), physical component score (PCS) scores on the SF-36 health survey questionnaires (physical function/bodily pain and general health), 6-min walking distance in meters (6 MWD), and US-measured SF depth (mm). The US measured depth was obtained before and after an external pneumatic compression device was inflated to 100 mmHg to facilitate aspiration by increasing available SF volumes under positive pressure [24].

The WOMAC score is a validated patient-self-administered index of knee osteoarthritis pain and functional capacity [27]. It consists of 24 separate items divided into three subcategories (pain, stiffness, and physical function) rated on a difficulty scale as either none, slight, moderate, very, or extreme. The PCS score is a composite score of 21 questions, which are related to four domains: physical functioning, role limitations due to physical health, pain, and general health. The maximum value of 100 would indicate no functional limitations, no pain, and excellent health scored using the following instrument: https://chiro.org/LINKS/How_to_score_the_SF-36.shtml, accessed on 5 July 2023 [28,29].

Lower values on the self-reported WOMAC scores and VAS indicate improved function or less pain, whereas higher PCS scores and greater distance on the 6 MWD indicate an improvement in function with less pain and an ability to ambulate further. We defined the subset of responders based upon OMERACT-OARSI definitions as those subjects who had either a 50% improvement in function on WOMAC scores or a 50% reduction in pain on VAS scores, or those with a 20% improvement in function on WOMAC scores and a 20% reduction in pain on VAS scores [30].

The SF depth was measured on the recorded US image (GE logiq e) as the largest anechoic region in mm of depth on either the lateral ($n = 30$) or medial ($n = 4$) infrapatellar compartment. All study data (demographics, medical history, prior treatments, screening criteria) and results were placed into the NJH REDCap^{TM} version 13.1.37 (Vanderbilt University, Nashville, TN, USA) web-based secure research database system for storage and subsequent statistical analysis.

2.5. Statistical Analysis

Statistical differences between baseline values and results at 3, 6, and 12 months were determined using a paired ANOVA test with $p < 0.05$ significance. SF and peripheral blood protein levels of each analyte between baseline and those at 3 months were also measured using paired ANOVA, with the cytokine concentration outcomes transformed into log10 with p-values < 0.05 considered significant and adjusted for the number of analytes using the Bonferroni method. If values were missing for an individual subject for a specific analyte, then that subject was excluded from statistical analysis for that specific analyte. For the purpose of calculations, samples that exceeded the upper limit of the analytical measurement range or those that were below the detection limit were assigned the upper limit value or lower limit value, respectively, for the respective cytokine, chemokine, MMP, or protein, as previously described [15].

A linear regression analysis of improvement on WOMAC scores was regressed against log10-transformed analyte concentrations to determine associations between clinical improvement and baseline cytokine concentrations. All modeling was performed in the R language [31]. Correlations were then performed to determine which baseline clinical features (age, gender, BMI, prior surgery, radiographic severity KL II vs. III, and serum or SF biomarker proteins) correlated best with IA HA responsiveness at 3, 6, and 12 months. Differences between paired serum OA biomarkers were analyzed using paired t tests. A non-paired t-test was used to compare differences in age and BMI between responders and non-responders, and Fisher's exact test was used for the other clinical variables.

3. Results

Thirty-six of the subjects had adequate aspirated SF volumes on their first visit and therefore received two IA HA injections and continued study enrollment. Figure 2 displays the study subject participation numbers and reasons for any withdrawals. No subjects were excluded from enrolling in this study based on the presence or absence of knee effusions on physical examination, including those with very small effusions observed on US imaging during their initial visit. Thirteen of the 49 enrolled subjects were ineligible to continue to participate since their aspirated SF volume was <0.5 mL. The average measured SF depth on US was only 3.2 ± 2.2 mm before the pneumatic device was inflated, even among those with a successful SF aspiration of ≥0.5 mL. On physical examination, only 1 of our 49 enrolled subjects had a clinically apparent effusion, whereas three others only had an effusion with a fluid bulge in the medial compartment during manual compression of the lateral compartment. Therefore, 92% of our patients had non-effusive knee OA.

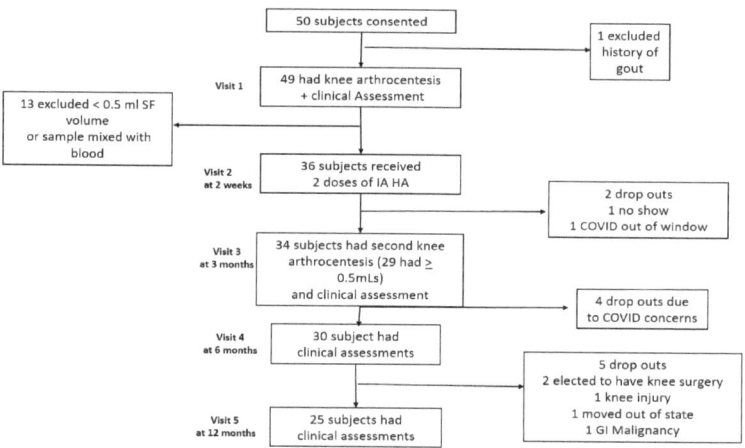

Figure 2. Subject participation, timeline of study visits, and reasons for withdrawals.

The results in Table 1 display the demographic and clinical features of 34 subjects who completed baseline and 3-month evaluations. An equal number of female and male patients, who also met the BMI inclusion criteria of <40, had their 3-month follow-up visits. No study subjects were excluded based on the size of the knee effusion or prior surgical interventions, except for total knee arthroplasty. There were slightly more subjects with a KL III severity score (56%) than those with a KL II rating (44%), whereas KL I or IV scores were exclusion criteria. We enrolled twelve subjects with the following prior surgical procedures on the aspirated knees: five with meniscectomies, three with ACL reconstruction, two with surgery for recurrent patella dislocations, and two with arthroscopic resurfacing/debridement procedures. Ten of the 12 subjects who received prior surgery returned for their 3-month follow-up visit and therefore were listed in Table 1. The mean age of those with prior surgery (58 years, range 35–71) was similar to that of those without surgery (60 years, range 39–78). The higher prevalence of the lateral (88%) vs. medial (12%) site of joint aspiration reflected the preferred site by the performing physician to reduce subject discomfort unless the medial joint site had a substantially larger joint effusion on US.

The clinical efficacy and measured SF depth results for the subjects who completed baseline, 3-, 6-, and 12-month visits are displayed in Table 2. Sustained clinical and statistically significant improvements compared to baseline values were observed on WOMAC scores and self-reported VAS at 12 months, with a 50% and 54% decrease, respectively ($p < 0.0001$). PCS scores also significantly increased over baseline scores by 24% at 12 months ($p < 0.0001$). The 6 MWD improved at 3 months by 7% ($p < 0.01$); however, the improved distance walked at 6 and 12 months was not statistically significant. In a subset of 18 of the 34 patients at 3 months with an adequate SF volume remaining for analysis and without blood contamination, the SF total WBC count fell 54% at 3 months from 199 ± 200 to 92 ± 70 cells/mm^3; however, this difference was not statistically significant ($p = 0.05$). While improvements in WOMAC, VAS, and PAS scores were observed at

3, 6, and 12 months, the measured SF volumes before or after inflation of the pneumatic compression device were slightly lower at 3 months. However, these differences did not achieve statistical significance. Only one study-related adverse event was observed (1 out of 72 injections), with one subject experiencing increased knee pain 4 h after her second IA HA injection with some knee swelling 24 h later, which resolved completely within one week, and then she was able to resume running.

Table 1. Clinical features and demographic information on 34 OA subjects who completed baseline and 3-month visits following intra-articular HA knee injections.

Age	60.8 years (35–78)
Gender	17 Male (50%)/17 Female (50%)
BMI kg/m^2	28 (20–39)
Prior knee surgery	10 (29%)
K-L grade	
II	15 (44%)
III	19 (56%)
Knee injected	
Right	18 (53%)
Left	16 (47%)
Lateral	30 (88%)
Medial	4 (12%)

Table 2. Subject's mean and standard deviation values with percentage change in four functional and pain instruments and synovial fluid depth measurements at baseline compared to values 3-, 6-, and 12-months post-IA HYADD4 injections with statistical significance in p-values.

	Baseline Mean ± SD n = 36	3-Month Mean ± SD n = 34	6-Month Mean ± SD n = 30	12-Month Mean ± SD n = 25
WOMAC score	771 ± 394	463 ± 358 40% decrease $p < 0.0001$	464 ± 352 40% decrease $p < 0.0001$	402 ± 333 50% decrease $p < 0.0001$
VAS score	4.9 ± 2.0	2.7 ± 1.7 45% decrease $p < 0.0001$	2.4 ± 1.9 51% decrease $p < 0.0001$	2.2 ± 1.73 54% decrease $p < 0.0001$
PCS score	64.7 ± 18.1	74.6 ± 18.7 15% increase $p < 0.0001$	76.5 ± 18.1 18% increase $p < 0.0001$	81.2 ± 11.9 24% increase $p < 0.0001$
6 MWD-Meters	404 ± 67	432 ± 83 7% increase $p < 0.007$	422 ± 75 5% increase NS	424 ± 69 5% increase NS
SF before inflation (mm)	3.2 ± 2.2	3.1 ± 2.2 3% decrease NS	4.0 ± 2.9 25% increase NS	4.2 ± 2.8 31% increase NS
SF after inflation (mm)	6.4 ± 3.7	5.2 ± 2.8 18% decrease NS	7.5 ± 4.0 17% increase NS	7.5 ± 3.4 17% increase NS

Legend: WOMAC score = Western Ontario and McMaster Universities Osteoarthritis Index; VAS = Visual Analog Pain score; PCS score = subset on SF 36 quality of life questionnaire; 6 MWD = 6-min walking distance; SF = depth of synovial fluid measured on ultrasound; NS = not significant values compared to baseline.

Table 3 displays the demographic and clinical features of the 30 subjects who met the criteria as responders compared to the six non-responder subjects. Twenty-four respondent subjects had both a 50% improvement in WOMAC scores and a 50% reduction in pain on the VAS. Four respondent subjects met criteria by having a 50% improvement in function on WOMAC scores or a 50% reduction in pain on the VAS scale. Only two subjects met responder criteria by having a 20% improvement in function on the WOMAC and a 20% reduction in pain on the VAS scale. There were no statistical differences between responders and non-responders in baseline demographic features of age and BMI using the unpaired *t*-test or based upon gender, prior surgical intervention, or KL ratings using the Fisher's exact test. Furthermore, no statistical differences were observed among responders vs. non-responders based upon baseline values on WOMAC, VAS, PCS score, 6 MWD, or the amount of SF measured by US.

Table 3. Clinical features, functional status, pain, and synovial fluid measurements at baseline between responders and non-responders with *p*-values.

Demographics	Responders n = 30	Non Responders n = 6	*p*-Values
Age mean and range	59 (19–78) years	62 (54–78) years	0.48
Gender and %	13 F (43%)/17 M (57%)	4 F (66%)/2 M (33%)	0.39
BMI mean and range	28.1 (19–39)	26.6 (21–32)	0.61
Prior Surgery and %	9 (30%)	3 (50%)	0.38
KL II or III and %	18 KL II (60%)/12 KL III (40%)	5 KL II (83%)/1 KL III (17%)	0.39
Functional Status, pain and US depth of SF			
WOMAC score	814	675	0.44
VAS (1–10 scale)	5.2	3.5	0.051
PCS score	64.1	64.6	0.96
6 MWD (meters)	406	428	0.49
US depth Before inflation	3.7 mm	4.3 mm	0.75
After inflation	7.7 mm	5.9 mm	0.37

The results of the OA serum biomarkers are presented in Table 4. The results of only those subjects with paired serum collected at baseline and 3 months later (34 of 36 subjects who received HA injections) were analyzed for statistical differences. While serum levels of C2C, CP II, and COMP were lower at 3 months compared to baseline values, these differences were not statistically significant. In contrast, HA levels were actually higher at 3 months, but those levels were also not statistically different from baseline values.

Table 4. Serum cartilage biomarker levels at baseline and 3 months after IA HA injection with *p*-values.

	Baseline Mean ± SD	3-Month Mean ± SD	% Increase or Decrease from Baseline	*p*-Values
	n = 34	n = 34		
C2C ng/mL	278 ± 48	263 ± 52	5% decrease	0.08
COMP ng/mL	828 ± 400	798 ± 435	4% decrease	0.36
HA ng/mL	41 ± 29	52 ± 58	27% increase	0.27
CPII ng/mL	1269 ± 508	1204 ± 549	5% decrease	0.32

Legend: C2C = collagen Type II cleavage product; COMP = cartilage oligomeric matrix protein; HA = hyaluronic acid; CPII = procollagen II C-Propeptide. *p*-values were calculated using paired *t*-tests.

The SF levels of various protein biomarkers 3 months after IA HA injections and percentage increases or decreases from baseline values are reported in Table 5. These SF protein levels are from paired samples analyzed on the Luminex platform using identical

19-plex, 3-plex, or 5-plex kits on the same day for each subject's paired samples. Due to the number of separate proteins analyzed and subsequent sample depletion as the assay needed to be validated during multiple prior runs, the number of paired SF samples available for final analysis was either 10 or 16 paired subjects, as reported in Table 5. While some analytes had large changes from baseline levels, including a 61% increase for IL-8 and an 87% decrease in IL-4 levels at 3 months, only the observed 16% reduction in MMP-10 levels at 3 months was statistically different from baseline values. p-values were calculated with a paired two-sided t-test on the log-concentrated levels in pg/mL.

Table 5. The mean values, standard deviation, percentage change, and p-values for each analyte at baseline and 3 months after IA HA injections.

Protein	Baseline Mean ± SD pg/mL	3-Month Mean ± SD pg/mL	% Increase or Decrease from Baseline	p-Values
IL-1ra $n = 16$	345 ± 332	518 ± 564	50% increase	0.127
IL-4 $n = 10$	1971 ± 5243	251 ± 107	87% decrease	0.395
IL-6 $n = 16$	60 ± 98	40 ± 44	33% decrease	0.905
IL-7 $n = 16$	7 ± 1	8 ± 2	14% increase	0.167
IL-8 $n = 16$	36 ± 41	58 ± 77	61% increase	0.273
IL-15 $n = 16$	6 ± 3	7 ± 4	17% increase	0.825
IL-18 $n = 16$	109 ± 63	103 ± 63	6% decrease	0.402
IGFBP-1 $n = 16$	6376 ± 9346	6707 ± 12,560	5% increase	0.406
IGFBP-3 $n = 16$	36,517 ± 49,159	40,790 ± 58,870	12% increase	0.808
MMP-1 $n = 10$	7971 ± 6827	8323 ± 9046	4% increase	0.541
MMP-2 $n = 10$	283,599 ± 218,875	249,307 ± 194,342	12% decrease	0.325
MMP-3 $n = 10$	245,119 ± 153,269	235,275 ± 175,421	4% decrease	0.293
MMP-8 $n = 10$	1354 ± 503	1729 ± 1899	28% increase	0.686
MMP-9 $n = 10$	5014 ± 4464	6375 ± 9225	27% increase	0.956
MMP-10 $n = 16$	238 ± 206	200 ± 208	16% decrease	0.0427

Legend: IL-1 ra = Interleukin 1 receptor antagonist, IL-4 = Interleukin 4, IL-6 = Interleukin 6, IL-7 = Interleukin 7, IL-8 = Interleukin 8, IL-18 = Interleukin 18, IL-15 = interleukin 15, IGFBP-1 Insulin-Like Growth Factor Binding Protein 1, IGFBP-3 = Insulin-Like Growth Factor Binding Protein 3, MMP-1 Matrix Metalloproteinase 1, MMP-2 = Matrix Metalloproteinase 2, MMP-3 = Matrix Metalloproteinase 3, MMP-8 = Matrix Metalloproteinase 8, MMP-9 = Matrix Metalloproteinase 9, MMP-10 = Matrix Metalloproteinase 10. p-values < 0.5 was only observed for MMP 10 levels.

To determine if baseline SF protein biomarker values predicted an improved response to IA HA injections at 3 months, linear regression statistics on each of these 15 biomarker protein levels in Table 5 were utilized to identify any significant correlations between baseline values from 26 separate subjects and subsequent changes in their total WOMAC scores at 3 months. No significant correlations were observed between baseline levels of any of these 15 SF proteins and changes in WOMAC scores at 3 months, with p-values ranging from 0.10 to 0.97.

4. Discussion

4.1. Injection and Aspiration Technique

We used US-visualized needle insertion and a pneumatic external compression device to ensure that the HA product was delivered with greater accuracy into the intra-synovial space. We also used an 18-gauge needle for aspiration since our prior study indicated that the very high SF viscosity on normal knees required a larger-bore needle for successful knee aspirations, even when performed under positive pressure using the pneumatic compression device [15]. We therefore confirmed with direct needle visualization on the US monitor that the aspirating and injecting needle was in the anechoic region. Prior studies using non-imaged guided knee IA injections indicate the intrasynovial space may be missed in 20–30% of attempts, depending upon the volume of SF and experience of the performing physician [22,32]. This error rate could be even higher among our OA patients since they had very small SF volumes measured by depth on US, with a mean of only 3.2 ± 2.2 mms. Our aspiration technique may also have facilitated a more successful aspiration of SF for biomarker analysis using a pneumatic compression device. This increases the amount of SF available after inflation, and SF is under positive pressure. In a report by Iqbal et al. using non-image-guided aspiration in a flexed knee aspiration technique in patients without large effusions, they were able to increase the successful knee aspiration rate from 41% to 75% using a pneumatic thigh cuff inflated to 100 mmHg [33]. Therefore, our ability to aspirate ≥ 0.5 mL in 74% of our patients on their initial visit probably reflects the benefit of utilizing the US-guided needle visualization technique with external compression [34].

The difference in our injection technique compared to landmarked guided injections might also explain the very low incidence of injection site product reactions (only 1 of 72 HA injections) and provide an explanation for the longer clinical benefit durability of 12 months. These durable clinical improvements occurred after a single series of two HA injections 7 days apart. Bisicchia et al. also reported clinical benefit in a prospective randomized study of IA HYADD4 at 26 weeks on WOMAC and VAS, which was superior to IA methylprednisolone; however, benefit above baseline scores was not observed at 52 weeks for either product using a non-image-guided injection technique [35]. In another knee OA study using the same IA HA product, Benazzo et al. reported improvements in WOMAC scores at 6 months in a prospective open-label study from a single series of two IA injections, and clinical benefit was maintained at 52 weeks following a repeat series of IA injections at 6 months without image guidance [36]. In a retrospective report using the ANTIAGE registry of clinicians who performed IA injections of HYADD4 using ultrasound on KL II–IV knee OA patients, Priano reported significant reductions in WOMAC and VAS scores among 74.5% of patients (698 of 937) at 6 months [21]. At 12 months, improvement in pain at rest and with movement was also reported as the only clinical outcome data available from 11% of patients (106 of 937) available for analysis.

Our observed clinical efficacy results and durability of response may also have been related to this specific HA product. In a meta-analysis of low vs. high molecular weight IA HA injection products, Hummer et al. reported clinically important improvements in pain reduction when high but not low molecular weight HA injection products were injected compared with placebo [37]. A review by Ferkel et al. also supports molecular weight and other differences in product manufacturing and composition as important factors in efficacy outcomes in clinical trials using different HA products [38].

4.2. SF Volume Measurements

Even though we observed significant improvements in WOMAC, VAS, and PCS scores at 3, 6, and 12 months, this was not associated with statistically significant changes in the amount of SF as determined by the measured depth of the anechoic region on US either before or after inflation of the external pneumatic compression device. Results of the Multicenter Osteoarthritis Knee Hyaluronic Acid Study (MOKHA) included 46 knee OA patients with very similar demographics as our study subjects regarding age and KL rating who also received IA HYADD4 injections [39]. They recorded an 18% reduction in knee effusions on MRI imaging at 6 months but not at 12 months. They also reported clinical benefit at 6 and 12 months on Knee Injury and Osteoarthritis Outcome Scores (KOOS); however, their subjects received a second series of IA HA injections at 6 months.

In another very ambitious prospective placebo-controlled study, McAlindon et al. performed a double-blinded knee OA efficacy study of normal saline vs. triamcinolone injections every 3 months for 2 years. They also reported no change in SF volumes quantitated on MRI at 2 years between these two groups or from baseline values [40]. They also reported no differences in functional outcomes between the two groups, despite the greater cartilage volume loss reported in the triamcinolone group. However, the suggestion that corticosteroids cause additional cartilage loss and thus progression of osteoarthritis has not been substantiated in other careful radiographic progression trials. Several studies have demonstrated no difference in the gold standard of radiographic progression of OA or cartilage turnover biomarkers between intra-articular corticosteroid treatment and placebo or intra-articular HA administration [41–44].

4.3. Serum and SF Biomarkers

Posey et al. have reviewed the role of serum COMP levels in various forms of arthritis [45]. Since levels are elevated in early but not advanced OA, we anticipated a fall in levels at 3 months following IA HYADD4 injections since all of our patients were KL II or III. They also reviewed the effect of weight-bearing exercise, which increases COMP levels; therefore, it is possible our observed 27% increase in levels at 3 months may have been related to an increase in ambulation related to less pain as documented on WOMAC, VAS, and PCS scores. We also documented an increase in 6 MWD at 3 months, as noted in Table 2. Our baseline and 3-month levels of COMP and C2C might have been higher than reported in other studies since our samples were obtained within 45 min of subjects completing their 6 MWD. While elevated serum HA levels correlate with the progression and severity of OA, we are not aware of serum HA measurements before and after IA HA injection [46].

Synovial fluid is potentially an ideal source of biomarkers to investigate the pathogenic mechanisms of cartilage damage in OA, characterize different disease endotypes, and identify potential therapeutic targets. SF biomarkers may also identify those at highest risk for disease progression as well as those most likely to respond to a specific therapeutic agent. SF is an ultrafiltrate of plasma due to the lack of a typical basement membrane within synovial tissue, and in OA, various inflammatory and catabolic proteins are released by synoviocytes. Since cartilage does not have a blood supply, the SF also provides nutritional support, and synoviocytes produce key SF proteins that help maintain cartilage health and preserve function, such as HA and lubricin, as well as proteinases, collagenases, and prostaglandins [47].

SF was available for SF biomarker analysis in a much smaller subset of our study subjects than planned, as only 18 of our 34 subjects had paired samples at 3 months since some subjects had smaller volumes at 3 months compared to their baseline visit, which made aspiration more difficult. Some of the patients with aspirated volumes of 0.5 to 1.0 mL were also contaminated with blood as determined by visual inspection and the SF WBC count and differential, and some were consumed during feasibility studies. We have observed from multiple prior SF quantitative protein assays on patients with various forms of knee arthritis that the accuracy of SF cytokine levels was not robust on SF volumes < 1.0 mL or when contaminated with peripheral blood arising from intra-synovial bleeding during needle insertion [15]. Therefore, we were only able to report results from a subset of 16 and 10 patients who had paired baseline and 3-month samples in

Table 5. Furthermore, the high viscosity of our SF sample matrix made sample processing and analysis, particularly with the Luminex multiplex bead arrays, challenging. Sample viscosity may have contributed to clogging of the Luminex fluidics system and poor bead recovery, therefore leading to uninterpretable results for some samples.

We observed that only 1 of 15 synovial fluid proteins (MMP 10 levels) had significant changes at 3 months following IA HA, even though the clinical improvement on WOMAC, VAS, PCS scores, and 6 MWD at this time was significant. Barksby et al. report that MMP 10 (also called stromelysin 2) is produced by synovial fibroblasts and articular chondrocytes and is expressed in diseased joint synovium, suggesting it is also an activator of procollagenases [48]. They also reported similar SF MMP-10 levels in patients with OA compared to those with rheumatoid arthritis and juvenile idiopathic arthritis. Therefore, a reduction in MMP-10 levels 3 months after IA HA suggests one potential mechanism of clinical efficacy if this protease is a major contributor to cartilage collagenolysis in OA. However, the roles of various MMPs in OA pathogenesis are very complex, and levels are also modulated by various cytokines and proteins within the SF, bone, and cartilage, as reviewed by Mehana and colleagues [49].

Our study with a small number of SF samples may have been underpowered to identify statistically different changes in some of these SF proteins and other biomarkers of inflammation. It is also possible that clinical improvement mediated by IA HA injections may result in changes in the inflammatory or catabolic proteins in cartilage that occur earlier than 3 months. Falcinelli et al. documented lower SF levels of IL-6, MMP-2, and MMP-13 when measured 7 days after IA administration of the same HA product (HYADD 4-G) [50]. It is also likely that the 54% lower SF WBC counts observed at 3 months might have achieved statistically significant differences if our sample size were larger.

In another study reporting SF protein biomarkers after a different IA HA product (1% sodium hyaluronate), after three weekly injections on 28 subjects, there was a greater reduction in SF TNF alpha levels at 6 months in adults < 65 years of age compared to adults > 65 years of age. However, the other inflammatory cytokines (IL-1 beta, IL-6, IL-8, and IL-12) and levels of IL-4, IL-10, IL-13, and monocyte chemotactic did not differ from baseline values [51]. In another interesting study of three weekly IA Hyaluronan injections in OA patients with clinical knee effusions, one week post-treatment, IL-6 levels were statistically lower in both normal saline-injected ($n = 19$) and HA-treated patients ($n = 22$), whereas TNF alpha and IL-8 levels did not change in either group [52].

Our open-label, non-blinded study did not include a placebo injection because the goal was not to determine the efficacy of IA HA compared to saline injection. Our objective was to determine if observed clinical benefit at 3, 6, or 12 months was associated with reductions in the amount of measured knee SF volumes or changes in SF WB counts, serum cartilage, and SF biomarkers at 3 months. We also wanted to identify if any baseline clinical and demographic features or SF biomarker profiles predicted clinical responsiveness to IA HA injections at 3 months. In a meta-analysis of 149 efficacy trials of various modes of delivery of placebo, Bannuru et al. described that the greatest placebo effect occurred when the placebo was delivered via an intra-articular route, but they also acknowledged the potential for therapeutic benefit from saline injections by diluting inflammatory mediators [53]. A reduction in SF IL-6 levels one week post-saline injection suggests a potential therapeutic benefit from knee aspiration or normal saline instillation into the intra-synovial space rather than exclusively a "placebo effect", since saline and HA-injected subjects had improved WOMAC scores, but higher values were observed in the IA HA-treated group [54]. Altman et al. reviewed the evidence in a meta-analysis of 38 randomized controlled trials and concluded that, given the substantial and uniform reduction of OA knee pain using IA saline, a potential therapeutic effect rather than solely due to a placebo effect may well account for some of the observed clinical improvement [55].

Our OA study population would have been more homogeneous if we had excluded those patients with prior knee surgery. However, since these are common orthopedic procedures among knee OA patients who receive therapeutic IA HA injections, they were not excluded. The overall mean age of the previously operated subjects was similar to that of the non-operated group, as noted in Table 1. Our inclusion of these subjects suggests that symptomatic knee OA, even among those with prior non-arthroplasty surgical procedures, may also display a durable response to this IA HA product when delivered via US guidance.

4.4. Strengths

The single-center study design ensured uniform adherence to study protocol and aspiration/injection technique, as well as SF sample handling, compared to a multicenter study. This is important since some of these cytokines are labile at room temperature and sensitive to degradation, whereas all of our samples were centrifuged and cryopreserved within 60 min of collection [56]. US guidance also allowed us to perform IA HA injections more accurately among OA patients with small effusions, unlike those reported by Sezgen with palpable effusions, which may represent a different OA endotype than our study patients [52]. It is also possible that our improved durability and clinical efficacy were also due to the removal of catabolic SF proteins prior to the first of two IA HA injections, as aspiration prior to glucocorticoid injections has a therapeutic benefit [54,55].

4.5. Study Limitations

We acknowledge that our small sample size and the small subset of SF samples available for final analysis at 3 months may have resulted in the lack of statistically significant changes in some protein biomarkers. While all 36 subjects had ≥ 0.5 mL of SF aspirated on their first study visit, 3 months later, many subjects had even smaller SF volumes, and therefore some of these subjects did not have adequate SF volumes for paired SF analysis.

It is also possible that those study subjects who dropped out between their 3-, 6-, or 12-month visits may have skewed the results in favor of a higher level of responders who remained in the study at 12 months than if there were fewer voluntary withdrawals. However, despite institutional COVID restrictions and subject hesitancy due to COVID, only 4 of 34 (12%) enrolled subjects at 3 months did not return at 6 months. The two athletic subjects who dropped out between 6 and 12 months decided to pursue elective orthopedic surgical interventions, whereas three others were unable to participate due to an unrelated sports injury, malignancy, or relocation out of state. Since there were only two withdrawals due to potential lack of continued efficacy, we suspect their inclusion in our final analysis would likely not have skewed the results since the differences were $p < 0.0001$ at 12 months on the WOMAC, PCS, and VAS efficacy scales.

5. Conclusions

While improvements in WOMAC, VAS scores, and PCS scores on the SF 36 were observed at 3, 6, and 12 months after US-guided knee injections with this HA product, a statistically significant reduction in US-measured SF volumes was not observed at these same time points. The 6 MWD improved at 3 months but not at 6 or 12 months. IA injections using US needle visualization confirmed that the product was delivered into the intra-synovial fluid space with improved accuracy, which may also have resulted in our very low incidence of observed post-IA injection reactions (1 out of 72 injections) as well as a greater durable clinical response lasting 12 months. Our baseline clinical features and SF biomarker panel did not predict responders vs. non-responders. A fall in MMP-10 levels was observed at 3 months, whereas the other fourteen SF proteins and four serum biomarkers were unchanged.

The sustained efficacy results in this study may not be comparable to IA injections using a different HA product if injected without US guidance or without an aspiration prior to the first HA injection. The current recommendation against the use of IA HA for knee osteoarthritis by the American College of Rheumatology and the American Academy of Orthopedic Surgeons reflects the small effect size of prior studies that delivered HA without image guidance [57–59]. In Europe, however, the 2020 EULAR recommendations support the use of IA HA injections for knee OA [60]. In addition, our results may not be generalizable to different OA phenotypes, including those with morbid obesity, more advanced KL grades, or large knee effusions.

We anticipate a larger study will be necessary to validate a SF-based biomarker panel to identify which individual OA patients will most likely receive the greatest benefit from HA or therapeutic IA injections. This information may also help identify if these agents reduce catabolic pro-inflammatory proteins, which cause irreversible cartilage loss, and discover more effective therapeutic targets to improve the quality of life for patients with knee OA.

Author Contributions: All authors were involved in conducting these studies, the drafting of this article, or critically revising for important intellectual content. R.T.M., E.A.R., C.M.C., M.D.G. and V.K. had full access to the SF cytokine and protein level results and took full responsibility for the integrity of the data and the accuracy of the data analysis. Conception and design: R.T.M., E.A.R., E.D.H. and V.K. Acquisition of data: R.T.M., M.T.G., I.A.A., L.M.K. and M.L.W. Analysis and interpretation of the data: R.T.M., E.A.R., E.D.H., C.M.C., M.T.G., J.L.C., G.J.C. and V.K. All authors have read and agreed to the published version of the manuscript.

Funding: This study was funded by an investigator-initiated OA SF biomarker Grant funded by Fidia Farmaceutici SpA, Abano Terme, Padova, Italy, and Fidia USA (Fidia ISS Project No. P005-NOV2018, HS 3179).

Institutional Review Board Statement: The study was conducted according to the guidelines of the Declaration of Helsinki and approved by the Institutional Review Board of National Jewish Health and BRANY for HS 3179 to have patients enrolled and consented for this study.

Informed Consent Statement: All subjects signed a National Jewish Health-approved subject consent form for HS 3179.

Data Availability Statement: The data used to generate Figure 1, Tables 1–3 were entered into REDCap database at National Jewish Health and contains personal health information (PHI) so is considered confidential except for access by the investigators and biostatistician James Crooks who performed the statistical analysis.

Acknowledgments: Support for this project was provided by funding from an Investigator-Initiated OA SF Biomarker Grant awarded to R. Meehan funded by Fidia (HS 3179, NCT 04093232). Saad Nasir of Fidia USA, provided valuable expertise in the initial design of this study. Janet L. Hueber performed serum cartilage biomarkers in the Biomarkers Core facility at the Duke Molecular Physiology Institute along with Virginia Kraus. Matthew Eggleston in the Complement ADX labs at NJH performed the Luminex-based SF biomarkers.

Conflicts of Interest: The pneumatic compression device (KneeTapTM) used in the study was granted US patent #7468048 to R. Meehan in 2008, with NJH as the owner. Subsequently, Arthroventions LLC was granted a license from NJH to commercialize this device. E. Hoffman and R. Meehan were co-founders of Arthroventions LLC. No other potential COI exists for any other authors, and this potential COI is managed each year by NJH VP/Chief Compliance Officer, Legal, and Regulatory Affairs, Alicia Christensen, JD, christensena@njhealth.org.

References

1. Katz, J.N.; Arant, K.R.; Loeser, R.F. Diagnosis and Treatment of hip and knee osteoarthritis A Review. *JAMA* **2021**, *325*, 568–578. [CrossRef]
2. US Bureau of Labor Statistics. Consumer Price Index for All Urban Consumers (CPI-U): U.S. City Average by Expenditure Cate-gory. Available online: https://www.bls.gov/news.release/cpi.t01.htm (accessed on 5 July 2023).
3. Schieker, M.; Conaghan, P.G.; Mindeholm, L.; Praestgaard, J.; Solomon, D.H.; Scotti, C.; Gram, H.; Thuren, T.; Roubenoff, R.; Ridker, P.M. Effects of interleukin-1β inhibition on incident hip and knee replacement: Exploratory analyses from a randomized, double-blind, placebo-controlled trial. *Ann. Intern. Med.* **2020**, *173*, 509–515. [CrossRef] [PubMed]
4. Heijman, M.W.J.; Fiolet, A.T.J.; Mosterd, A.; Tijssen, J.G.P.; van den Bemt, B.J.F.; Schut, A.; Eikelboom, J.W.; Thompson, P.L.; van den Ende, C.H.M.; Nidorf, S.M.; et al. Association of low-dose colchicine with incidence of knee and hip replacements. *Ann. Intern. Med.* **2023**, *176*, 732–742. [CrossRef] [PubMed]
5. Zhu, K.Y.; Acuna, A.J.; Samuel, L.T.; Grits, D.; Kamath, A.F. Hyaluronic acid injections for knee osteoarthritis, has utilization among Medicare beneficiaries changed between 2021 and 2018? *J. Bone Jt. Surg. Am.* **2022**, *104*, e43. [CrossRef] [PubMed]

6. Loeser, R.F.; Goldring, S.R.; Scanzello, C.R.; Goldring, M.B. Osteoarthritis: A disease of the joint as an organ. *Arthritis Rheum.* **2012**, *64*, 1697–1707. [PubMed]
7. Ene, R.; Sinescu, R.D.; Ene, P.; Cirstoiu, M.M.; Cirstoiu, F.C. Synovial inflammation in patients with different stages of knee osteoarthritis. *Rom. J. Morphol. Embryol.* **2015**, *56*, 169–173.
8. Benito, M.J.; Veale, D.J.; FitzGerald, O.; van den Berg, W.B.; Bresnihan, B. Synovial tissue inflammation in early and late osteoarthritis. *Ann. Rheum. Dis.* **2005**, *64*, 1263–1267. [CrossRef]
9. Roemer, F.W.; Guermazi, A.; Felson, D.T.; Niu, J.; Nevitt, M.C.; Crema, M.D.; Lynch, J.A.; Lewis, C.E.; Torner, J.; Zhang, Y. Presence of MRI-detected joint effusion and synovitis increases the risk of cartilage loss in knees without osteoarthritis at 30 months follow up: The MOST study. *Ann. Rheum. Dis.* **2011**, *70*, 1804–1809. [CrossRef]
10. Wojdasiewicz, P.; Poniatowski, L.A.; Szukiewicz, D. The Role of inflammatory and anti-inflammatory cytokines in the pathogenesis of osteoarthritis. *Mediat. Inflamm.* **2014**, *2014*, 561459. [CrossRef]
11. Goldring, M.B.; Otero, M.; Plumb, D.A.; Dragomir, C.; Favero, M.; El Hachem, K.; Hashimoto, K.; Roach, H.I.; Olivotto, E.; Borzi, R.M.; et al. Roles of inflammatory and anabolic cytokines in cartilage metabolism: Signals and multiple effectors converge upon MMP-13 regulation in osteoarthritis. *Eur. Cell Mater.* **2011**, *21*, 202–220. [CrossRef]
12. Mobasheri, A.; Bay-Jensen, A.C.; van Spil, W.E.; Larkin, J.; Levesque, M.C. Osteoarthritis year in review 2016: Biomarkers (biochemical markers). *Osteoarthr. Cartil.* **2017**, *25*, 199–208.
13. Bay-Jenson, A.C.; Thudium, C.S.; Mobasheri, A. Development and use of biochemical markers in osteoarthritis: Current update. *Cur. Opin. Rheumatol.* **2018**, *30*, 121–128. [CrossRef] [PubMed]
14. Lotz, M.; Martel-Pelletier, J.; Christiansen, C.; Brandi, M.L.; Bruyere, O.; Chapurlat, R.; Collette, J.; Cooper, C.; Giacovelli, G.; Kanis, J.A.; et al. Republished: Value of biomarkers in osteoarthritis: Current status and perspectives. *Postgrad. Med. J.* **2014**, *90*, 171–178.
15. Meehan, R.T.; Regan, E.A.; Hoffman, E.D.; Wolf, M.L.; Gill, M.T.; Crooks, J.L.; Parmar, P.J.; Scheuring, R.A.; Hill, J.C.; Pacheco, K.A.; et al. Synovial fluid cytokines, chemokines and MMP levels in osteoarthritis patients with knee pain display a profile similar to many Rheumatoid arthritis patients. *J. Clin. Med.* **2021**, *10*, 5027. [CrossRef] [PubMed]
16. Nelson, A.E. Osteoarthritis year in review 2017: Clinical. *Osteoarthr. Cartil.* **2018**, *26*, 319–325. [CrossRef] [PubMed]
17. Altman, R.D.; Mango, A.; Forefinger, A.; Nazi, F.; Nicholls, M. The mechanism of action for hyaluronic acid treatment in the osteoarthritic knee: A systemic review. *BMC Musculoskelet. Discord.* **2015**, *16*, 321–331. [CrossRef]
18. Altman, R.; Beda, A.; Mango, A.; Nazi, F.; Shaw, P.; Meese, P. Anti-Inflammatory effects of intra-articular hyaluronic acid: A systemic review. *Cartilage* **2019**, *10*, 43–52. [CrossRef]
19. Moreland, L.W. Intra-articular hyaluronic (hyaluronic acid) in Humans? For treatment of osteoarthritis: Mechanisms of action. *Arthritis Res. Ther.* **2003**, *5*, 54–67. [CrossRef]
20. Bonnevie, E.D.; Galesso, D.; Secchieri, C.; Bonassar, L.J. Frictional characterization of injectable hyaluronic acid is more predictive of clinical outcomes than traditional rheological or viscoelastic characterization. *PLoS ONE* **2019**, *14*, e0216702.
21. Priano, F. Early efficacy of intra-articular HYADDR4 (HymovisR) injections for symptomatic knee osteoarthritis. *Joints* **2017**, *5*, 79–84.
22. Berkoff, D.J.; Miller, L.E.; Block, J.E. Clinical utility of ultrasound guidance for intra-articular knee injections: A review. *Clin. Interv. Aging* **2012**, *7*, 89–95. [PubMed]
23. Wu, T.; Dong, Y.; Song, H.x.; Fu, Y.; Li, J.H. Ultrasound-guided versus landmark in knee arthrocentesis: A systemic review. *Semin. Arthritis Rheum.* **2016**, *45*, 627–632. [CrossRef] [PubMed]
24. Meehan, R.; Wilson, C.; Hoffman, E.; Altimier, L.; Kaessner, M.; Regan, E.A. Ultrasound measurement of knee synovial fluid during external pneumatic compression. *J. Orthop. Res.* **2019**, *37*, 601–608. [CrossRef] [PubMed]
25. Kellgren, J.H.; Lawrence, J.S. Radiological assessment of osteo-arthrosis. *Ann. Rheum. Dis.* **1957**, *16*, 494–503. [CrossRef] [PubMed]
26. Kraus, V.B.; Collins, J.E.; Hargrove, D.; Losina, E.; Nevitt, M.; Katz, J.N.; Wang, S.X.; Sandell, L.J.; Hoffman, S.C.; Hunter, D.J. Predictive validity of biochemical biomarkers in knee osteoarthritis: Data from the FNIH OA biomarkers consortium. *Ann. Rheum. Dis.* **2017**, *76*, 186–195. [CrossRef] [PubMed]
27. Bellamy, N.; Buchanan, W.W.; Goldsmith, C.H.; Campbell, J.; Stitt, L.W. Validation study of WOMAC: A health status instrument for measuring clinically important patient relevant outcomes to antirheumatic drug therapy in patients with osteoarthritis of the hip or knee. *J. Rheumatol.* **1988**, *15*, 1833–1840.
28. Ware, J.E.; Snow, K.; Klosinski, M.; Gandek, B. *SF 36 Health Survey*; Manual and Interpretations Guide; The Health Institute New England Medical Centre: Boston, MA, USA, 1993.
29. Patel, A.A.; Donegan, D.; Albert, T. The 36-Item Short. *J. Am. Acad. Orthop. Surg.* **2007**, *15*, 126–134. [CrossRef]
30. Pham, T.; van der Heijde, D.; Altman, R.D.; Anderson, J.J.; Bellamy, N.; Hochberg, M.; Simon, L.; Strand, V.; Woodworth, T.; Dougados, M. OMERACT-OARSI Initiative: Osteoarthritis Research Society International set of responder criteria for osteoarthritis clinical trials revisited. *OsteoArthritis Cartil.* **2004**, *12*, 389–399. [CrossRef]
31. R Core Team. *R: A Language and Environment for Statistical Computing*; R Foundation for Statistical Computing: Vienna, Austria, 2020. Available online: https://www.R-project.org (accessed on 5 July 2023).
32. Maricar, N.; Parkes, M.J.; Callaghan, M.J.; Felson, D.T.; O'Neill, T.W. Where and how to inject the knee—A systemic review. *Semin. Arthritis Rheum.* **2013**, *43*, 195–203. [CrossRef]

33. Iqbal, A.; Brahmabhatt, S.; Muruganandam, M.; Trost, J.R.; Farshami, F.J.; Cisneros, D.R.; Kiani, A.N.; McElwee, M.K.; Hayward, W.A.; Haseler, L.J.; et al. Extraction of Synovial fluid from the non-effusive pathologic knee with pneumatic compression. *Authorea* **2022**. [CrossRef]
34. Bhavsar, T.B.; Sibbitt, W.L.; Band, P.A.; Cabacungan, R.J.; Moore, T.S.; Salayandia, L.C.; Fields, R.A.; Kettwich, S.K.; Roldan, L.P.; Emil, N.S.; et al. Improvement in diagnostic and therapeutic arthrocentesis via constant compression. *Clin. Rheumatol.* **2018**, *37*, 2251–2259. [CrossRef] [PubMed]
35. Bisicchia, S.; Bernardi, G.; Tudisco, C. HYADD4 versus methylprednisolone acetate in symptomatic knee osteoarthritis: A single-centre single blind prospective randomized controlled clinical study with a 1 year follow up. *Clin. Exp. Rheumatol.* **2016**, *34*, 857–863. [PubMed]
36. Benazzo, F.; Perticarnini, L.; Padolino, A.; Castelli, A.; Gifuni, P.; Lovato, M.; Manzini, C.; Giordan, N. A multi-centre, open label, long-term follow-up study to evaluate the benefits of a new viscoelastic hydrogel (HymovisR) in the treatment of knee osteoarthritis. *Eur. Rev. Med. Pharmacol. Sci.* **2016**, *20*, 959–968.
37. Hummer, C.D.; Angst, F.; Ngai, W.; Whittington, C.; Yoon, S.S.; Duarte, L.; Manitt, C.; Schemitsch, E. High molecular weight intraarticular hyaluronic acid for the treatment of knee osteoarthritis: A network meta-analysis. *BMC Musculoskelet. Disord.* **2020**, *21*, 702. [CrossRef] [PubMed]
38. Ferkel, E.; Manjoo, A.; Martins, D.; Bhandari, M.; Sethi, P.; Nicholls, M. Intra-articular Hyaluronic acid treatments review of product properties. *Cartilage* **2023**. [CrossRef]
39. Henrotin, Y.; Bannuru, R.; Malaise, M.; Ea, H.K.; Confavreux, C.; Bentin, J.; Urbin-Choffray, D.; Conrozier, T.; Brasseur, J.P.; Thomas, P.; et al. Hyaluronan derivative HYMOVISR increases cartilage volume and Type II collagen turnover in osteoarthritic knee: Data from MOKHA study. *BMC Musculoskelet. Disord.* **2019**, *20*, 293. [CrossRef]
40. McAlindon, T.E.; LaValley, M.P.; Harvey, W.F.; Price, L.L.; Driban, J.B.; Zhang, M.; Ward, R.J. Effect of Intra-articular triamcinolone vs saline on knee cartilage volume and pain in patients with knee osteoarthritis, a randomized clinical trial. *JAMA* **2017**, *317*, 1967–1975. [CrossRef]
41. Latourte, A.; Rat, A.C.; Omorou, A.; Ngueyon-Sime, W.; Eymard, F.; Sellam, J.; Roux, C.; Ea, H.K.; Cohen-Solal, M.; Bardin, T.; et al. Do glucocorticoid injections increase the risk of knee osteoarthritis progression over 5 Years? *Arthritis Rheumatol.* **2022**, *74*, 1343–1351. [CrossRef]
42. Bucci, J.; Chen, X.; LaValley, M.; Nevitt, M.; Torner, J.; Lewis, C.E.; Felson, D.T. Progression of knee osteoarthritis with use of intraarticular glucocorticoids versus hyaluronic acid. *Arthritis Rheumatol.* **2022**, *74*, 223–226. [CrossRef]
43. Klocke, R.; Levasseur, K.; Kitas, G.D.; Smith, J.P.; Hirsch, G. Cartilage turnover and intra-articular corticosteroid injections in knee osteoarthritis. *Rheumatol. Int.* **2018**, *38*, 455–459. [CrossRef]
44. Raynauld, J.P.; Buckland-Wright, C.; Ward, R.; Choquette, D.; Haraoui, B.; Martel-Pelletier, J.; Uthman, I.; Khy, V.; Tremblay, J.L.; Bertrand, C.; et al. Safety and efficacy of long-term intraarticular steroid injections in osteoarthritis of the knee: A randomized, double-blind, placebo-controlled trial. *Arthritis Rheum.* **2003**, *48*, 370–377. [CrossRef]
45. Posey, K.L.; Hecht, J.T. The role of cartilage oligomeric matrix protein (COMP) in skeletal disease. *Curr. Drug Targets* **2008**, *9*, 869–877. [CrossRef]
46. Sasaki, E.; Tsuda, E.; Yamamoto, Y.; Maeda, S.; Inoue, R.; Chiba, D.; Fujita, H.; Takahashi, I.; Umeda, T.; Nakaji, S.; et al. Serum hyaluronic acid concentration predicts the progression of joint space narrowing in normal knees and established knee osteoarthritis—A five year prospective cohort study. *Arthritis Res. Ther.* **2015**, *17*, 283–293. [CrossRef] [PubMed]
47. Nygaard, G.; Firestein, G.S. Restoring synovial homeostasis in rheumatoid arthritis by targeting fibroblast-like synoviocytes. *Nat. Rev. Rheumatol.* **2020**, *16*, 316–333. [CrossRef] [PubMed]
48. Barksby, H.E.; Milner, J.M.; Patterson, A.M.; Peak, N.J.; Hui, W.; Robson, T.; Lakey, R.; Middleton, J.; Cawston, T.E.; Richards, C.D.; et al. Matrix Metalloproteinase 10 promotion of collagenolysis via procollagenase activation. *Arthritis Rhem.* **2006**, *54*, 3244–3253. [CrossRef] [PubMed]
49. Mehana, E.S.E.; Khafaga, A.F.; El-Blehi, S.S. The role of matrix metalloproteinases in osteoarthritis pathogenesis: An updated review. *Life Sci.* **2019**, *234*, 116786. [CrossRef]
50. Falcinelli, E.; Giordan, N.; Luccioli, F.; Piselle, E.; La Paglia, G.M.C.; Momi, S.; Mirabelli, G.; Petito, E.; Alunno, A.; Gresele, P.; et al. Randomized Trial of HymovisR versus SynviscR on Matrix Metalloproteinase in Knee osteoarthritis. *Muscles Ligaments Tendons J.* **2020**, *10*, 553–561. [CrossRef]
51. Vincent, H.K.; Percival, S.S.; Conrad, B.P.; Seay, A.N.; Montero, C.; Vincent, K.K. Hyaluronic acid (HA) Viscosupplementation on synovial fluid inflammation in knee osteoarthritis: A Pilot study. *Open Orthop. J.* **2013**, *7*, 378–384. [CrossRef]
52. Sezgin, M.; Demirel, A.C.; Karaca, C.; Ortancil, O.; Ulkar, G.B.; Kanik, A.; Cakci, A. Does Hyaluronan affect inflammatory cytokines in knee osteoarthritis? *Rheumatol. Int.* **2005**, *25*, 264–269. [CrossRef] [PubMed]
53. Bannuru, R.R.; McAlindon, T.E.; Sullivan, M.C.; Wong, J.B.; Kent, D.M.; Schmid, C.H. Effectiveness and implications of alternative placebo treatments, a systemic review and network meta-analysis of osteoarthritis trials. *Ann. Intern. Med.* **2015**, *163*, 365–372. [CrossRef]
54. Weitoft, T.; Uddenfeld, P. Importance of synovial fluid aspiration when injecting intra-articular corticosteroids. *Ann. Rheum. Dis.* **2000**, *59*, 233–235. [CrossRef] [PubMed]

55. Altman, R.D.; Devji, T.; Bhandari, M.; Fierlinger, A.; Niazi, F.; Christensen, R. Clinical benefit of intra-articular saline as a comparator in clinical trials of knee osteoarthritis treatments: A systemic review and meta-analysis of randomized trials. *Semin. Arthritis Rheum.* **2016**, *46*, 151–159. [CrossRef]
56. Knight, V.; Long, T.; Meng, Q.H.; Linden, M.A.; Roads, D.D. Variability in the Laboratory Measurement of Cytokines: A Longitudinal Summary of a College of American Pathologists Proficiency Testing Survey. *Arch. Pathol. Lab. Med.* **2020**, *144*, 1230–1233. [CrossRef] [PubMed]
57. Kolasinski, S.L.; Neogi, T.; Hochberg, M.C.; Oatis, C.; Guyatt, G.; Block, J.; Callahan, L.; Copenhaver, C.; Dodge, C.; Felson, D.; et al. 2019 American College of Rheumatology/Arthritis Foundation guideline for the management of osteoarthritis of the hand, hip, and knee. *Arthritis Rheumatol.* **2020**, *72*, 220–233. [CrossRef] [PubMed]
58. Jevsevar, D.S.; Brown, G.A.; Jones, D.L.; Matzkin, E.G.; Manner, P.A.; Mooar, P.; Schousboe, J.T.; Stovitz, S.; Sanders, J.O.; Bozic, K.J.; et al. American Academy of Orthopaedic Surgeons evidence-based guideline on treatment of osteoarthritis of the knee, 2nd edition. *J. Bone Jt. Surg. Am.* **2013**, *95*, 1885–1886. [CrossRef]
59. Johansen, M.; Bahrt, H.; Altman, R.D.; Bartels, E.M.; Juhl, C.B.; Bliddal, H.; Lund, H.; Christensen, R. Exploring reasons for the observed inconsistent trial reports on intra-articular injections with hyaluronic acid in the treatment of osteoarthritis: Meta-regression analyses of randomized trials. *Semin. Arthritis Rheum.* **2016**, *46*, 34–48. [CrossRef]
60. Pendleton, A.; Arden, N.; Dougados, M.; Doherty, M.; Bannwarth, B.; Bijlsma, J.; Cluzeau, F.; Cooper, C.; Dieppe, P.; Gunther, K.; et al. EULAR recommendations for the management of knee osteoarthrtitis: A report of a task force of the standing committee for the international clinical studies including therapeutic trials (ESCISIT). *Ann. Rheum. Dis.* **2000**, *59*, 936–944. [CrossRef]

Disclaimer/Publisher's Note: The statements, opinions and data contained in all publications are solely those of the individual author(s) and contributor(s) and not of MDPI and/or the editor(s). MDPI and/or the editor(s) disclaim responsibility for any injury to people or property resulting from any ideas, methods, instructions or products referred to in the content.

MDPI AG
Grosspeteranlage 5
4052 Basel
Switzerland
Tel.: +41 61 683 77 34

Journal of Clinical Medicine Editorial Office
E-mail: jcm@mdpi.com
www.mdpi.com/journal/jcm

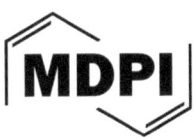

Disclaimer/Publisher's Note: The title and front matter of this reprint are at the discretion of the Guest Editor. The publisher is not responsible for their content or any associated concerns. The statements, opinions and data contained in all individual articles are solely those of the individual Editor and contributors and not of MDPI. MDPI disclaims responsibility for any injury to people or property resulting from any ideas, methods, instructions or products referred to in the content.

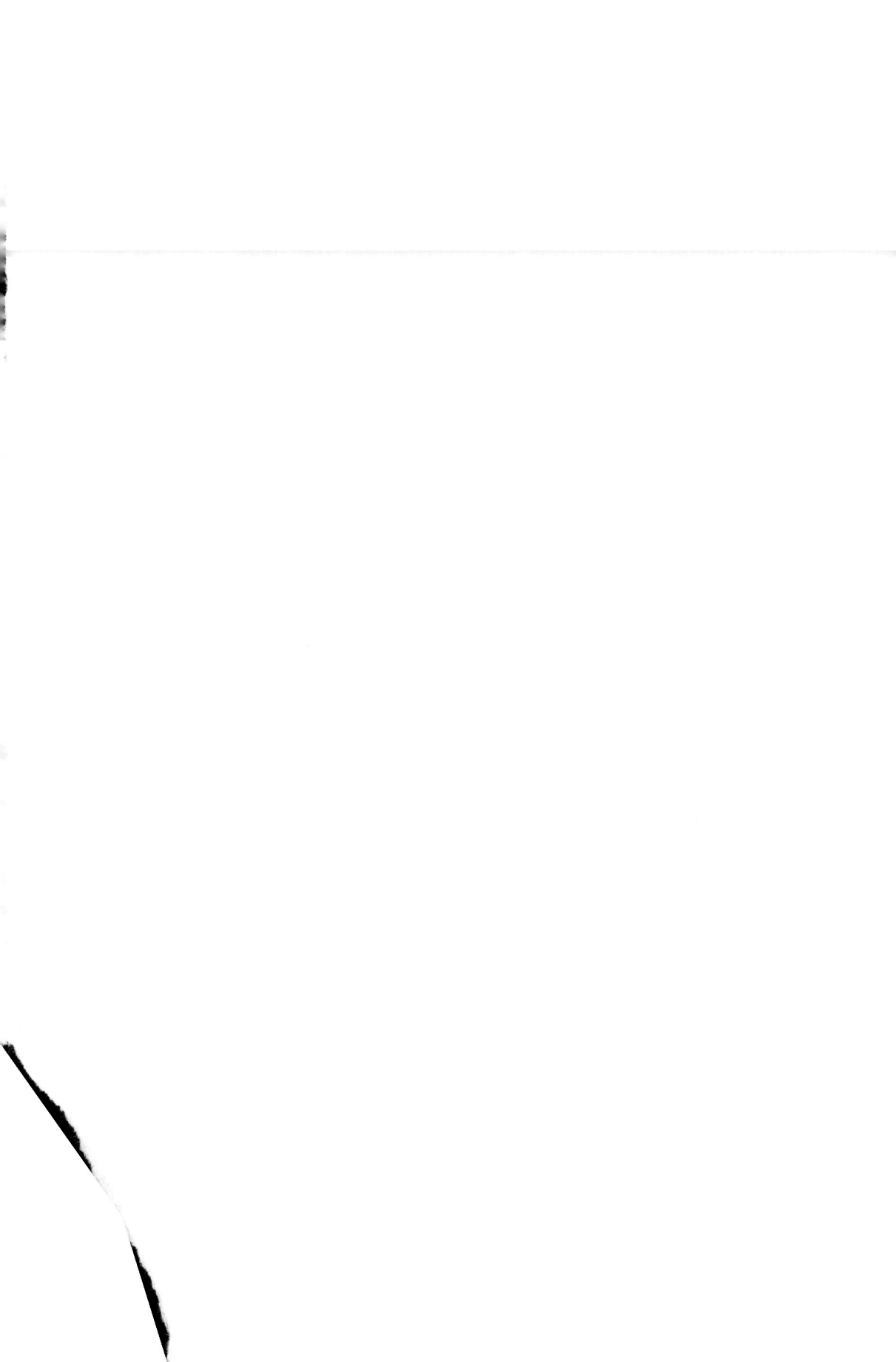

www.ingramcontent.com/pod-product-compliance
Lightning Source LLC
LaVergne TN
LVHW070000100526
838202LV00019B/2588